Dr. Naomi Demp

Hematology Board Review
Blueprint Study Guide and Q&A

Editors

Francis P. Worden, MD
Professor of Medicine
Director of the Hematology/Oncology Fellowship Program
University of Michigan Medical School
Ann Arbor, Michigan

Rami N. Khoriaty, MD
Assistant Professor
Department of Internal Medicine, Division of Hematology/Oncology
University of Michigan Medical School
Ann Arbor, Michigan

Kathleen A. Cooney, MD, MACP
H.A. and Edna Benning Presidential Endowed Chair
Professor and Chair
Department of Internal Medicine
University of Utah School of Medicine
Huntsman Cancer Institute
Salt Lake City, Utah

Michael W. Deininger, MD, PhD
Chief
Division of Hematology and Hematologic Malignancies
M.M. Wintrobe Professor of Medicine
Senior Director of Transdisciplinary Research
University of Utah School of Medicine
Huntsman Cancer Institute
Salt Lake City, Utah

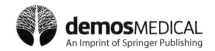

demosMEDICAL
An Imprint of Springer Publishing

Visit our website at www.springerpub.com

ISBN: 9780826137821
ebook ISBN: 9780826137838

Acquisitions Editor: David D'Addona
Compositor: Exeter Premedia Services Private Ltd.

Medicine is an ever-changing science. Research and clinical experience are continually expanding our knowledge, in particular our understanding of proper treatment and drug therapy. The authors, editors, and publisher have made every effort to ensure that all information in this book is in accordance with the state of knowledge at the time of production of the book. Nevertheless, the authors, editors, and publisher are not responsible for errors or omissions or for any consequences from application of the information in this book and make no warranty, expressed or implied, with respect to the contents of the publication. Every reader should examine carefully the package inserts accompanying each drug and should carefully check whether the dosage schedules mentioned therein or the contraindications stated by the manufacturer differ from the statements made in this book. Such examination is particularly important with drugs that are either rarely used or have been newly released on the market.

Library of Congress Cataloging-in-Publication Data

Names: Worden, Francis P., editor. | Khoriaty, Rami N., editor. | Cooney, Kathleen A., editor. | Deininger, Michael W., editor.
Title: Hematology board review : blueprint study guide and Q&A / editors, Francis P. Worden, Rami N. Khoriaty, Kathleen A. Cooney, Michael W. Deininger.
Description: New York : Demos Medical Publishing/Springer Publishing Company, [2018] | Includes bibliographical references and index.
Identifiers: LCCN 2018003818 | ISBN 9780826137821 (alk. paper) | ISBN 9780826137838 (e-book)
Subjects: | MESH: Hematologic Diseases | Hematology—methods | Examination Questions
Classification: LCC RC633 | NLM WH 18.2 | DDC 616.1/50076—dc23
LC record available at https://lccn.loc.gov/2018003818

Printed in the United States of America.
19 20 21 22 /6 5 4 3

Hematology Board Review

Contents

Contributors

Asra Ahmed, MD, Assistant Professor, Department of Internal Medicine, Division of Hematology/Oncology, University of Michigan Medical School, Ann Arbor, Michigan

Emily Bellile, MS, Senior Statistician, Center for Cancer Biostatistics, Department of Biostatistics, University of Michigan School of Public Health, Ann Arbor, Michigan

Dale Bixby, MD, PhD, Associate Professor, Department of Internal Medicine, Division of Hematology/Oncology, University of Michigan Medical School, Ann Arbor, Michigan

Paula L. Bockenstedt, MD, Associate Professor, Department of Internal Medicine, Division of Hematology/Oncology, University of Michigan Medical School, Ann Arbor, Michigan

Patrick Burke, MD, Clinical Lecturer, Department of Internal Medicine, Division of Hematology/Oncology, University of Michigan Medical School, Ann Arbor, Michigan

Erica Campagnaro, MD, Associate Professor, Department of Internal Medicine, Division of Hematology/Oncology, University of Michigan Medical School, Ann Arbor, Michigan

Shannon Carty, MD, Assistant Professor, Department of Internal Medicine, Division of Hematology/Oncology, University of Michigan Medical School, Ann Arbor, Michigan

Daniel Couriel, MD, MS, Professor of Medicine, Director, Bone Marrow Transplant Program, Department of Internal Medicine, University of Utah School of Medicine, Division of Hematology and Hematologic Malignancies, Huntsman Cancer Institute, Salt Lake City, Utah

Michael W. Deininger, MD, PhD, Chief, Division of Hematology and Hematologic Malignancies, M.M. Wintrobe Professor of Medicine, Senior Director of Transdisciplinary Research, University of Utah School of Medicine, Huntsman Cancer Institute, Salt Lake City, Utah

Sumana Devata, MD, Assistant Professor, Department of Internal Medicine, Division of Hematology/Oncology, University of Michigan Medical School, Ann Arbor, Michigan

Radhika Gangaraju, MD, Assistant Professor, Department of Medicine, Division of Hematology and Oncology, University of Alabama at Birmingham School of Medicine, Birmingham, Alabama

Kyle Greene, MD, Hematology/Oncology Fellow, Department of Internal Medicine, Divisions of Hematology and Oncology, University of Utah School of Medicine, Huntsman Cancer Institute, Salt Lake City, Utah

Monalisa Ghosh, MD, Assistant Professor, Department of Internal Medicine, Division of Hematology/Oncology, University of Michigan Medical School, Ann Arbor, Michigan

J. Matthew Hancock, MD, Fellow, Department of Internal Medicine, Division of Hematology/Oncology, University of Michigan Medical School, Ann Arbor, Michigan

Morgan Jones, MD, PhD, Fellow, Department of Internal Medicine, Division of Hematology/Oncology, University of Michigan Medical School, Ann Arbor, Michigan

Rami N. Khoriaty, MD, Assistant Professor, Department of Internal Medicine, Division of Hematology/Oncology, University of Michigan Medical School, Ann Arbor, Michigan

Darren King, MD, Fellow, Department of Internal Medicine, Division of Hematology/Oncology, University of Michigan Medical School, Ann Arbor, Michigan

Richard King, MD, Fellow, Department of Internal Medicine, Division of Hematology/Oncology, University of Michigan Medical School, Ann Arbor, Michigan

Catherine Lee, MD, Assistant Professor, Department of Internal Medicine, University of Utah School of Medicine, Division of Hematology and Hematologic Malignancies, Huntsman Cancer Institute, Salt Lake City, Utah

Thomas Michniacki, MD, Fellow, Department of Pediatrics, University of Michigan Medical School, Ann Arbor, Michigan

Andy Nguyen, MD, Bone Marrow Transplant Team, Department of Hematology/Oncology, LDS Hospital, Intermountain Healthcare, Salt Lake City, Utah

Charles J. Parker, MD, Professor of Medicine, Department of Internal Medicine, University of Utah School of Medicine, Division of Hematology and Hematologic Malignancies, Huntsman Cancer Institute, Salt Lake City, Utah

Brian Parkin, MD, Assistant Professor, Department of Internal Medicine, Division of Hematology/Oncology, University of Michigan Medical School, Ann Arbor, Michigan

Alexander T. Pearson, MD, PhD, Assistant Professor, Department of Internal Medicine, Division of Hematology/Oncology, University of Chicago, Chicago, Illinois

Tycel J. Phillips, MD, Assistant Professor, Department of Internal Medicine, Division of Hematology/Oncology, University of Michigan Medical School, Ann Arbor, Michigan

Austin Poole, MD, Hematology/Oncology Fellow, Department of Internal Medicine, Divisions of Hematology and Oncology, University of Utah School of Medicine, Huntsman Cancer Institute, Salt Lake City, Utah

Josef T. Prchal, MD, The Charles A. Nugent, MD; Margaret Nugent Endowed Chair, Professor of Medicine, Adjunct Professor, Human Genetics, Adjunct Professor, Pathology, Department of Internal Medicine, University of Utah School of Medicine; Division of Hematology and Hematologic Malignancies, Huntsman Cancer Institute, Salt Lake City, Utah

Angel Qin, MD, Fellow, Department of Internal Medicine, Division of Hematology/Oncology, University of Michigan Medical School, Ann Arbor, Michigan

Albert Quiery, MD, Assistant Professor, Department of Internal Medicine, Division of Hematology/Oncology, University of Michigan Medical School, Ann Arbor, Michigan

Sabarinath Venniyil Radhakrishnan, MD, Visiting Instructor, Department of Internal Medicine, University of Utah School of Medicine, Division of Hematology and Hematologic Malignancies, Huntsman Cancer Institute, Salt Lake City, Utah

Melissa A. Reimers, MD, Fellow, Department of Internal Medicine, Division of Hematology/Oncology, University of Michigan Medical School, Ann Arbor, Michigan

John C. Reneau, MD, Fellow, Department of Internal Medicine, Division of Hematology/Oncology, University of Michigan Medical School, Ann Arbor, Michigan

Mary Mansour Riwes, DO, Assistant Professor, Department of Internal Medicine, Division of Hematology/Oncology, University of Michigan Medical School, Ann Arbor, Michigan

Lyndsey Runaas, MD, Instructor, Department of Internal Medicine, Division of Hematology/Oncology, Medical College of Wisconsin, Milwaukee, Wisconsin

Jordan K. Schaefer, MD, Fellow, Department of Internal Medicine, Division of Hematology/Oncology, University of Michigan Medical School, Ann Arbor, Michigan

Maryann Shango, MD, Staff Physician, Swedish Cancer Institute, Edmonds, Washington

Brittany Siontis, MD, Fellow, Department of Internal Medicine, Division of Hematology/Oncology, University of Michigan Medical School, Ann Arbor, Michigan

Suman L. Sood, MD, Assistant Professor, Department of Internal Medicine, Division of Hematology/Oncology, University of Michigan Medical School, Ann Arbor, Michigan

Tsewang Tashi, MD, Assistant Professor, Department of Internal Medicine, University of Utah School of Medicine, Division of Hematology and Hematologic Malignancies, Huntsman Cancer Institute, Salt Lake City, Utah

Jessica Thibault, MD, Hematology/Oncology Fellow, Department of Internal Medicine, Divisions of Hematology and Oncology, University of Utah School of Medicine, Huntsman Cancer Institute, Salt Lake City, Utah

Nguyen H. Tran, MD, Fellow, Department of Internal Medicine, Division of Hematology/Oncology, University of Michigan Medical School, Ann Arbor, Michigan

Kelly Walkovich, MD, Assistant Professor, Department of Pediatrics and Communicable Diseases, University of Michigan Medical School, Ann Arbor, Michigan

Ryan A. Wilcox, MD, PhD, Assistant Professor, Department of Internal Medicine, Division of Hematology/Oncology, University of Michigan Medical School, Ann Arbor, Michigan

Jedrzej Wykretowicz, MD, PhD, Fellow, Department of Internal Medicine, Division of Hematology/Oncology, University of Michigan Medical School, Ann Arbor, Michigan

Sarah Yentz, MD, Fellow, Department of Internal Medicine, Division of Hematology/Oncology, University of Michigan Medical School, Ann Arbor, Michigan

Preface

Preparation for board examinations can be a daunting and an overwhelming process for many of us. As trainees, we are often busy with research projects, manuscripts, and a large clinical volume, making it difficult to find time to study for board examinations. As practicing physicians, we find it hard to keep up on material needed for board recertification.

Questions on the board examinations are drawn from well-established, validated medical literature and widely accepted clinical guidelines. With this said, the University of Michigan Hematology and Oncology fellowship program and the University of Utah Hematology/Oncology fellowship program have designed this board review book to be an excellent resource for individuals who are preparing for their hematology boards as well as for hematologists or oncologists needing a refresher in practice or in preparation for maintenance of certification (MOC). This book is not intended to be an all-encompassing review. Rather, it is intended to help summarize the important facts that one might need to know for one's examination, similar to taking notes of relevant information that one would like to memorize. We created each chapter to cover all topics listed by the American Board of Internal Medicine (ABIM) as material one should know for the Hematology Board Examination.

In this review, we provide the most accurate and up-to-date information, including well-established treatment regimens for a variety of blood disorders, iron disorders, bone marrow failure syndromes, platelet and megakaryocytic disorders, hemostasis, thrombosis, and hematologic malignancies as well as indications, risks, and complications for transfusion medicine and hematopoietic cell transplantation (HCT).

We hope that fellows, practicing hematologists, and practicing medical oncologists preparing for their certification or recertification will find the *Hematology Board Review* as a useful tool. Our goal is to help our readers summarize and solidify many important clinical facts and to help them build confidence in their exam preparation about their knowledge.

As the hematology/oncology fellowship program director at the University of Michigan (Ann Arbor, MI) and as the Chair of Internal Medicine at the University of Utah, we engaged our fellows and faculty to develop the *Hematology Board Review*. Each chapter is written by a fellow and edited by an expert faculty member or an ancillary staff clinician at the University of Michigan or University of Utah. The book is similarly formatted to the *Oncology Boards Review, 2nd Edition* with approximately five questions, answers, and rationales provided at the end of each chapter so that individuals preparing for the boards will be able to assess their readiness for all key topics that they will find on the actual exam.

Finally, we dedicate this book to Michelle Reinhold for her continued devotion and immeasurable service to the University of Michigan Hematology / Oncology Fellowship Program as program coordinator.

Francis P. Worden, MD
Rami N. Khoriaty, MD
Kathleen A. Cooney, MD, MACP
Michael W. Deininger, MD, PhD

Normal Hematopoiesis

1

Kyle Greene and Tsewang Tashi

DEVELOPMENTAL HEMATOPOIESIS

1. Where and when does the earliest hematopoiesis occur in humans?

- Earliest hematopoiesis occurs in the yolk sac starting with primitive erythropoiesis at around 3 to 5 weeks of gestation, followed soon in the aorta-gonad-mesonephros (AGM). Many cells from AGM also express cell surface markers that are in common with endothelial cells, suggesting that hematopoietic and endothelial cells share a common precursor, called "hemangioblast."

2. What are the embryonic hemoglobin types?

- Hemoglobin Gower (Gower 1 and 2) and hemoglobin Portland (Portland I and II)

3. Where does hematopoiesis take place in the developing fetus?

Hematopoietic Organ	Timeline
Yolk sac	3 to 5 weeks of gestation until about 3 months
Aorta-gonad-mesonephros (AGM)	4 to 6 weeks of gestation
Liver and spleen	Starts at about 2 months until 6 months; *embryonic hemoglobin switch to fetal hemoglobin*
Bone marrow	Starts around 4 months and continues onward into postnatal life

4. Where does hematopoiesis take place after birth?

- In children, it occurs mostly in the marrow of the long bones, such as femur and tibia, while in adults, the majority of hematopoiesis occurs in the vertebrae and pelvis. Sternum, cranium, ribs, femur, and tibia develop the rest.

5. How is fetal hemoglobin (HbF) different?

- HbF is made of $\alpha2\gamma2$ and has higher oxygen affinity than adult hemoglobin A ($\alpha2\beta2$).

HEMATOPOIETIC STEM CELLS

1. What is the difference between hematopoietic stem cells (HSCs) and progenitor cells (HPCs)?

- The difference between HSC and HPC is not very clear-cut. However, while HSCs are the pluripotent undifferentiated cells that can replenish the whole blood system, HPCs are those that have somewhat started to differentiate and commit toward a specific lineage. Both HSCs and HPCs are morphologically indistinguishable. The ambiguous term hematopoietic stem/progenitor cells (HSPCs) is still widely used.

Hematopoietic Stem Cell (HSC)	Progenitor Cell (HPC)
Undifferentiated and has ability to self-renew	Progressively lose self-renewal capacity as they become more differentiated
Pluripotent—can replenish the entire blood system	Oligopotent—can replenish the lineage specific cells
Usually in quiescent state (G0 phase)	More inclined to divide and proliferate
Can undergo unlimited cell divisions	Can undergo limited cell divisions
Usually resistant to cytokines	More responsive to cytokines

2. How do you identify a HSC?

- There is no unique immunophenotype marker for HSC, because progenitor cells and cells that have started to differentiate toward a specific lineage also express many of the cell surface markers that are found on HSCs. It is the absence of any lineage-specific marker that defines a bona fide HSC. Some predominant cell surface markers on HSC are
  - CD34: mediates cell adhesion to marrow stroma
  - CD117, also called stem cell factor receptor (SCF receptor) or C-kit receptor: promotes stem cell survival and proliferation
  - CD133: develops and maintains cell membrane protrusions
  - CD110 also called c-MPL or thrombopoietin receptor: promotes stem cell growth

3. What are colony forming assays?

- Colony forming assays are in vitro techniques to test for hematopoietic stem cell and progenitor cell (HSPC) function. When HSPCs are cultured in a semisolid methylcellulose medium, they form discrete colonies of lineage-committed cells, all arising from a single progenitor cell. Depending on the committed lineage, they are called colony forming unit-erythroid (CFU-E), CFU-granulocytes/macrophage, (CFU-GM), burst forming unit-erythroid (BFU-E), and CFU-granulocytes/erythroid/macrophages/megakaryocytes (CFU-GEMM).

HEMATOPOIETIC MICROENVIRONMENT

1. What is the function of bone marrow stroma?

- Bone marrow stromal matrix includes fibroblasts, osteoclasts, osteoblasts, adipocytes, mesenchymal cells, endothelial cells, and macrophages. They provide an environment or a "niche," conducive for hematopoietic stem cells to maintain, self-renew, grow, and differentiate, regulated by multiple signals mediated through various growth factors and cytokines produced by the stromal matrix.

2. **How is hematopoiesis regulated?**
   - Hematopoiesis is mainly regulated by a complex network of growth factors and transcription factor signaling pathways. Other cells, such as neurons from the sympathetic nervous system, also play a role in the regulation of hematopoietic stem cells (HSCs), mainly by diurnal modulation of HSC homeostasis.

3. **What is HSC "homing"?**
   - HSC "homing" is the phenomenon by which a transplanted HSC migrates to take up its residence in the bone marrow (engraftment). Various receptors and chemokines play an important role in "homing." One such chemokine is the stromal derived factor-1 (SDF-1) and its receptor CXCR4 is expressed on HSC. Plerixafor is a CXCR4 receptor antagonist that is clinically used in mobilizing and collecting stem cells prior to a stem cell transplant.

4. **Which are the major growth factors involved in hematopoiesis?**
   - Examples of growth factors include various cytokines, erythropoietin, thrombopoietin, stem cell factor (SCF), granulocyte colony stimulating factor (G-CSF), and granulocyte/macrophage colony stimulating factor (GM-CSF).

Growth Factor	Source of Production	Target Cells
Erythropoietin (EPO)	Renal peritubular cells	Erythroid progenitors
Thrombopoietin (TPO)	Liver, kidney, marrow stromal cells	Stem cell, megakaryocyte progenitors
G-CSF	Marrow stromal cells	Granulocytes
GM-CSF	Marrow stromal cells	Granulocytes, macrophages
M-CSF	Marrow stromal cells	Monocyte progenitors
SCF (C-kit ligand)	Marrow stromal cells	Stem cells
Cytokines (interleukins), chemokines	Marrow stromal cells	Multipotent precursor cells of myeloid and lymphoid lineage

5. **Give a few examples of the clinical use of growth factors.**
   - Recombinant erythropoietin (EPO), such as darbepoetin and epoetin, are used in anemia due to cancer chemotherapy, anemia of chronic kidney disease, and myelodysplastic syndromes (MDS).
   - Granulocyte colony stimulating factor (G-CSF) and granulocyte/macrophage colony stimulating factor (GM-CSF) are used in chemotherapy-induced neutropenia.
   - G-CSF and plerixafor (CXCR4 receptor inhibitor) are used in stem cell collection prior to stem cell transplant.

6. **What are the major transcription factors (TFs) involved in hematopoiesis?**
   - Examples of TFs include *Hox, GATA1, GATA2, RUNX1, MLL, CEBPa, PAX5, Ikaros,* and *PU.1,* among many others. Mutations in the genes of these TFs can be pathogenic and lead to many hematological malignancies such as acute leukemia and lymphomas.

7. **What are the two main lineage progenitors arising from HSCs?**
   - Common myeloid progenitor (CMP) and common lymphoid progenitor (CLP)
   - Myeloid progenitors are committed to myeloid lineage and give rise to all the myeloid lineage cells, including granulocytes (*neutrophils, eosinophils, basophils*), monocytes, erythrocytes, and megakaryocytes
   - Lymphoid progenitors are committed to lymphoid lineage and give rise to all lymphoid cells, including B cells, T cells, and NK cells.

8. **Where do myelopoiesis and lymphopoiesis occur?**
   - Myelopoiesis originates from the common myeloid progenitor and occurs in the bone marrow. Myelopoiesis includes erythropoiesis, granulopoiesis, and megakaryopoiesis.
   - Early lymphopoiesis occurs in the bone marrow, but naïve lymphocytes migrate to the peripheral lymph nodes (B cells) or the thymus (T cells) for maturation and then become activated once they are "trained" and "learn" to recognize antigens. They then circulate between the lymphatic system and blood circulation, scanning for any foreign antigens. Plasma cell is a terminally differentiated B cell, which produces immunoglobulins. NK cells originate and mature in the bone marrow.

ASSESSMENT OF HEMATOPOIESIS

1. **How is hematopoiesis assessed?**
   - By complete blood count (CBC)
   - By bone marrow aspirate and biopsy

2. **How do you assess for hematopoiesis on a bone marrow biopsy and aspirate?**
   - By assessing the bone marrow cellularity—which is the "nonfat" portion of the marrow—for erythropoiesis, granulopoiesis, and megakaryopoiesis (commonly called the "trilineage hematopoiesis"). Cellularity is age dependent and is commonly measured as 100 – age = cellularity.

3. **Why does bone marrow cellularity decrease with aging?**
   - HSCs and the surrounding stroma undergo several changes with aging, including an increase in adipocytes, increased level of reactive oxygen species (ROS) production, altered HSC mobilization, and decrease in self-renewal capacity of the HSCs.

QUESTIONS

1. **Which of the following statements about hematopoiesis is incorrect?**
   A. Early hematopoiesis occurs in the yolk sac, starting with primitive granulopoiesis.
   B. Embryonic hemoglobin switching to fetal hemoglobin takes place during the liver hematopoiesis.
   C. Hematopoietic and endothelial cells arise from a common progenitor, the "hemangioblast."
   D. The spleen is a site of extramedullary hematopoiesis in chronic myeloproliferative neoplasm (MPN) patients.

2. A 24-year-old male is referred for anemia by his primary care provider. His complete blood count (CBC) shows white blood cell (WBC) of 5.4 K/mcL, hemoglobin (Hb) of 12.5 g/dL, mean corpuscular volume (MCV) 89 FL, and platelet count of 299 K/mcL. Iron studies were normal. High-performance liquid chromatography (HPLC) shows HbA = 80%, HbA2 = 3%, and fetal hemoglobin (HbF) = 17%. Which of the following is correct?
    A. Presence of HbF will shift the Hb-oxygen dissociation curve to the right.
    B. The patient likely has hereditary persistence of fetal hemoglobin (HPFH) and his P50 is likely to be decreased.
    C. Globin genotyping is likely to reveal an absence of beta-globin.
    D. He is likely to have hepatosplenomegaly due to extramedullary hematopoiesis.

3. A 65-year-old man is admitted to the hospital due to a 2-week history of upper respiratory infection (URI)-like symptoms and complete blood count (CBC) at the emergency department (ED) showing white blood cell (WBC) 35 K/mcL, hemoglobin (Hb) 9.5 g/dL, and platelet count 35 K/mcL. Differential count shows 75% blasts and 20% neutrophils. A bone marrow biopsy and aspirate was done, and flow cytometry revealed an immunophenotype positive for CD13, CD33, CD34, CD117, and HLA-DR, but negative for CD15, CD64, and CD11b. Which of the following statements is incorrect?
    A. This patient has acute myeloid leukemia, most likely arising from mutations in the hematopoietic stem cells (HSCs) and progenitor cells.
    B. Progenitor cells progressively lose self-renewal capacity as they differentiate.
    C. HSCs can be identified from the in vitro colony forming assays.
    D. HSCs and progenitor cells are morphologically indistinguishable.

4. Which of the following statements is incorrect?
    A. Erythropoietin is produced by the peritubular cells in the kidney.
    B. Thrombopoietin is produced by the liver only in response to low platelet counts.
    C. Mutations in granulocyte colony stimulating factor (G-CSF) receptor can be found in chronic neutrophilic leukemia.
    D. Eltrombopag is a thrombopoietin (TPO) mimetic, which can be used for treating idiopathic thrombocytopenic purpura (ITP).

ANSWERS

1. **A. Early hematopoiesis occurs in the yolk sac, starting with primitive granulopoiesis.** Primitive hematopoiesis originates in the yolk sac, starting with erythropoiesis, to deliver oxygen to other parts of the developing embryo.

2. **B. The patient likely has hereditary persistence of fetal hemoglobin (HPFH) and his P50 is likely to be decreased.** HbF has higher Hb-oxygen affinity, which will shift the oxygen dissociation curve to the left. P50 is the partial pressure of oxygen when hemoglobin is 50% saturated, and with higher oxygen affinity, P50 will be decreased. An asymptomatic patient with mild anemia and a normal MCV with elevated HbF most likely has HPFH. Absence of beta-globin is seen in beta-thalassemia major, and HPLC would show complete absence of HbA. Hepatosplenomegaly associated with extramedullary hematopoiesis is typically found in thalassemia major and chronic myeloproliferative neoplasms.

3. **C. HSCs can be identified from the in vitro colony forming assays.** HSCs cannot be isolated or identified, as they are morphologically indistinguishable from progenitor cells and do not have any specific cell surface markers.

4. **B. Thrombopoietin is produced by the liver only in response to low platelet counts.** TPO is produced constitutively by the liver and is inactivated by binding to the TPO receptor (c-MPL) on circulating platelets. Therefore, it is the level of platelets that regulates availability of thrombopoietin to megakaryocytes.

Red Blood Cell Production Disorders

Jessica Thibault and Josef T. Prchal

Nutritional Deficiencies

EPIDEMIOLOGY

1. **What is the incidence of anemia secondary to nutritional deficiencies?**
   - Iron deficiency anemia affects 10% to 15% of adults worldwide.
   - The exact incidence of B12 and folate deficiency are unknown.

ETIOLOGY AND RISK FACTORS

1. **What is the etiology of nutritional deficiency–related anemia?**
   - Lack of dietary intake or malabsorption: B12, folate, and iron; also pica (rare cause of iron deficiency); infection of *diphyllobothrium latum* interferes with B12 absorption, that is, chronic hemolysis requires more folate; chronic bleeding and intravascular hemolysis are causes of iron deficiency.

2. **What are the common risk factors?**
   - Menstruating women
   - Pregnancy and lactation
   - Inflammatory gastrointestinal disease
   - Bariatric surgery
   - Medications including methotrexate, trimethoprim, pyrimethamine, phenytoin, valproate, and carbamazepine can increase risk of folate deficiency
   - Severely limited diets such as in the case of some alcoholics
   - Increasing age is a risk factor for B12 deficiency
   - Clinical or subclinical chronic blood loss

SIGNS AND SYMPTOMS

1. **What are the common signs and symptoms of nutritional deficiency–related anemia?**
   - Fatigue
   - Dyspnea
   - Pallor
   - Weakness
   - Headache
   - Angina
   - Decreased exercise tolerance

- Restless leg syndrome
- Pica
- Neuropsychiatric symptoms with B12 deficiency

DIAGNOSTIC WORKUP/CRITERIA

1. What tests are included in the diagnostic workup?

- Complete blood count with differential
- Creatinine, BUN, liver function tests
- Reticulocyte count
- Iron studies including ferritin, serum iron, total iron binding capacity (TIBC), and transferrin saturation
- B12 and folate
- If iron deficiency anemia is diagnosed, a full workup to rule out blood loss is indicated

2. What are the diagnostic criteria for iron deficiency anemia?

- Microcytic anemia (note; microcytosis in moderate to severe iron deficiency anemia but may not be present in mild iron-deficient anemia
- Low serum iron (but also decreases with inflammation); low transferrin saturation (typically <20%)
- Increased serum transferrin or TIBC
- Low ferritin is more sensitive and specific than iron and TIBC but low ferritin may not be present; ferritin is an acute phase reactant, so normal or even high ferritin does not rule out iron deficiency
- If above scenario is a possibility, reticulocyte hemoglobin concentration (readily available by automatic blood counters), soluble transferrin receptor index (ratio of soluble transferrin receptor and ferritin), and marrow iron studies can be helpful
- Staining of the bone marrow aspirate smear for iron used to be the gold standard, but it is not required in most scenarios; then reticulocyte hemoglobin concentration and soluble transferrin receptor index are good substitutes

3. What are the diagnostic criteria for folate deficiency?

- Macrocytic anemia
- Serum folate level below 2 ng/mL but it reflects recent folate intake; better measurement of folate stores is red cell folate
- Serum folate values between 2 and 4 ng/mL are equivocal and can be further worked up with methylmalonic acid and homocysteine levels. Normal methylmalonic acid and elevated homocysteine is indicative of folate deficiency. Methymalonic acid may occasionally be elevated in folic acid deficiency as well

4. What are the diagnostic criteria for B12 deficiency?

- Macrocytic anemia
- Serum B12 less than 200 pg/mL is diagnostic
- Serum B12 between 200 and 300 pg/mL is equivocal. Elevated methylmalonic acid and elevated homocysteine is diagnostic of B12 deficiency in this situation

- Pernicious anemia may be identified by testing for autoantibodies to intrinsic factor

TREATMENT

1. **What is the treatment for iron deficiency anemia?**
   - Transfusion of red blood cells if the patient is severely symptomatic or has evidence of end-organ damage
   - Replacement dose is based on the calculated iron deficit (mg) = body weight $\times$ (14 − Hgb) $\times$ (2.145), but replenishment of iron stores is also needed
   - Oral or intravenous (IV) iron can be used depending on the underlying cause of iron deficiency, availability, cost, and the patient's compliance and ability to tolerate oral iron
     - Oral preparations: ferrous fumarate, ferrous gluconate, ferrous sulfate, ferrous succinate, ferric citrate, ferrous ascorbate, and polysaccharide iron complex. Dose is dependent on patient age and estimated iron deficit, but typically is ~200 mg of elemental iron per day; ferrous sulfate is cheapest and well absorbed. Coated preparations should not be used, as >90% of iron is absorbed in duodenum.
     - New data suggests that once-daily dosing of oral iron may increase absorption and be sufficient to correct iron deficits.
     - IV preparations: ferric carboxymaltose, iron sucrose, iron dextran, ferric gluconate, and ferric carboxymaltose. Each can cause hypotension and allergic reaction. Largest single dose (2 g of iron) can be administered as iron dextran.

2. **What is the treatment for folate deficiency?**
   - With 1 to 5 mg of oral folic acid daily for 2 to 4 months, plasma is corrected immediately and normal erythropoiesis is restored but replenishments of stores (stores last ~3 months for normal erythropoiesis) requires several weeks of therapy or indefinitely if there is not a reversible cause.
   - IV folic acid can be given in those unable to receive oral replacement or those with large small-bowel resections or pathology.
   - Of note, treatment with folic acid can mask symptoms of B12 deficiency.

3. **What is the treatment for vitamin B12 deficiency?**
   - For pernicious anemia: 1,000 mcg (intramuscular [IM] or subcutaneous) once per week for 4 weeks followed by 1,000 mcg per month
   - Dietary deficiency: 1,000 mcg parenterally or orally once per week until the deficiency is corrected and then once per month or every other month

Anemia of Chronic Disease

EPIDEMIOLOGY

1. **How common is anemia of chronic disease?**
   - Anemia of chronic disease is the second most common cause of anemia. The exact incidence is unknown.

ETIOLOGY AND RISK FACTORS

1. **What is the etiology of anemia of chronic disease?**
   - Anemia of chronic disease is caused by inflammatory states (increased cytokines, interleukin [IL]-1, and IL-6) that cause increased hepcidin production in the liver. This, in turn, leads to reduced absorption of iron and trapping of iron in macrophages and subsequent decreased hemoglobin synthesis. There is also a relative increase in hepcidin production mediated by low erythroferrone and an inability to increase erythropoietin in response to anemia.

2. **What are the common underlying diseases for anemia of chronic disease?**
   - Infections (acute infections, HIV, etc.)
   - Autoimmune diseases
   - Malignancy
   - Inflammatory bowel disease
   - Heart failure
   - Diabetes
   - Chronic kidney disease
   - Chronic obstructive pulmonary disease (COPD)

SIGNS AND SYMPTOMS

1. **What are the common signs and symptoms of anemia of chronic disease (ACD)?**
   - Fatigue mediated by both inflammatory cytokines and anemia
   - Symptoms of anemia: dyspnea, pallor, decreased exercise tolerance angina

DIAGNOSTIC WORKUP/CRITERIA

1. **What are the most common presenting signs/symptoms in essential thrombocythemia (ET)?**
   - Many patients present with a mild normocytic, normochromic anemia. In ~25% of cases, the anemia is microcytic.
   - Red cell distribution width is nonspecific and can be normal to increased.
   - Mean corpuscular hemoglobin (MHC) is normal to low in a proportion of cases.
   - Absolute reticulocyte count is often low.
   - Serum iron and TIBC are low. Transferrin saturation can be low or normal.
   - Peripheral smear may be normal or show signs of an underlying inflammatory condition (toxic granulation, left shift, malignant cells, etc.)

2. **How is the diagnosis of ACD made?**
   - There is no specific diagnostic test. The diagnosis is suspected when the following are present:
     - Ferritin is normal or high.
     - Serum iron and TIBC are low.

- ○ Transferrin saturation may be normal or low.
- ○ Erythrocyte sedimentation rate (ESR) and *C-reactive protein* (CRP) may be elevated.
- ○ Low iron and elevated hepcidin is the hallmark (if hepcidin assay available).

TREATMENT

1. What is the preferred treatment for ACD?

- The primary treatment is correction of the underlying disorder.

2. What are additional treatment options?

- Red cell transfusions
- Use of erythropoietin analogues if the patient is symptomatic and has not responded to treatment of the underlying disorder; darbepoetin alfa is the most convenient preparation. Erythropoietin decreases hepcidin; thus, it immediately releases iron from the stores, permitting productive erythropoiesis
- Supplemental iron to achieve transferrin saturation of ≥20% and serum ferritin ≥100 ng/mL

Red Cell Aplasia

EPIDEMIOLOGY

1. What is the median age at diagnosis?

- Red cell aplasia can affect patients at any age, but more commonly it affects adolescents and adults.

2. What is the incidence of red cell aplasia?

- This varies by subtype, but overall is very rare.

ETIOLOGY AND RISK FACTORS

1. What are the common risk factors for red cell aplasia?

- Thymoma
- Subcutaneous erythropoietin administration in patients with chronic kidney disease is a risk factor for anti-erythropoietin antibody–mediated red cell aplasia, which is almost no longer seen with newer erythropoietin preparations

PATHOLOGY—CLASSIFICATION

1. What are the causes of pure red cell aplasia?

- Most common cause in an adult is idiopathic
- Thymoma
- Congenital form: Diamond-Blackfan syndrome
- Large granular lymphocyte leukemia/lymphoma
- Anti-erythropoietin antibodies
- Drugs including phenytoin, isoniazid, valproic acid, chloramphenicol, azathioprine, and mycophenolate

- T-cell and B-cell lymphoproliferative disorders
- ABO-incompatible hematopoietic cell transplant
- Infection including parvovirus B10, mumps, hepatitis, Epstein-Barr virus (EBV), and HIV

SIGNS AND SYMPTOMS

1. What are the common signs and symptoms?

- Symptoms of anemia: fatigue, dyspnea, pallor, decreased exercise tolerance, angina
- Complete blood count (CBC) shows anemia that is often severe, normocytic, and normochromic. White blood cells and platelets are unaffected
- Reticulocyte count is markedly decreased

DIAGNOSTIC WORKUP/CRITERIA

1. What is the diagnostic workup?

- Bone marrow aspiration and biopsy confirms diagnosis
- CT or MRI of the chest to rule out thymoma
- Viral studies as indicated
- Peripheral smear
- Additional tests when an underlying hematologic condition is suspected

2. What are the diagnostic criteria?

- An absolute reticulocyte count <10,000/microL
- Normal white blood cell and platelet counts
- Normocellular bone marrow, few or no erythroid precursors but normal white cell and platelet precursors
- Anemia that is normocytic (rarely macrocytic) and normochromic

PROGNOSIS

1. What is the prognosis for red cell aplasia?

- Overall survival (OS) in most studies is 10 to 20 years for idiopathic red cell aplasia.
- OS is lower in patients with underlying malignancy.
- Up to 15% of patients may have spontaneously remitting disease.

TREATMENT

1. What is the initial management for red cell aplasia?

- Red cell transfusions for symptomatic anemia
- Search for an underlying cause or offending drug and treat accordingly
- A short period of observation is reasonable for idiopathic red cell aplasia since some cases will spontaneously remit. If it does not resolve, treatment with glucocorticoids, glucocorticoids and cyclosporine, or glucocorticoids and cyclophosphamide are all reasonable initial treatments. There have been no randomized trials comparing these treatments

- Patients with recurrent or refractory disease can be treated with intravenous immunoglobulin (IVIG), plasmapheresis, azathioprine, rituximab, alemtuzumab, or daclizumab. Hematopoietic stem cell transplantation may be indicated in select cases.

Sideroblastic Anemia

EPIDEMIOLOGY

1. **What is the median age at diagnosis?**
   - Sideroblastic anemia can affect patients at any age. The median age at diagnosis varies depending on the underlying etiology.

ETIOLOGY AND RISK FACTORS

1. **What is the cause of sideroblastic anemia?**
   - Sideroblastic anemias are due to inherited or acquired abnormalities in heme synthesis and mitochondrial function.
     - The specific mitochondrial pathways that are typically affected include heme synthesis, iron–sulfur cluster production, and mitochondrial protein synthesis.

2. **What are the common congenital and acquired causes of sideroblastic anemia?**
   - Congenital
     - X-linked, X-linked with ataxia
     - Glutaredoxin 5 deficiency
     - Erythropoietic protoporphyria
     - Mitochondrial defects
     - Pearson marrow-pancreas syndrome
     - Thiamine-responsive megaloblastic anemia
   - Acquired
     - Clonal acquired sideroblastic anemias—myeloid neoplasms with ring sideroblasts
     - Alcoholism (the most common cause)
     - Drugs including isoniazid, chloramphenicol, linezolid, and cycloserine
     - Copper deficiency (secondary to zinc toxicity or from malabsorption typically after gastrointestinal [GI] surgery)
     - Lead poisoning

3. **What are the risk factors for sideroblastic anemia?**
   - Family history
   - Alcoholism
   - Males are more likely to inherit X-linked recessive types of sideroblastic anemia
   - No racial predominance is known

SIGNS AND SYMPTOMS

1. **What are the common clinical features of sideroblastic anemia?**
   - Pallor
   - Fatigue
   - Dyspnea
   - Hepatosplenomegaly
   - Congenital forms often present with microcytic or normocytic anemia
   - Acquired forms often present with normocytic or macrocytic anemia

DIAGNOSTIC WORKUP/CRITERIA

1. **What is the diagnostic workup when sideroblastic anemia is suspected?**
   - CBC and blood smear
   - Iron studies
   - Erythrocyte folate level
   - Plasma copper and ceruloplasmin levels
   - Bone marrow aspirate and biopsy
   - Genetic testing

2. **What are the diagnostic criteria?**
   - Anemia—may be microcytic, normocytic, or macrocytic
   - Ring sideroblasts on the bone marrow aspirate smear
   - Ring sideroblasts are erythroblasts with iron-loaded mitochondria. With Prussian blue staining, they appear as a ring of blue granules surrounding the nucleus
   - Genetic testing if applicable

PROGNOSTIC FACTORS

1. **What is the prognosis for sideroblastic anemia?**
   - The prognosis varies depending on the underlying cause
   - Patients with acquired sideroblastic anemia who have a reversible cause typically have no long-term sequela of the disease
   - Sideroblastic anemia with MDS has a median survival of 38 months
   - Thrombocytosis is a good prognostic sign
   - Transfusion dependence is a poor prognostic sign

2. **What are the major causes of death in sideroblastic anemia?**
   - Secondary hemochromatosis—organ failure
   - Leukemia

TREATMENT

1. **What is the treatment for congenital sideroblastic anemia?**
   - For patients with non-syndromic forms, treatment is aimed at relieving the symptoms of anemia and preventing organ damage from iron overload. Periodic transfusions are appropriate to treat symptomatic anemia, but they should be minimized when possible to prevent iron overload.

- For patients with syndromic forms, treatment is dictated by other features of their disease and symptom management.
- Patients should be referred to genetics.

2. **What is the treatment for acquired sideroblastic anemia?**
- Remove offending drug, toxin, and so forth. For isoniazid-induced sideroblastic anemia, vitamin B6 can be given while continuing the drug.
- In cobalt deficiency, remove excessive zinc and/or administer IV iron.
- Treatment of MDS is discussed in a later chapter.

Congenital Dyserythropoietic Anemias (CDA)

EPIDEMIOLOGY

1. **Congenital dyserythropoietic anemias are rare. There are three known subtypes.**

ETIOLOGY AND RISK FACTORS

1. **What is the etiology of type I CDA?**
- Type I CDA is caused by mutations in the *CDAN1* gene, encoding codanin-1, a cell cycle–regulated protein involved in the histone assembly. It is inherited in an autosomal recessive pattern. Homozygosity is often associated with consanguinity. In a number of patients, only one or no *CDAN1* mutated allele is identified. Other causative genes, such as *C15ORF41*, may be responsible.

2. **What is the etiology of type II CDA?**
- Type II CDA is also known by its acronym HEMPAS (*h*ereditary *e*rythroblastic *m*ultinuclearity associated with a *p*ositive *a*cidified *s*erum test).
- It is inherited in an autosomal recessive pattern. It is due to mutations in *SEC23B* gene, which encodes a component of the coat protein complex II (COPII), responsible for the biogenesis of endoplasmic reticulum–derived vesicles, a component of the cis-Golgi.

3. **What is the etiology of type III CDA?**
- Autosomal dominant inheritance due to mutations in *KIF23* gene encoding mitotic kinesin-like protein 1, critical for cytokinesis

4. **There are several rare types of CDA that do not conform to types I to III.**

SIGNS AND SYMPTOMS

1. **What are the common presenting features of type I CDA?**
- Moderately severe macrocytic anemia
- Hepatomegaly and cholelithiasis are common
- Splenomegaly is common and increases with age
- Dysmorphic skeletal features may be present, typically affecting hands and feet. Less common are small stature, almond-shaped blue eyes, hypertelorism, and micrognathia

- Iron overload from erythroferrone-mediated low hepcidin may be the major cause of morbidity and mortality in adulthood

2. **What are the common presenting features of type II CDA?**
   - Anemia varies from mild to severe.
   - Moderate-to-marked anisocytosis, poikilocytosis, anisochromia, and contracted spherocytes are present in the peripheral blood.
   - Gaucher-like cells and ring sideroblasts may be found in the marrow.
   - More than 10% of mature bi- and multinucleated red cell precursors is a morphologic hallmark.

3. **What are the common presenting features of type III CDA?**
   - Most patients are asymptomatic with mild-to-moderate anemia, mild jaundice, and commonly cholelithiasis.
   - Intravascular hemolysis is common.
   - Some macrocytes may be extremely large. The marrow has marked erythroid hyperplasia, with large multinucleate erythroblasts with big lobulated nuclei, and giant multinucleate erythroblasts.

DIAGNOSTIC WORKUP

1. **What is the diagnostic workup for CDA?**
   - Laboratory studies including complete blood count with differential, completed metabolic panel, reticulocyte count, iron studies
   - Bone marrow biopsy
   - Gene mutation testing

TREATMENT

1. **What is the treatment for CDA?**
   - Red cell transfusions may be necessary; iron chelation should be instituted when the ferritin level exceeds 500 to 1,000 mcg/L.
   - There may be a partial benefit with splenectomy; this is less effective in type II CDA.
   - Interferon alfa is effective in most patients with type II CDA.
   - Stem cell transplantation has been used in few patients and should be considered early before iron overload develops.
   - Type III CDA generally does not require treatment.

Inefficient Erythropoiesis in Thalassemias

DEFINITION

1. **What is thalassemia?**
   - A group of disorders, each resulting from an inherited defect in the rate of synthesis of one or more globin chains

- Resultant imbalance of globin chain production may cause ineffective erythropoiesis, defective hemoglobin production, red cell hemoglobin precipitates, hemolysis, and anemia of variable degree

ETIOLOGY

1. **What is the etiology of ineffective erythropoiesis in thalassemias?**
   - In homozygous β-thalassemia, β-globin synthesis is absent or greatly reduced, resulting in hypochromic microcytic red cells. As excess α-chains are incapable of forming viable hemoglobin tetramers, they precipitate in red cell precursors, resulting in intramedullary destruction of the abnormal erythroid cells (ineffective erythropoiesis) and hemolysis.
   - In heterozygous β-thalassemia, there is usually only mild hypochromic microcytic anemia with elevated HbA_2. Some are more severe because of poor heme-binding properties and instability, with red cell inclusions containing precipitated β-chains as well as excess α-chains. These are sometimes described as "hyperunstable hemoglobins."
   - In α-thalassemias, defective α-chain production manifests in both fetal and adult life, as α-chains are present in both fetal and adult hemoglobins. The defect in hemoglobin synthesis leads to hypochromic, microcytic cells.
   - Severe anemia and the high oxygen affinity of HbF in homozygous β-thalassemia produce severe tissue hypoxia.
   - Erythropoietin production and consequent expansion of marrow leads to deformities of skull with frequent sinus and ear infections, porous long bones, and pathologic features.
   - Constant exposure of the spleen to red cells of precipitated globin chains leads to "work hypertrophy" of the spleen, ultimately leading to splenomegaly. The enlarged spleen may sequester red cells and expand plasma volume, exacerbating anemia.
   - Iron overload from erythroferrone-mediated low hepcidin may be the major cause of morbidity and mortality in adulthood.

SIGNS AND SYMPTOMS

1. **What are the signs and symptoms of ineffective erythropoiesis in thalassemias?**
   - Microcytic anemia
   - Peripheral smear shows marked anisopoikilocytosis, hypochromia, target cells, basophilic stippling, large poikilocytes, nucleated red cells, and inclusions of Hb in hypochromic red cells
   - Bone marrow shows marked erythroid hyperplasia, abnormal erythroblasts with stippling, increased sideroblasts, and markedly increased storage iron
   - Symptoms of anemia: fatigue, dyspnea, pallor, decreased exercise tolerance, angina
   - Skeletal deformities if not treated adequately
   - Failure to thrive in early childhood

DIAGNOSTIC WORKUP

1. How is thalassemia worked up?

- CBC with differential
- Hemoglobin electrophoresis
- Bone marrow biopsy in some cases

TREATMENT

1. What is the treatment?

- Transfusion of packed red blood cells that have been washed, filtered, and frozen to maintain hemoglobin between 9.5 and 14 g/dL
- Iron chelation for all patients with regular transfusion requirements
- Hematopoietic stem cell transplantation with human leukocyte antigen (HLA)-matched sibling donor is very effective if performed early

QUESTIONS

1. A 68-year-old man with a history of alcoholism and poor nutrition presents with several months of shortness of breath and fatigue. Physical examination is unremarkable. Laboratory values include the following:

Laboratory test	Patient's value (reference range)
White blood cell count	4×10^9/L (4×10^9–10×10^9/L)
Hemoglobin	6 g/dL (13–16 g/dL)
Mean corpuscular volume (MCV)	116 fL (80–100 fL)
Platelet count	180×10^9/L (150×10^9–400×10^9/L)
Reticulocyte count	1.0% (0.7%–2.07%)
Ferritin	110 ng/mL (35–150 ng/mL)
Total iron binding capacity (TIBC)	243 mcg/dL (240–450 mcg/dL)
Transferrin saturation	13% (20%–50%)
Vitamin B12	220 pg/mL (211–911 pg/mL)
Folate	3 ng/mL (≥3 ng/mL)
Methylmalonic acid	2.8 mcg/dL (0–4.7 mcg/dL)
Homocysteine	77 µmol/L (<11 µmol/L)

Which of the following most likely accounts for the patient's anemia?
A. Folate deficiency
B. B12 deficiency
C. Erythropoietin deficiency
D. Iron deficiency

2. A 49-year-old woman is evaluated in the clinic for progressive dyspnea on exertion, pallor, and fatigue. She has a history of congestive heart

failure, diabetes mellitus, and latent tuberculosis for which she is taking isoniazid. Her laboratory data is as follows:

Laboratory test	Patient's value (reference range)
White blood cell count	3.8×10^9/L (4×10^9–10×10^9/L)
Hemoglobin	8.2 g/dL (13–16 g/dL)
Mean corpuscular volume (MCV)	102 fL (80–100 fL)
Platelet count	310×10^9/L (150×10^9–400×10^9/L)
Ferritin	72 ng/mL (35–150 ng/mL)
Total iron binding capacity (TIBC)	273 mcg/dL (240–450 mcg/dL)
Transferrin saturation	27% (20%–50%)
Vitamin B12	240 pg/mL (211–911 pg/mL)
Folate	5 ng/mL (≥3 ng/mL)

A bone marrow biopsy reveals ringed sideroblasts. What is the appropriate next step in the care of this patient?
A. Refer for genetic testing
B. Stop isoniazid
C. Start vitamin B6
D. Start vitamin B12

3. All of the following statements are true regarding vitamin B12 deficiency except
   A. B12 deficiency leads to ineffective erythropoiesis and pancytopenia
   B. High-dose oral B12 can be used to treat deficiency
   C. High levels of methyl malonic acid (MMA) always indicate B12 deficiency
   D. Folic acid supplementation alone in patients with B12 deficiency can worsen neurologic symptoms

4. All are true about anemia of chronic disease (ACD) except
   A. ACD occurs due to the sequestration of iron in the macrophages and decreased absorption from intestine
   B. It is characterized by high hepcidin levels and low expression of ferroportin
   C. It is characterized by low transferrin saturation, high iron binding capacity, and high ferritin
   D. Management of the underlying disorder is the treatment of choice

5. A 54-year-old lady with a history of chronic kidney disease (CKD) Stage 5 presents to the clinic for evaluation of anemia. She has exertional shortness of breath and fatigue but denies any bleeding source. Physical exam is positive for elevated jugular venous pressure (JVP), pedal edema, and bibasilar crackles in the lung.

White blood cell count	5.0×10^9/L (4×10^9–10×10^9/L)
Hemoglobin	8.0 g/dL (13–16 g/dL)
Mean corpuscular volume (MCV)	84 fL (80–100 fL)
Platelet count	280×10^9/L (150×10^9–400×10^9/L)
Ferritin	72 ng/mL (35–150 ng/mL)
Total iron binding capacity (TIBC)	220 mcg/dL (240–450 mcg/dL)
Transferrin saturation	17% (20%–50%)
Erythropoietin	20 mU/mL (2.6–18.5 mU/mL)

What is the best treatment option for this patient?

A. No active intervention
B. Darbepoetin supplementation
C. Oral iron supplementation
D. Combined darbepoetin and intravenous iron supplementation

ANSWERS

1. **A. Folate deficiency.** The patient presents with macrocytic anemia and an equivocal serum folate level. When the folate is between 2 and 4 ng/mL, methylmalonic acid and homocysteine levels are used to diagnose or rule out a deficiency. An elevated homocysteine level and normal methylmalonic acid is consistent with folic acid deficiency. Poor nutrition with a lack of vegetable and vegetables compounded by moderate alcohol interference with folate metabolism is a risk factor for folate deficiency. However, it is seen in those drinking only hard liquor and wine (no folate content; but it is not seen in beer drinkers [rich in folate]). The patient also has functional iron deficiency (transferrin saturation <20%); however, this does not explain the patient's macrocytic anemia.

2. **C. Start vitamin B6.** This patient has sideroblastic anemia, which is likely acquired from the isoniazid that she is taking for latent tuberculosis. Isoniazid-induced sideroblastic anemia is unique in that you can continue treatment and supplement with vitamin B6.

3. **C. High levels of methyl malonic acid (MMA) always indicate B12 deficiency.** Mild elevations in methylmalonic acid (MMA) can occur in patients with renal disease or small-bowel bacterial overgrowth and so should not be used as the only parameter to diagnose B12 deficiency. In B12 deficiency, MMA and homocysteine are both elevated compared to homocysteine alone in folic acid deficiency.

4. **C. It is characterized by low transferrin saturation, high iron binding capacity, and high ferritin.** In anemia of chronic disease, there is a functional iron deficiency with low transferrin saturation and low total iron binding capacity with high ferritin. In contrast, in iron deficiency anemia there is a low transferrin saturation but associated with high total iron binding capacity and low ferritin.

5. **D. Combined darbepoetin and intravenous iron supplementation.** Even though the erythropoietin level is above the normal range, it is relatively low for the level of anemia. Patients with renal failure have a functional iron deficiency, and the best results are obtained when intravenous (IV) iron is given in addition to erythropoietin. The goal of therapy is to keep Hb between 10 and 12 g%.

Sabarinath Venniyil Radhakrishnan and Charles J. Parker

Warm Antibody Hemolytic Anemia

EPIDEMIOLOGY

1. **What is the incidence of warm antibody hemolytic anemia (WAHA)?**
   - The incidence of WAHA is ~1 in 80,000. The disease can occur at all ages, but the peak incidence is in the seventh decade, probably due to the accompanying increase in the incidence of lymphoproliferative diseases in this age group.

ETIOLOGY AND RISK FACTORS

1. **What is the pathophysiology of WAHA?**
   - The autoantibodies are almost always of the immunoglobulin G (IgG) class (IgA-mediated WAHA is fleetingly rare and IgM antibodies are almost invariably cold agglutinins) and bind to red cells optimally at 37°C.
   - These antibodies bind to common antigens on the red cells, resulting in panreactivity when tested for antigen specificity. Approximately 50% bind to Rh complex constituents and the other 50% bind to non-Rh blood group antigens.
   - Fc receptors, complement C3 receptors, or both on reticuloendothelial cells bind opsonized red cells coated with antibodies, activation/degradation products of C3, or both, and trap the *red blood cells* (RBCs) primarily in the spleen. Splenic macrophages phagocytose opsonized red cells, and if the phagocytic event produces partial loss of the membrane, microspherocytes are formed. *The presence of microspherocytes observed in the peripheral blood film is a defining feature of WAHA.*

2. **What are the secondary causes of WAHA?**
   - Lymphoproliferative disorders, including chronic lymphocytic leukemia (CLL), Hodgkin, and non-Hodgkin lymphoma
   - Autoimmune diseases, including connective tissue disorders, particularly systemic lupus erythematosus (SLE)
   - Drug induced, including cephalosporins and quinine/quinidine
   - Non-lymphoid neoplasia, including ovarian cancer

SIGNS AND SYMPTOMS

3. **What are the clinical features of WAHA?**
   - Onset can be insidious or acute.
   - Patients may present with pallor, icterus, and symptoms of anemia.

4. What are the laboratory features of WAHA?

- Macrocytic anemia, due to compensatory reticulocytosis (reticulocytes are macrocytic)
- Signs of extravascular hemolysis, including unconjugated hyperbilirubinemia, low serum haptoglobin, elevated serum lactate dehydrogenase (LDH)
- Hemoglobinuria is a feature of intravascular hemolysis and is rare in WAHA
- Direct antiglobulin test (direct Coombs test) is positive for immunoglobulin G (IgG), C3, or both in 90% to 95% of cases

5. What is direct antiglobulin test (DAT)-negative WAHA?

- The density of immunoglobulin G (IgG) on the surface of red cells required to produce a positive DAT varies with the commercial reagent used. Generally, a density of >150 molecules of IgG or complement C3/red cells will produce a positive DAT. Normal red cells have 30 to 60 molecules of IgG nonspecifically bound to their surface.
- The presenting symptoms and signs (including microspherocytes and reticulo-cytosis) and treatment responses are similar in DAT-positive and DAT-negative patients.
- Proposed causes of DAT-negative WAHA include the following:
  - The density of IgG or C3 on the red cell surface is below the detection threshold of the commercially available Coombs reagent
  - Low-affinity IgG antibodies that dissociate from the surface during washing steps used to prepare cells for the DAT
  - Non-IgG antibodies, usually IgA antibodies (the Coombs reagent used for initial screening in the DAT has antibodies against only IgG and complement C3)

DIAGNOSTIC CRITERIA

1. What is the differential diagnosis for DAT-negative hemolytic anemia?

- Hereditary spherocytosis: HS is usually manifested at a younger age, but mild cases may not produce clinically significant anemia until later in life
- Wilson disease: The oxidative damage of hemoglobin by copper leads to hemo-lytic anemia, and the cells appear contracted with small irregular projections representing Heinz bodies
- Acute hemolysis due to toxins such as lecithinase-C produced by clostridium perfringens. In this case, evidence of sepsis would likely be apparent
- Zieve syndrome: due to recent heavy alcohol intake, accompanied by fatty liver, hyperlipidemia, and hemolytic anemia
  - Paroxysmal nocturnal hemoglobinuria (PNH is a non-spherocytic hemo-lytic anemia)
  - Delayed transfusion reactions

2. How will you transfuse red cells for patients with WAHA and what are the caveats?

- Identification of a compatible donor is rare, as nearly all antibodies in WAHA are panagglutinins (e.g., they bind to all donor red cells).

- The presence of coexisting alloantibodies must be excluded. This process is accomplished by using the patient's red cells to absorb all of the autoantibody. If residual antibody is found after absorption, it can be tested for specificity so that donor red cells expressing the particular alloantigen can be avoided.
- As perfectly compatible donor cells are almost never available because of the panagglutinin nature of the autoantibody, the blood bank will provide the least incompatible blood for transfusion (i.e., the blood that gives the weakest reaction in cross-match testing).
- In general, transfusion is safe in patients with WAHA, and transfusion should not be withheld because a completely compatible donor cannot be found. However, transfusion should be limited to the amount of blood necessary to prevent symptoms or to protect the patient against untoward effects of anemia such as coronary ischemia, high-output heart failure, or tissue hypoxia.

TREATMENT

1. What is the treatment for WAHA?

- Glucocorticoids are first-line treatment and induce responses in about 80% of patients, but approximately half of these patients will relapse within a year (typically during the steroid taper). The dosing differs between institutions but usually starts with prednisone at 1 mg/kg body weight per day.
- This dosage is maintained for 3 to 4 weeks and tapered at a rate of 10 mg/week.
- Care should be taken to more slowly taper the prednisone, once doses of 20 to 30 mg per day are reached. There are no guidelines on how to taper steroids and some groups continue the dose of 15 to 20 mg/d for 2 to 3 months after remission of disease and then slowly taper over another 1 to 2 months. Others continue to taper the dose once it reaches 20 mg/d over 4 to 8 weeks. During this time, hemoglobin should be monitored weekly and the patient should be supplemented with folic acid, 1 mg/d.
- As long as the dose of prednisone is ≥20 mg/d, patients should receive prophylactic *pneumocystis jiroveci* pneumonia (PJP) therapy.
- The goal of treatment is amelioration of symptoms and transfusion independence. *These goals can be achieved despite persistence of a positive direct antiglobulin test (DAT). Therefore, DAT negativity is not essential for successful treatment.*

2. What are the indications for second-line treatment?

- Need for prednisone dose of more than 0.1 mg/kg per day or 0.15 mg/kg every other day
- Fall in hemoglobin to less than 10 gm% with continued evidence of hemolysis (the acceptable hemoglobin concentration depends on the functional capacity of the patient)
- Inability to tolerate steroids

3. What are the second-line treatment options in WAHA?

- Rituximab: 375 mg/m^2 of rituximab given weekly for four doses; the overall response rate is in the range of 70% to 90%, but about 50% relapse with a mean duration of response of 20 months.

- Splenectomy: response rate of 60% to 90%, but about one third will have early relapse (within 1–2 months of surgery). Prolonged remissions are observed in approximately 40% to 50% of patients, but late relapses can occur. Patients who relapse after splenectomy often respond to low-dose glucocorticoids. Patients should be vaccinated against encapsulated organisms (pneumococcus, *Haemophilus influenzae* type B, and meningococcus), ideally at least 14 days prior to splenectomy.
- **Immunomodulatory agents** including azathioprine, cyclophosphamide, cyclosporine, mycophenolate mofetil, and danazol. A common feature of these second-line treatments is a delayed response. Therefore, if tolerated, treatment should be continued for 3 to 4 months before considering it a failure in the unresponsive patient.

Cold Agglutinin Disease (CAD)

EPIDEMIOLOGY

1. What is the epidemiology of CAD?

- Prevalence of ~14 per million people; occurs in women more than men, with the primary CAD mostly found in older people with a median age at diagnosis of 72 years
- The median overall survival is 10.6 years after diagnosis

2. What is the pathophysiology of CAD?

- The cold agglutinins in primary CAD are monoclonal autoantibodies, almost exclusively immunoglobulin M (IgM), directed against the carbohydrate antigen I or i on red cells. These antibodies are able to bind and agglutinate red cells below body temperature. Autoagglutination occurs because of the pentameric structure of the IgM molecule.
- *Red blood cell* (RBC) agglutination occurs optimally at 0°C to 5°C, and agglutination in vivo leads to blood flow impediment and resulting vascular symptoms, predominately acrocyanosis affecting exposed areas, including the nose, the ear, and the hands and fingers.
- IgM antibodies can activate complement on the red cell surface that leads to extravascular hemolysis due to phagocytosis by reticuloendothelial cells (particularly those in the liver) that have receptors for activation and degradation products of complement C3. The activation of complements occurs at higher temperatures of 20°C to 25°C, and once complement C3 is covalently bound to the red cells, hemolysis occurs independent of whether or not the agglutinin is still bound to the red cells, as there are no reticuloendothelial receptors for IgM. Complement activation can cause direct (intravascular) lysis of red cells, but it is uncommon for clinically significant intravascular hemolysis to occur due to the presence of complement activation inhibitors in the plasma and on red cell surface.
- The highest temperature at which the agglutinin can bind to red cells is called its thermal amplitude. The higher the thermal amplitude, the more likely the disease will be symptomatic, as complement activation is initiated at 20°C to 25°C and is optimal at 37°C.

STAGING

1. What are the clinical features of CAD?

- Chronic hemolysis or episodic cold-induced acute hemolysis
- Vascular manifestations include acrocyanosis, livedo reticularis, and Raynaud's phenomenon. These processes occur due to agglutination of red cells in the microvasculature of areas of the body that are exposed to cold

DIAGNOSTIC CRITERIA

1. What are the laboratory features of CAD?

- In addition to anemia, reticulocytosis, and other features of hemolysis, the mean corpuscular volume (MCV) may be falsely elevated due to clumping of red cells.
- Similarly, the blood film exhibits red blood cell (RBC) autoagglutination that can be prevented by processing blood at 37°C prior to slide preparation.
- DAT is positive for C3 but the antibody is not detected because the DAT reagent does not contain anti-immunoglobulin M (anti-IgM).
- A cold agglutinin titer above 1:64 is needed for diagnosis, but a titer of 1:512 is generally considered clinically significant even though lower titers can also cause hemolysis. In addition, the thermal amplitude should be determined for the cold agglutinin.
- Serum protein electrophoresis usually reveals a monoclonal IgM protein.
- Complement levels are low because of chronic consumption, but some of the complement proteins are acute phase reactants and during stress, their levels can increase, thereby exacerbating hemolysis.
- Bone marrow shows erythroid hyperplasia and may show lymphoplasmacytic aggregates, which can be clonal.

2. What are the secondary causes of CAD?

- Autoimmune disease
- Lymphoma/CLL
- Infection, particularly *Mycoplasma pneumoniae* (anti-I) and infectious mononucleosis (anti-i). The antibodies are polyclonal and self-limiting
- *All patients with CAD should undergo a bone marrow biopsy and imaging studies to investigate for an underlying lymphoproliferative neoplasm*

TREATMENT

1. How do you treat CAD?

- Avoiding cold by wearing protective clothing or moving to a warmer climate may be the only treatment required for patients with mild disease.
- In secondary CAD, treatment of the primary diseases such as lymphoma will usually lead to improvement in CAD symptoms.
- Treatment is indicated in symptomatic anemia with disabling vascular symptoms or transfusion-dependent hemolytic anemia.
- *Splenectomy and corticosteroids are rarely effective in the treatment of CAD.*

- If the degree of anemia warrants blood transfusion, then washed *red blood cells* (RBCs; to remove complement component from contaminating plasma) infused through an in-line blood warmer should be given.
- As immunoglobulin M (IgM) can easily be removed from plasma, if the cold agglutinin needs to be removed urgently as in critically ill patients or in preparation for surgical procedures such as cardiothoracic bypass surgery, plasma exchange with albumin replacement can be used, but the benefits are transient.
- Operating room precautions to keep the patient warm should be in place to prevent agglutination and hemolysis.
- In patients with chronic symptomatic hemolysis, rituximab 375 mg/m^2 weekly for 4 weeks produces a 50% response rate. In case of relapse after a durable response, rituximab at the same dose can be repeated.
- Rituximab with fludarabine achieves higher (70%) and longer responses (median 66 months), but toxicity is problematic.
- Rituximab with bendamustine is also effective with 71% response, including 40% complete response (CR) with a median observed response duration of 32 months and is better tolerated than rituximab-fludarabine.

2. **What are the types of drug-induced hemolytic anemia?**

- **Hapten or drug adsorption mechanism**
  - This mechanism is classically described for penicillin-induced hemolytic anemia.
  - Affected patients have usually received high doses of penicillin (10–30×10^6 units per day for 7–10 days or more).
  - IgG antibody against penicillin is implicated. The antibodies bind to penicillin-coated red cells and induce a positive DAT for IgG. This mechanism produces extravascular hemolysis mediated by binding of the Fc portion of the anti-penicillin IgG to specific receptors on reticuloendothelial cells.
  - Indirect Coombs test performed with antibody from the sera or eluate from the red cell surface is *only positive when tested against penicillin-coated red cells*.
  - The process abates in a few days after discontinuation of the drug.
  - This mechanism is also seen with cephalosporins, semisynthetic penicillins, tetracyclines, and tolbutamide.
- **Ternary complex mechanism**
  - The drug-dependent antibody binds to a neoantigen that is formed by the interaction between the drug and a red cell membrane constituent.
  - Antibodies are IgG or IgM and activate complement on the red cell surface and can lead to *severe intravascular hemolysis*. Extravascular hemolysis mediated by phagocytosis of the opsonized red cell by macrophages is also observed.
  - The DAT is usually positive only for C3 as the loosely bound immunoglobulins are washed off during lab processing of the sample being tested.
  - The indirect Coombs test to detect the drug-induced antibody is *positive only if the drug is added to all steps of the reaction*.

- ○ Quinidine is the prototypic example of this type of drug-induced WAHA, but other drugs including cephalosporin can cause immune-mediated hemolysis through this mechanism.
- **Autoantibody mechanism**
  - ○ The most commonly implicated drug is methyldopa, an antihypertensive that is rarely used in the United States currently.
  - ○ The clinical picture is characterized by IgG-mediated extravascular hemolysis similar to primary autoimmune hemolytic anemia.
  - ○ The indirect Coombs test is positive from the eluate or the serum in the absence of the drug.
  - ○ Autoimmune processes induced by methyldopa occur about 3 to 6 months after start of treatment.
  - ○ Patients with CLL treated with fludarabine, cladribine, and pentostatin can also develop autoimmune hemolytic anemia.

Paroxysmal Nocturnal Hemoglobinuria

EPIDEMIOLOGY

1. **What is the epidemiology of paroxysmal nocturnal hemoglobinuria (PNH)?**
   - The estimated prevalence is ~2–4 cases/million population, classifying PNH as an ultra-orphan disease.
   - Most common age of presentation is between 30 and 59 years with perhaps a slight female predominance.

ETIOLOGY AND RISK FACTORS

1. **What is the etiology and pathogenesis of PNH?**
   - Absence of glycosylphosphatidylinositol-anchored proteins (GPI-APs) due to somatic mutation in the *PIGA* gene located on the X chromosome (males and females are equally effective because males have one X chromosome and females have one functioning X chromosome in somatic tissues due to X inactivation).
   - As the mutations occur in hematopoietic stem/early progenitor cells (HSPCs), all hematopoietic lineages (erythrocytes, platelets, granulocytes, monocytes, and lymphocytes) derived from the mutant clone are deficient in all GPI-APs.
   - PNH is an acquired, clonal disorder, and patients can have more than one *PIGA*-mutant clone with discrete mutations among the clones, but usually one clone is dominant.
   - CD55 and CD59 are GPI-APs that are important in protecting the red cells from the steady state low-grade activation of the alternative pathway of complement (APC). CD55 or decay acceleration factor (DAF) regulates the formation and stability of the C3 and C5 convertases of the APC. CD59 or membrane inhibitor of reactive lysis (MIRL) inhibits the formation of the C5b–C9 membrane attack complex and also inhibits the activity of the APC C3/C5 convertase.

- The mechanisms that account for the clonal selection and clonal expansion of the *PIGA*-mutant HSPCs are incompletely understood with different hypotheses attributing clonal selection to a survival advantage for the GPI-negative cells in the setting of immune-mediated attack on the bone marrow (particularly aplastic anemia), and clonal expansion due to mutations in genes other than *PIGA* that provide a growth/survival advantage.
- Unlike other acquired clonal process, PNH does not lead to replacement of the normal hematopoiesis. Therefore, PNH is a clonal disease but not a malignant disease.
- Bone marrow failure in PNH is not due to the PNH clone but is caused by autoimmune destruction of HSPC by T cells; hence, the close association of PNH with aplastic anemia and immune-mediated myelodysplastic syndrome. The *PIGA*-mutant HSPCs survive the immune attack because of deficiency of one or more GPI-APs, but the exact mechanism underlying the survival advantage of the *PIGA*-mutant, GPI-AP deficient HSPC in the setting of immune attack is speculative.

SIGNS AND SYMPTOMS

1. What are the clinical features of PNH?

- Anemia
  - Non-spherocytic intravascular hemolysis characterized by abnormally high serum lactate dehydrogenase (LDH; due to intravascular hemolysis) and a negative DAT test. Reticulocytosis is present but is usually lower than expected for the degree of anemia because there is always an element of bone marrow failure in PNH.
  - PNH can be associated with aplastic anemia (approximately 50% of patients with aplastic anemia have a detectable PNH clone) and low-grade myelodysplastic syndrome (approximately 15% of cases).
- **Thrombosis**
  - Mostly venous but arterial thrombosis can occur
  - Unusual locations including hepatic veins, leading to Budd Chiari syndrome, mesenteric, cerebral, and dermal veins
  - The etiology of thrombophilia in PNH is incompletely understood and has been attributed to a variety of mechanisms including intravascular hemolysis and platelet activation by complement
  - Thrombosis is the most common cause of mortality in patients with PNH
- **Smooth muscle dystonia**
  - The intravascular hemolysis of PNH red cells releases free hemoglobin. This free hemoglobin is normally bound by haptoglobin and hemopexin, but once their binding capacity is exceeded, the free hemoglobin binds and depletes nitric oxide, resulting in smooth muscle dystonia leading to esophageal spasm and erectile dysfunction.
- **Nocturnal hemoglobinuria** is a presenting symptom in only 25% of patients.

2. Other symptoms

- Constitutional symptoms including fatigue and lethargy dominate the clinical picture in patients with classic PNH.

- As already noted, esophageal spasm, male impotence, and thromboembolic events may complicate PNH.

DIAGNOSTIC CRITERIA

1. How is PNH diagnosed?

- All patients have some degree of bone marrow failure that is manifested by varying combinations of anemia, thrombocytopenia, and leukopenia
- Features of intravascular hemolysis (often with markedly elevated serum lactate dehydrogenase [LDH])
- Can have iron deficiency due to hemoglobinuria
- Peripheral blood flow cytometry for detection of surface expression of GPI-APs on RBCs, granulocytes, and monocytes using monoclonal antibodies against CD55 and CD59 or fluorescein-labeled proaerolysin (FLAER) that binds to the glycan portion of GPI-APs. The FLAER assay cannot be used for RBCs, as the reagent does not bind to GPI-APs on red cells.
- Bone marrow studies are not required for the diagnosis of PNH but are useful in determining the characteristics of the bone marrow, as PNH is often seen in association with aplastic anemia and low-risk myelodysplastic syndrome (MDS). Nonrandom karyotypic abnormalities are uncommon.

2. When to suspect PNH?

- Non-spherocytic, DAT-negative hemolytic anemia
- Aplastic anemia
- Low-risk myelodysplastic syndrome (MDS) including refractory anemia or refractory cytopenia with multilineage dysplasia. PNH is not seen in conjunction with high-grade MDS such as MDS with excess blasts
- Venous thrombosis in unusual sites such as the hepatic vein and intra-abdominal and cerebral veins

3. What is the incidence of PNH clone in aplastic anemia and MDS?

- Fifty percent of aplastic anemia and 15% of patients with low-risk MDS have a PNH clone. In many cases, the PNH clones are less than 1% and are too small to produce biochemical evidence of hemolysis (called subclinical PNH); however, there are exceptions with clones large enough to produce evidence of hemolysis (called PNH in the setting of bone marrow failure). The presence of a PNH clone may be a surrogate marker for immune-mediated bone marrow failure as patients with aplastic anemia and low-risk MDS with a PNH clone have a higher probability of responding to immunosuppressive therapy compared to patients without a PNH clone.

STAGING

1. What is phenotypic mosaicism in PNH?

- Phenotypic mosaicism is a hallmark of PNH.
- Patients with PNH have either two or three types of red cells.
- PNH I cells have normal expression of GPI-Aps (these are the residual normal cells), PNH II cells have partial deficiency of GPI-APs, and PNH III cells have complete absence of GPI-APs.

- The phenotypic mosaicism is due to genotypic mosaicism arising from multiple clones with discrete *PIGA* mutations. In patients with type III cells, the mutation completely inactivates the enzymatic function of the *PIGA* protein (a glycosyl transferase essential for the biosynthesis of the GPI anchor). In patients with type II cells, the mutation causes partial inactivation of the enzyme such that the cells express about 10% of the normal amount of GPI-APs.
- Thus, the peripheral blood of patients is a mosaic of normal and abnormal cells and the size of the PNH clone or clones varies greatly among patients. Patients can have all three types of cells or have a combination of either PNH I and PNH II or PNH I and PNH III, the latter being the most common phenotype.

PROGNOSTIC FACTORS

1. **Why should PNH flow studies be done on both RBCs and granulocytes?**
   - Because hemolysis eliminates PNH III cells, flow cytometry on RBCs will underestimate the PNH clone size. Granulocyte survival is normal in PNH and therefore more accurately reflects the size of the PNH clone.
   - But flow studies on granulocytes are not helpful in categorizing the three types of PNH cells, so phenotyping should be done on RBCs.
   - Phenotypic analysis of cells is important as the type II cells are relatively resistant to spontaneous complement-mediated hemolysis and patients with high percentage of these cells typically have a more benign clinical course.

2. **Does the PNH clone increase with age?**
   - PNH clones can expand, disappear, or remain stable over time. In most cases, the clone remains stable.
   - The clone size should be measured yearly.
   - There is no evidence that patients with subclinical PNH progress to clinical PNH.

3. **How is PNH classified clinically?**
   - Subclinical PNH
     - Small PNH clone of <10% (usually <1%)
     - No biochemical evidence of intravascular hemolysis
     - Seen in the setting of bone marrow failure syndromes
   - PNH in the setting of another bone marrow failure (BMF) syndrome
     - Evidence of mild hemolysis
     - Presence of a concomitant BMF syndrome
     - PNH clone usually <50%
   - Classic PNH
     - Evidence of florid hemolysis
     - No concomitant BMF syndrome
     - PNH clone >50% (often greater than 90%)

TREATMENT

1. When should patients with PNH be treated?

- Clinically significant hemolysis resulting in constitutional symptoms, symptomatic anemia, or both
- Thrombotic event

2. How is PNH treated?

- The need for treatment depends on the presence of PNH-related symptoms, degree of hemolysis, episodes of thrombosis, and the size of the PNH clone.
- Eculizumab is a humanized monoclonal antibody that binds to complement C5 and prevents its conversion to C5b, thereby blocking formation of the cytolytic membrane attack complex.
- Treatment with eculizumab improves the anemia, reduces transfusion requirements, and ameliorates constitutional symptoms.
- *Eculizumab does not address the underlying cause of PNH and therefore must be administered indefinitely.*

3. What are the reasons for failure of eculizumab therapy?

- As the maintenance dosing of eculizumab is not weight based, breakthrough hemolysis can occur, and increasing the dose or reducing the interval between treatments can restore the response.
- As eculizumab does not affect the increased formation and stability of the C3 convertase, activation and degradation products of C3 deposited on the red cells can initiate extravascular hemolysis. Rituximab and splenectomy are not useful as the opsonization is C3 mediated, resulting in extravascular hemolysis that occurs predominantly in the liver.
- A polymorphism in C5 found in some Asian patients (particularly Japanese patients) prevents binding of eculizumab to C5.

4. What is the role of anticoagulation in PNH?

- No indication for prophylactic anticoagulation in PNH patients on eculizumab if they have never had a thromboembolic event prior to starting treatment with eculizumab
- All patients who have a thrombotic episode should be anticoagulated for life, including those on eculizumab
- If the PNH clone is more than 50% but the patient has no indication for eculizumab, he or she should be prophylactically anticoagulated with Coumadin. Studies using other anticoagulants, including direct oral anticoagulants, have not been reported for patients with PNH

Paroxysmal Cold Hemoglobinuria

EPIDEMIOLOGY

1. What is the epidemiology of paroxysmal cold hemoglobinuria (PCH)?

- Data is limited, but most PCH occurs in children less than 5 years old. There appears to be a male predominance.

- PCH associated with congenital syphilis accounted for 90% of cases in the past but is rare now due to reduction in syphilis as a result of effective antimicrobial therapy.
- PCH in adults has been associated with viral infections and with lymphoproliferative disorders.

2. What is the pathophysiology of PCH?

- Polyclonal IgG antibodies against the P antigen on the red cells lead to activation of the classical pathway of complement, resulting in intravascular hemolysis.
- The IgG antibody, called the Donath-Landsteiner antibody, has biphasic properties. It binds to the P antigen at cold temperatures and remains bound to the red cells at temperatures sufficient to activate the classical pathway of complement.
- IgG in PCH is able to bind the surface of the red cells in cold temperatures such as those that are encountered in the extremities. When the IgG-coated red cells flow to core areas of the body where the temperature is optimal for complement activation, the red cells undergo brisk complement-mediated intravascular hemolysis.

3. What are the clinical manifestations of PCH?

- Usually transient hemolysis. May be accompanied by hemoglobinuria, chills and rigors, myalgia, back and pelvic pain, nausea, fatigue, and jaundice. In severe cases, acute renal failure can occur as a result of massive hemoglobinuria.
- In chronic PCH, episodes of hemolysis are precipitated by exposure to cold temperatures.
- Physical exam reveals anemia and jaundice without either splenomegaly or lymphadenopathy.

4. What are the laboratory features of PCH?

- Signs of intravascular hemolysis as evidenced by high serum LDH, reduced haptoglobin, high levels of free plasma hemoglobin, hemoglobinuria, and hemosiderinuria, and indirect hyperbilirubinemia
- Anemia is normocytic or macrocytic
- Unlike cold agglutinin disease, there is no red cell agglutination seen in the peripheral blood film as the antibody in PCH is an IgG (IgM in cold agglutinin disease)
- A classic blood smear finding is neutrophil erythrophagocytosis
- The DAT test is usually positive for C3 and negative for IgG
- The Donath-Landsteiner test is specific for PCH. Patient serum is cooled to 4°C and incubated with P antigen–positive RBCs. At 4°C, the Donath-Landsteiner IgG antibody binds to the RBCs, and when the sample is warmed to 37°C, the classical pathway of complement is activated and the cells undergo complement-mediated hemolysis

TREATMENT

1. What is the treatment for PCH?

- Hemolysis is usually self-limiting and transient.

- Supportive measures such as keeping the patient warm and avoiding cold exposure are recommended.
- Blood transfusion if anemia is severe. Most donors are P antigen positive, so P-negative donor blood may not be available. Therefore, transfusion with P-positive blood may be the only option. Transfusion with P antigen–positive blood is usually safe as long as a blood warmer is used and the patient is kept warm.
- As PCH is usually transient, immunosuppression is not usually required.
- Plasmapheresis can be used in severe cases, but the response is short-lived because the IgG antibody in the extravascular space reequilibrates with the plasma.
- Rituximab can be given to treat refractory PCH.
- As the hemolysis is due to activation of complement, eculizumab could also be used to treat refractory patients.

Metabolic Enzyme Deficiency Hemolytic Anemia

1. How is enzyme deficiency hemolytic anemia classified?
The enzyme deficiencies that can lead to hemolytic anemia can be divided into three groups:

- Disorders of the enzymes involved in the antioxidant pathway necessary to protect RBC proteins and hemoglobin from oxidation
- Disorders of anaerobic glycolysis that is the source of ATP
- Disorders of nucleotide purine and pyrimidine metabolism

Most of the enzyme disorders are autosomal recessive except for G6PD deficiency, which is X linked.

GLUCOSE 6 PHOSPHATE DEHYDROGENASE DEFICIENCY

- Glucose 6 phosphate dehydrogenase B (G6PD B) is the normal wild-type enzyme and is not associated with hemolysis.
- It has a half-life of 62 days, providing sufficient enzyme activity to protect red cells from oxidative damage throughout their life span.

1. What are the different variants of G6PD deficiency?

- **World Health Organization (WHO) classification of G6PD deficiency variants:**
  - Class I: severe enzyme deficiency with less than 10% activity characterized clinically by chronic hemolysis
  - Class II: severe enzyme deficiency, but characterized clinically by intermittent hemolysis precipitated by drugs, infection, or chemicals. G6PD Mediterranean [B (−) genotype], the mutant form that causes favism, has a half-life that is measured in hours. Therefore, the enzyme activity is markedly reduced in all red cells irrespective of their age and leads to severe disease. Favism (caused by eating fava beans) occurs most frequently in children under 5 years of age and can be fatal

- Class III: moderate deficiency with 10% to 60% activity. Hemolysis only with precipitating factors and is usually limited to older red cells. G6PD A- is found in 10% to 15% of African Americans and is primarily responsible for primaquine sensitivity and typically causes only mild hemolysis. Its half-life is ~13 days and so the older red cells are particularly susceptible to oxidative damage
- Class IV: no enzyme activity deficiency. G6PD A+ has normal enzyme function and does not cause hemolysis
- Class V: mutants with increased enzyme activity

2. **What is the inheritance of G6PD deficiency?**
- The gene that encodes G6PD is located on the X chromosome. Therefore, males who inherit the mutant X chromosome from their mothers are affected. Females who inherit the mutant X chromosome will be mosaics because of X inactivation in somatic tissues. Females can be affected clinically depending upon the degree of skewing of X inactivation.
- Most of the mutations are missense mutations that impact enzymatic activity variably, explaining the heterogeneity of the disease.

3. **What is the pathophysiology of G6PD deficiency?**
- G6PD catalyzes the first step in the hexose monophosphate pathway that converts glucose-6-phosphate to 6-phosphogluconate, and in the process, reduces NADP to NADPH.
- NADPH is important for maintaining glutathione in the reduced state.
- Glutathione is the major antioxidant in the red cell. Therefore, when G6PD activity is deficient, hemoglobin and other red cell proteins are oxidized, leading to precipitation of the damaged proteins. Binding of the precipitated proteins to the cytoskeleton distorts the red cell, reducing its life span.
- The oxidized, denatured hemoglobin forms insoluble complexes that attach to the membrane, creating Heinz bodies that are seen as membrane blebs on Wright stain and visualized specifically with methyl violet staining.
- The oxidized hemoglobin also undergoes cross-linking that leads to puddling of hemoglobin in the cytoplasm, forming the bite cells that are characteristic of G6PD deficiency seen in the Wright-stained peripheral blood film.
- Oxidation also causes disulfide bond formation between membrane and cytoskeletal proteins that makes the red cells rigid and leads to destruction within the spleen.

4. **What are the clinical features of G6PD deficiency?**
- Most are asymptomatic and without biochemical evidence of hemolysis or anemia at baseline.
- Only individuals with the Class I variant have ongoing, chronic hemolytic anemia.
- Episodes of acute hemolysis are precipitated by drugs, infections, or certain foods including fava beans (favism is an imprecise alternative name for G6PD deficiency).

- The hemolysis can be both intravascular and extravascular and lead to a fall in hemoglobin concentration and onset of jaundice in 2 to 4 days of occurrence of the precipitating event.
- In cases due to G6PD A− with the onset of reticulocytosis, the symptoms abate as the reticulocytes have near-normal G6PD activity, but in G6PD Mediterranean and other Class II variants, the anemia is usually more severe and longer lasting, persisting even after the precipitating event has passed.
- Many drugs can precipitate an acute attack, including antimalarials, aspirin, nitrofurantoin, nonsteroidal anti-inflammatory drugs, quinine, quinidine, and sulfa drugs.

TREATMENT

1. Who should be tested for G6PD deficiency?

- Testing is appropriate before starting medications such as dapsone and rasburicase that can cause severe hemolysis in patients with G6PD deficiency.
- Testing can be omitted in patients starting on sulfonylurea or antibiotics such as nitrofurantoin that cause only mild hemolysis.

2. When to test for G6PD deficiency?

- During an episode of acute hemolysis, the G6PD-deficient red cells are lysed, and therefore the results of testing for enzyme deficiency can be falsely negative, especially in patients with Class III variants. Testing 3 months after the inciting event is recommended in order to eliminate false-negative results.
- The basic principle of all screening and confirmatory testing in G6PD deficiency is assessment of reduction of NADP to NADPH by the enzyme.
- The fluorescent spot test is the most sensitive and reliable initial assay, and for confirmation, NADPH production is assessed quantitatively by spectrophotometry.
- Confirmation of the diagnosis by molecular studies is available but not routinely done as the information does not affect management decisions.

3. How do we manage G6PD deficiency?

- Avoid fava beans and drugs that can precipitate a hemolytic crisis.
- Red blood transfusion is safe and indicated in acute, severe hemolysis.
- Adequate hydration and good urine output should be maintained to prevent renal insufficiency as a consequence of hemoglobinuria.
- As acute, severe hemolysis is mostly intravascular, splenectomy is not effective.

PYRUVATE KINASE DEFICIENCY

- Although the disease is rare, pyruvate kinase (PK) deficiency is the most common cause of congenital non-spherocytic, chronic hemolytic anemia.
- Inheritance is autosomal recessive.
- PK deficiency leading to hemolytic anemia is due to mutation in the LR (liver, red cell) isoform of the protein, leading to marked reduction of enzyme activity in red cells.

DIAGNOSTIC CRITERIA

1. **What is the mechanism of hemolysis in pyruvate kinase (PK) deficiency?**
   - The mechanism of hemolysis in PK deficiency is incompletely understood. Decrease in ATP production alone has not been clearly shown to be causative.
   - As the deficiency leads to a block in the glycolytic pathway, 2,3 DPG levels are increased, consequently shifting the oxygen dissociation curve to the right. This increase in 2,3 DPG improves oxygen delivery, thereby ameliorating the effects of the anemia.

SIGNS AND SYMPTOMS

1. **What are the clinical features of PK deficiency?**
   - The severity of hemolysis is variable, from mild compensated anemia to transfusion-dependent anemia to hydrops detalis.
   - Patients present with typical signs of extravascular hemolysis including pallor, icterus, splenomegaly, reticulocytosis and symptoms related to anemia.
   - Peripheral smear may show contracted echinocytes, but there are no specific diagnostic morphological findings.
   - The diagnosis is made by assaying the PK enzyme activity in red blood cells and detecting gene mutations in the PK LR gene.

TREATMENT

1. **What is the treatment for hemolytic anemia due to PK deficiency?**
   - Splenectomy is beneficial in patients with severe symptomatic anemia by ameliorating hemolysis and decreasing transfusion requirements.
   - Folic acid should be given to all patients.
   - Hematopoietic stem cell transplantation is an option in patients with severe disease.

PYRIMIDINE 5′ NUCLEOTIDASE (P5′N-1) DEFICIENCY

- P5′N-1 deficiency is an autosomal recessive disorder characterized by accumulation of pyrimidine nucleotides in the red cells.
- The characteristic morphologic feature on review of the peripheral blood film is *coarse basophilic stippling* due to precipitation of nondegraded RNA.
- Similar findings are observed in lead poisoning, as lead is an inhibitor of the enzyme.

Red Cell Membrane Defects

HEREDITARY SPHEROCYTOSIS

1. **What is the inheritance pattern and prevalence of hereditary spherocytosis (HS)?**
   - The most common mode of inheritance is autosomal dominant, accounting for 75% of HS.

- De novo mutations or autosomal recessive mutations account for the remaining 25% of cases.
- The severe forms of HS due to mutations in α-spectrin are autosomal recessive.
- HS is the most common inherited hemolytic anemia among people of Northern European ancestry with a prevalence of 1 in 2,000.

2. What is the pathophysiology of HS?

- Defect in proteins that are important in the vertical linkage of the lipid membrane to the underlying membrane skeleton is the cause of spherocytosis.
- Defects in ankyrin, spectrin, band 3, and protein 4.2 can lead to the formation and release of microvesicles from the lipid bilayer, which leads to the generation of microspherocytes.
- These spherocytes are not able to deform and negotiate the interendothelial fenestrations separating the red pulp and the sinuses of the spleen.
- In addition, HS red cells are trapped in an environment with low nutrients and low pH that lead to their eventual phagocytosis by splenic macrophages.
- Some of these conditioned red cells remain viable, escape the spleen, and contribute to the tail seen in the osmotic fragility test.

3. What are the different protein defects that lead to HS?

- β-spectrin defects account for 15% to 30% of HS patients, and they typically have mild-to-moderate disease and are transfusion independent.
- α-spectrin defects account for 5% of patients with HS. α-spectrin is normally produced in amounts that are three to four times greater than the amount of β-spectrin. Therefore, HS due to defects in α-spectrin is usually autosomal recessive. Patients can be compound heterozygotes or homozygotes, and in these cases, the clinical manifestations are usually severe.
- The most common cause of HS is a combined spectrin and ankyrin deficiency, accounting for 40% to 65% of HS patients of Northern European descent.
- Ankyrin primarily mediates binding of the cytoskeleton to the lipid moiety of the red cell membrane by linking band 3 to spectrin. Ankyrin deficiency leads to a proportional decrease in spectrin assembly in spite of normal production of the latter.
- Band 3 deficiency accounts for 33% of HS and presents with mild-to-moderate disease that follows an autosomal dominant inheritance pattern. Mushroom-shaped red cells are characteristically seen on review of the peripheral blood film.
- Protein 4.2 defects are usually autosomal recessively inherited and are a common cause of HS in Japan but rare in other populations.
- Rh proteins along with the Rh-associated glycoproteins interact with ankyrin and link the membrane cytoskeleton to the lipid bilayer of the red cell. Absence or deficiency of these proteins can produce the HS phenotype.

DIAGNOSTIC CRITERIA

1. **What are the clinical features of HS?**
   - Clinical manifestations can be divided into asymptomatic trait, and mild, moderate, and severe disease.
   - Patients in the same family usually have similar disease manifestations unless complicated by additional mutations.
   - Patients with HS trait have normal hemoglobin concentration, normal peripheral blood morphology, and no biochemical evidence of hemolysis. On testing, a slight increase in osmotic fragility may be observed if the red cells are incubated for 18 to 24 hours in nutrient-poor medium prior to osmotic fragility testing. The eosin 5'-maleimide (EMA) binding test is usually negative.
   - Mild HS is seen in 20% to 30% of patients. These patients have evidence of compensated hemolysis with normal hemoglobin, mild splenomegaly, mild reticulocytosis (usually less than 6%), and infrequent spherocytes observed in the peripheral blood film.
   - Moderate HS is seen in 60% to 70% of patients. They usually present during childhood but can manifest disease signs and symptoms at any age. They present with mild-to-moderate anemia, splenomegaly, intermittent indirect hyperbilirubinemia, and reticulocytosis. Patients may have fatigue and mild pallor secondary to the anemia or they may be asymptomatic.
   - Patients with severe HS have evidence of florid hemolysis and require intermittent or regular blood transfusion to treat the anemia.

SIGNS AND SYMPTOMS

1. **What are the complications of HS?**
   - Gall bladder disease due to bilirubinate stones
   - Leg ulcers and chronic dermatitis
   - Aplastic crisis due to viral infections, most commonly parvovirus B19 Infection
   - Megaloblastic crisis due to folate deficiency as a consequence of increased folate demand as in pregnancy or recovery from an aplastic crisis
   - Thrombosis, especially after splenectomy

2. **What are the laboratory features of HS?**
   - The degree of anemia depends on the severity of the HS defect. Mean corpuscular hemoglobin concentration (MCHC) can be increased due to cellular dehydration.
   - Depending on the severity of the disease, spherocytes with varying degree of anisopoikilocytosis with bizarre-shaped red cells are observed in the most severe forms. Pincer- or mushroom-shaped cells are typically seen in band 3 defects and spherocytic acanthocytes can be seen in β-spectrin defects.
   - Markers of hemolysis including elevated LDH, indirect hyperbilirubinemia, reticulocytosis, and decreased haptoglobin may be present depending upon the severity of the disease.
   - Eosin 5'-maleimide (EMA): EMA is a fluorescent dye that binds to red cell membrane proteins including band 3, Rh protein, Rh glycoprotein, and CD47.

Irrespective of the underlying defect, most patients with HS exhibit decreased binding of EMA. But decreased binding of EMA is also seen in patients with hereditary elliptocytosis, hereditary pyropoikilocytosis, some red cell enzymopathies, and congenital dyserythropoeitic anemia II.

- The most commonly used diagnostic assay for HS is the osmotic fragility test, wherein red cells are incubated in test tubes containing solutions of incrementally decreasing saline concentration. Because of the decreased relative surface area of spherocytes, they undergo osmotic lysis at a higher saline concentration than normal red cells. The osmotic fragility test is not specific for HS, as spherocytes in patients with warm antibody autoimmune hemolytic anemia also produce an abnormal result. The osmotic fragility test can be negative in HS patients with few spherocytes, recent blood transfusion, iron deficiency, or in the recovery phase from an aplastic crisis.
- As noted earlier, the incubated osmotic fragility test may be more sensitive and specific for detection of HS compared to the standard osmotic fragility test.
- The reduced red cell surface area can be measured by ektacytometry, but this test is available only in a few research labs.
- Other tests that may have more sensitivity and specificity include the acidified glycerol lysis test and the cryohemolysis test.
- To characterize the molecular defect in HS is challenging due to the multiple gene mutations that can produce the same phenotype.
- As a first step, erythrocyte proteins can be subjected to analysis by sodium dodecyl sulfate polyacrylamide gel electrophoresis (SDS-PAGE). Using this method, quantitative abnormalities in red cell cytoskeletal proteins can be identified in 75% to 93% cases.
- The gene encoding the abnormal protein can then be sequenced to identify the molecular abnormality.

TREATMENT

1. How is HS diagnosed clinically?

- Positive family history (however, 15%–25% of cases arise de novo)
- Hemolytic anemia with spherocytes and negative DAT
- Positive screening test such as the eosin 5'-maleimide (EMA)-binding assay or the incubated osmotic fragility test

2. What is the treatment for HS?

- The indications for splenectomy include patients who have transfusion-dependent anemia and patients who have symptomatic anemia including growth failure, leg ulcers, and extramedullary hematopoietic tumors.
- As the red cells are sequestered and destroyed in the spleen, splenectomy will improve the anemia in most patients with HS, rendering the red cell life span to near-normal duration. Splenectomy does not change the morphology of the peripheral blood red cells.
- Splenectomy also decreases the incidence of gallstones. If patients have symptomatic gallstones causing acute cholecystitis or biliary obstruction, a combined cholecystectomy and splenectomy can be performed.

- As the risk of post-splenectomy sepsis is high in patients with immature immune systems, the procedure should be delayed until the patient reaches the age of 5 to 9 years.
- Delay beyond 10 years of age increases the risk of cholelithiasis significantly.
- Immunization against encapsulated organisms including pneumococcus, *Haemophilus influenzae*, and meningococcus should be administered at least 2 weeks before splenectomy. Penicillin prophylaxis is controversial; some physicians give penicillin V for at least 5 years after splenectomy while others treat for the lifetime of the patient.
- Splenectomy failure is uncommon, but an accessory spleen can develop in 15% to 40% of patients and would be accompanied by the absence of Howell-Jolly bodies in the peripheral blood film.

OTHER RED CELL MEMBRANE DEFECTS

1. ### What is hereditary elliptocytosis (HE)?
   - Incidence 1 in 2,000 to 4,000, it is more common in individuals of West African descent as it may confer resistance to malaria
   - Pathophysiology is due to defective interaction between the horizontal components of the membrane cytoskeleton
   - Mutations in spectrin (most common), protein 4.1, and glycophorin lead to HE

2. ### What is hereditary pyropoikilocytosis (HPP)?
   - A subtype of HE in which the spectrin mutation is present in the homozygous or compound heterozygous state, and the mutations lead to abnormality of both the horizontal interaction due both to defects in spectrin self-association and to abnormalities of the vertical interactions due to spectrin deficiency
   - This combination leads to severe poikilocytosis with bizarre shapes and fragmentation, microspherocytes, and clinically significant hemolysis
   - Splenectomy is indicated to reduce transfusion requirements

3. ### What is spur cell anemia?
   - Seen in severe liver disease, where abnormal lipoproteins and excess cholesterol is produced in the liver. The abnormal and excess lipids are acquired by red cells and lead to an increase in the cellular surface area. After passage through the spleen, the red cells acquire projections seen as exaggerated forms of acanthocytes called spur cells because of the resemblance of the projections to spurs.
   - Patients present with hemolytic anemia with spur cell acanthocytes in the peripheral blood and signs of florid liver failure.
   - Treatment should focus on the liver failure, which is usually end stage when the spur cell anemia develops.

QUESTIONS

1. ### Which of the following statements is true about warm antibody hemolytic anemia (WAHA)?
   A. The direct antiglobulin test (DAT) is always positive in WAHA.

    B. The DAT can be positive for immunoglobulin G (IgG), IgA, IgM, or complement C3.

    C. The DAT can be positive for IgG, complement C3, or both.

    D. Splenectomy has no role in the management of WAHA.

2. **Which of the following statements is false about paroxysmal nocturnal hemoglobinuria (PNH)?**

    A. The gene that is somatically mutated in PNH is called *PIGA*.

    B. PNH is inherited in an autosomal recessive pattern.

    C. The hemolysis of PNH is mediated by the alternative pathway of complement.

    D. The peripheral blood of patients with PNH is a mosaic of normal and abnormal cells.

3. **Which of the following statements is true about cold agglutinin disease (CAD)?**

    A. The antibody that mediates the hemolysis of CAD is called the Donath-Landsteiner antibody.

    B. Glucocorticoids are considered the standard of care for treatment of CAD.

    C. The DAT is positive for C3 and IgM.

    D. The DAT is positive for C3 only.

4. **Which of the following statements is true about hereditary spherocytosis (HS)?**

    A. The inheritance pattern is invariably autosomal dominant.

    B. The osmotic fragility test is specific for HS.

    C. The gene that is mutated in HS is invariably α-spectrin.

    D. When splenectomy is required, it is best to wait until the patient is 5 to 9 years old to allow the immune system to mature and to avoid sufficient time for formation of bilirubinate gallstones.

5. **Which of the following statements is true about paroxysmal cold hemoglobinuria (PCH)?**

    A. The gene that is mutated in PCH is ankyrin.

    B. The Donath-Landsteiner antibody is an immunoglobulin M (IgM) antibody directed against the P antigen.

    C. The hemolysis of PCH is intravascular and mediated by the classical pathway of complement.

    D. Red cell agglutination is a characteristic feature of PCH.

6. **Which of the following statements is false with respect to glucose 6 phosphate dehydrogenase (G6PD) deficiency?**

    A. It is an X-linked disorder that is more common in areas in which malaria is endemic.

    B. Splenectomy is the treatment of choice.

    C. G6PD enzyme levels can be normal in red blood cells (RBCs) at the time of a hemolytic crisis.

    D. Ingestion of fava beans in patients with G6PD deficiency can precipitate acute hemolysis.

7. **All of the following are false with respect to paroxysmal nocturnal hemoglobinuria (PNH) treatment except**
   A. Eculizumab is indicated in all patients with PNH with a clone size greater than 10%.
   B. Eculizumab treatment predisposes to meningococcal infections.
   C. Anticoagulation can be discontinued in patients with thrombosis if they are treated with eculizumab.
   D. All patients with a PNH clone size more than 10% should be antico-agulated irrespective of whether they have a history of thrombosis.

8. **Which of the following is true with respect to cold agglutinin disease?**
   A. Hemolysis is mostly intravascular, mediated by complement.
   B. Splenectomy is the treatment of choice for refractory disease.
   C. Hemolysis is mainly extravascular and is mediated primarily by reticu-loendothelial cells in the liver.
   D. Role of rituximab in the treatment is controversial.

9. **All the following statements are false except**
   A. Donath-Landsteiner antibody leads to autoagglutination of red cells on the peripheral blood film.
   B. Corticosteroids are the first-line treatment in cold agglutinin disease.
   C. Direct antiglobulin test (DAT)-negative warm antibody hemolytic anemia (WAHA) can be immunoglobulin A (IgA) mediated.
   D. Positive DAT in spite of stable hemoglobin indicates treatment failure in WAHA.

10. **Which of the following statements is true?**
   A. Low-level paroxysmal nocturnal hemoglobinuria (PNH) clones are seen in patients with high-risk myelodysplastic syndrome (MDS).
   B. Immunomodulatory drugs such as mycophenolate mofetil may need to be continued for 4 to 5 months to see a response in warm anti-body hemolytic anemia (WAHA).
   C. Congenital syphilis is the most common cause of paroxysmal cold hemoglobinuria (PCH).
   D. The eosin 5'-maleimide (EMA) flow assay is a specific diagnostic test for hereditary spherocytosis (HS).

ANSWERS

1. C. The DAT can be positive for IgG, complement C3, or both.

2. B. PNH is inherited in an autosomal recessive pattern.

3. D. The DAT is positive for C3 only.

4. D. When splenectomy is required, it is best to wait until the patient is 5 to 9 years old to allow the immune system to mature and to avoid sufficient time for formation of bilirubinate gallstones.

5. C. The hemolysis of PCH is intravascular and mediated by the classical pathway of complement.

6. B. Splenectomy is the treatment of choice.

7. B. Eculizumab treatment predisposes to meningococcal infections.

8. C. Hemolysis is mainly extravascular and is mediated primarily by reticuloendothelial cells in the liver.

9. C. Direct antiglobulin test (DAT)-negative warm antibody hemolytic anemia (WAHA) can be immunoglobulin A (IgA) mediated.

10. B. Immunomodulatory drugs such as mycophenolate mofetil may need to be continued for 4 to 5 months to see a response in warm antibody hemolytic anemia (WAHA).

The Sickle Cell Syndromes

4

Sarah Yentz and Albert Quiery

DEFINITIONS AND NOMENCLATURE

1. **Recognize the genetic basis and the spectrum of clinical syndromes associated with the sickle cell gene:**
   - Hemoglobin S arises from a DNA point mutation, resulting in a single amino acid substitution, valine to glutamic acid, at the sixth amino acid of beta globin.
   - Hemoglobin S is codominant with hemoglobin A1 and other hemoglobin variants.
   - Heterozygosity for hemoglobin S alone is known as sickle cell trait.
   - Sickle cell disease (SCD) is defined as homozygosity for hemoglobin S or hemoglobin S in the compound heterozygote state with another pathologic beta globin variant (C, D, E) or when associated with beta thalassemia.

DEMOGRAPHICS

1. **Describe the frequency of sickle cell trait in the United States and worldwide.**
   - SCD is the most common inherited blood disorder worldwide
   - In endemic regions, heterozygosity for hemoglobin S confers partial protection from falciparum malaria infection, resulting in a survival advantage among carriers
   - Heterozygosity for the sickle cell gene is found in approximately
     - 20% of individuals from sub-Saharan Africa, regions in Saudi Arabia, and in India
     - 0.6% of Hispanics
     - 5% of individuals from the Mediterranean Basin (Sicily, Greece, and Southern Turkey)
   - Sickle cell disease occurs in approximately 1 of every 365 African American and in 1 of every 16,300 Hispanic births
   - There are an estimated 100,000 Americans living with SCD

2. **What is the median overall survival of a patient with SCD?**
   - The estimated median survival for SCD in developed nations is ~60 years.
   - The infant and childhood mortality decreased substantially with the introduction of the pneumococcal vaccine.

- Although death related to organ failure does occur in SCD, most deaths occur during a vaso-occlusive crisis related to acute chest syndrome, stroke, or venous thromboembolism (VTE).
- Elevated hemoglobin F levels are associated with improved outcomes.
- Coinheritance of alpha thalassemia reduces risk of stroke in SCD.

PATHOPHYSIOLOGY

1. **What effect does the sickle cell mutation have on red blood cells?**
   - When deoxygenated, the hemoglobin S molecule undergoes a conformational change that results in decreased solubility and polymerization. This is made worse by reduced oxygen tension and acidosis.

2. **What is the mechanism of anemia in sickle cell disease?**
   - Sickled cells undergo hemolysis leading to a chronic hemolytic anemia.
   - Average life span of a sickle cell is 17 days (~1/7 that of a normal red blood cell [RBC]).

3. **What causes the acute vaso-occlusive pain crisis typical of sickle cell disease?**
   - Entrapment of erythrocytes and leukocytes in the microcirculation leads to vascular obstruction and tissue ischemia.

4. **What factors contribute to the pathophysiology of vaso-occlusion?**
   - Impaired RBC deformability (hemoglobin polymerization and sickling)
   - Red cell adhesion to endothelial cells
   - Endothelial cell damage
   - Prothrombotic state (thrombin activation)
   - Leukocytosis and other inflammatory mediators

THE SICKLE CELL SYNDROMES

1. **What factors determine the clinical manifestations and disease severity in SCD?**
   - The beta globin genotype (AS, S-beta thalassemia, SC, and SS; see table in the Diagnosis section)
   - Higher concentration of hemoglobin F reduces severity (hereditary persistence of fetal hemoglobin [HPFH] or Hydrea)
   - Coexisting alpha thalassemia reduces the severity of some disease manifestations (1 or 2 gene deletions) for select sickle cell haplotypes
   - Based on anthropological and molecular data, there are five separate founder mutations resulting in distinct beta globin haplotypes. The Central African haplotype has the worst disease severity

2. **What is the role of coinherited hemoglobin C in sickle cell disease?**
   - Hemoglobin C substitution of lysine for glutamic acid at the sixth amino acid of the beta globin gene
   - Hemoglobin C carrier state (AC) is asymptomatic

- Homozygosity for hemoglobin C (CC) results in mild anemia and splenomegaly with minimal associated symptoms
- Compound heterozygosity for hemoglobin C and hemoglobin S results in a symptomatic sickle cell syndrome

3. **What is the role of coinherited beta thalassemia in sickle cell disease?**
   - Beta thalassemia represents a variety of genetic mutations that result in decreased beta globin production. The severity ranges from a mild/moderate decrease in beta globin production (beta + thalassemia) to a complete absence of beta globin production (beta 0 thalassemia).
   - Impaired production of beta globin chains leads to a relative excess of alpha globin chains that may be unstable and precipitate.
   - Compound heterozygosity for hemoglobin S and beta thalassemia results in a symptomatic sickle cell syndrome.

DIAGNOSIS

1. **List the various sickle cell syndromes.**
   - Sickle cell trait (heterozygous hemoglobin S; AS)
   - Sickle cell anemia (homozygous hemoglobin S; SS)
   - Hemoglobin S-C disease (SC)
   - Sickle beta (+) thalassemia
   - Sickle beta (0) thalassemia

2. **How is sickle cell disease diagnosed?**
   - Hemoglobin electrophoresis, isoelectric focusing, or high-performance liquid chromatography allows the identification and quantification of the various beta hemoglobin variants. These methods are not diagnostic for alpha thalassemia trait (loss of 2/4 alpha chains) or alpha thalassemia silent carrier state (loss of 1/4 alpha chains).

Syndrome Name	Genotype	Beta Globin Variant	Severity of Disease
Sickle cell trait	AS	60% A, 40% S	Largely asymptomatic
Sickle cell anemia	SS	>90% S	Most severe disease
Hemoglobin S-C disease	SC	50% S, 50% C	Severe
Sickle beta (+) thalassemia	S-Beta+	>50% S, < 50% A	Intermediate
Sickle beta (0) thalassemia	S-Beta 0	>90% S	Most severe disease
Sickle cell anemia with HPFH	SS-HPFH	65%–85% S 15%–35% F	Intermediate—less severe

3. **What can be seen on the peripheral smear?**
   - Polychromasia due to reticulocytosis
   - Howell-Jolly bodies due to hyposplenia

- Drepanocytes (sickle-shaped cells) in syndromes with >50% hemoglobin S
- Codocytes (target cells) in thalassemia
- Codocytes and hemoglobin crystals in hemoglobin C disease

4. What is hemoglobin A2?

- Normal and minor variant of hemoglobin A
- Hemoglobin A2 is increased in beta thalassemia and sickle beta thalassemia
- Hemoglobin A2 is composed of two alpha and two delta chains ($\alpha2\delta2$) as compared to hemoglobin A1, which is composed of two alpha and two beta chains ($\alpha2\beta2$)
- Sickle beta (0) thalassemia will have higher levels of hemoglobin A2 on hemoglobin electrophoresis and can thereby be distinguished from homozygous sickle cell disease

CAVEATS IN THE CLINICAL PRESENTATION OF THE VARIOUS SICKLE CELL SYNDROMES

1. Describe the clinical presentation of sickle cell trait

- Sickle cell trait is typically asymptomatic, except with extreme physical exertion such as in military recruits.
- Sickle cell trait can be associated with gross hematuria due to papillary necrosis, which may be precipitated by dehydration and/or physical exertion.
- Sickle cell trait is associated with increased risk for renal medullary carcinoma.

2. Which sickle cell syndromes have the most severe clinical symptoms?

- Homozygous SS disease and sickle beta (0) thalassemia are most severe.

3. List two symptoms that are more common in sickle cell (SC) disease

- Retinopathy and avascular necrosis are more common in SC disease.

4. What are the most common manifestations of a vaso-occlusive crisis?

- Bone pain
- Stroke
- Acute chest syndrome
- Dactylitis, primarily in children
- Priapism

5. Patients with SCD are at higher risk for what types of infections?

- Bacteremia with encapsulated organisms (*Streptococcus pneumoniae, Haemophilus influenzae, Neisseria meningitidis*), *Escherichia coli*, staphylococcal species, and *Salmonella*
- Pneumonia with *Mycoplasma, Chlamydia,* and *Legionella*
- Osteomyelitis with *Staphylococcus aureus* and *Salmonella*

6. Why is infection a major cause of morbidity/mortality for patients with SCD?

- Functional hyposplenism/asplenia

- o Of note, SCD commonly results in functional asplenia, although splenic sequestration crisis may still occur in adult patients with hemoglobin SC disease
- Decreased tissue perfusion
- Indwelling catheters
- Skin ulceration/bone infarction

7. **List several of the chronic complications that occur in patients with SCD:**
   - Avascular necrosis
   - Cognitive and educational delay related to cerebral infarctions
   - HTN
   - Chronic restrictive lung disease
   - Chronic renal failure
   - Osteoporosis
   - Heart failure
   - Proliferative retinopathy

Management of Acute Episodes

MANAGEMENT OF ACUTE CHEST SYNDROME

1. **Define acute chest syndrome**
   - Acute illness characterized by fever and/or respiratory symptoms, accompanied by a new pulmonary infiltrate on chest x-ray (CXR)

2. **What percentage of patients with sickle cell disease will have an episode of acute chest syndrome in their lifetimes?**
   - Fifty percent

3. **List common presenting symptoms in acute chest syndrome**
   - Fever, cough, chest pain, and shortness of breath

4. **List potential triggers for acute chest syndrome**
   - Infection, pulmonary embolism, bone marrow or fat embolism, fluid overload, and opiate narcosis with hypoventilation

5. **List tests in the diagnostic workup of acute chest syndrome**
   - CXR, complete blood count (CBC), comprehensive metabolic panel, type and screen, blood cultures, and respiratory viral panel; consider CT angiogram if clinically appropriate

6. **List general treatment measures for acute chest syndrome**
   - Antibiotics, incentive spirometry, supplemental oxygen, intravenous fluids, pain control, and simple or automated exchange transfusion

7. **What treatment has been shown to decrease the frequency of acute chest syndrome?**
   - Hydroxyurea

MANAGEMENT OF VASO-OCCLUSIVE PAIN CRISIS

1. **Describe the management of vaso-occlusive pain crises**
   - Prompt administration of pain medication and hydration

2. **What two treatments have been shown to decrease the frequency of acute pain crisis?**
   - Hydroxyurea
     - The 1995 Multicenter Study of Hydroxyurea in Sickle Cell Anemia (MSH) randomly assigned 299 adults with sickle cell anemia (Hemoglobin SS disease) and at least three painful episodes in a year to receive placebo or hydroxyurea. Compared with controls, the hydroxyurea-treated individuals had a decrease in painful events (median annualized rate, 4.5 vs. 2.5 events).
   - L-glutamine
     - The FDA approved in 2017 based on a randomized trial of 230 patients. Patients were randomized to daily treatment with L-glutamine (0.3 g/kg orally twice per day in powder form; maximum daily dose 30 g) or placebo. Those who received glutamine had fewer acute pain events (3 versus 4), fewer hospitalizations (2 versus 3), fewer days in the hospital (7 versus 11), and fewer episodes of acute chest syndrome (9 versus 23) (clinical trial number NCT01179217).

PREVENTIVE CARE IN SCD

1. **What are the recommendations for infectious prophylaxis in children with SCD?**
   - Administer oral penicillin prophylaxis twice daily until age 5 years in all children with sickle cell anemia (Hemoglobin SS disease) to reduce the risk for pneumococcal infections.
   - Vaccinate against *Streptococcus pneumoniae*.

2. **Describe the data and recommendations for stroke screening in children with sickle cell anemia.**
   - Children should be screened annually with transcranial Doppler beginning at age 2 years and continuing until age 16 years.
   - Data is from the Stroke Prevention Trial in Sickle Cell Anemia (STOP). Children were screened for elevated velocities in the distal internal carotid artery or proximal middle cerebral artery. One hundred and thirty children with elevated velocities were randomly assigned to either receive transfusions to maintain hemoglobin S (HbS) concentrations of less than 30% or remain on standard supportive care with transfusion only when clinically indicated. There were 10 cerebral infarctions and 1 intracerebral hematoma in the standard care group, as compared with 1 infarction in the transfusion group—a 92% difference in the risk of stroke ($p < 0.001$). This result led to the early termination of the trial.

3. **What is the treatment for the secondary prevention of recurrent stroke?**
   - Monthly simple or exchange transfusions

4. **In addition to standard screening for hypertension, what should SCD patients who are >10 years of age be annually evaluated for?**
   - Proteinuria
   - Dilated eye exam to evaluate for retinopathy

5. **List the benefits of hydroxyurea.**
   - Improved overall survival
   - Decrease in the frequency and severity of vaso-occlusive crises
   - Decrease in the incidence of acute chest syndrome

6. **What is the effect of hydroxyurea?**
   - Increases levels of hemoglobin F
   - Lowers the number of circulating leukocytes and reticulocytes and alters the expression of adhesion molecules, all of which contribute to vaso-occlusion
   - Raises RBC volume (higher mean corpuscular volume [MCV]) and improves cellular deformability and rheology, which increases blood flow and reduces vaso-occlusion

7. **List side effects of hydroxyurea.**
   - Myelosuppression, nausea, diarrhea, skin ulcers, mouth sores, and hair thinning

8. **How long does it take for hydroxyurea to lead to a clinical response?**
   - May take up to 3 to 6 months
   - A 6-month trial is recommended prior to declaring treatment failure
   - Monitor MCV, reticulocyte count, and WBCs for index of adherence, response, and dosing

TRANSFUSIONS IN SICKLE CELL DISEASE

1. **What are the benefits of exchange transfusion for patients with sickle cell disease?**
   - Increases the percent of normal (donor) hemoglobin A containing RBCs
   - Permits transfusion of increased volumes of donor blood without increasing blood viscosity
   - Reduces rate of iron accumulation

2. **What are the risks of exchange transfusion?**
   - Increased alloimmunization risk
   - Higher cost
   - Need for permanent venous access

3. **What are indications for chronic exchange/prophylactic transfusions in SCD?**
   - Secondary prevention of stroke, recurrent acute chest syndrome despite hydroxyurea, severe vaso-occlusive crisis not responsive to hydroxyurea, recurrent priapism, and pulmonary hypertension (HTN) not responsive to hydroxyurea

4. **What is the hemoglobin S goal in patients undergoing chronic exchange/prophylactic transfusions in SCD?**
   - Reduce the hemoglobin S to <30%

5. **What are the indications and data for preoperative transfusions in patients with SCD?**
   - Transfuse RBCs to bring the hemoglobin level to 10 g/dL prior to undergoing a surgical procedure involving general anesthesia.
   - Transfusion Alternatives Preoperatively in Sickle Cell Disease (TAPS) trial randomized 70 patients with SCD to no preoperative transfusion or preoperative transfusion with a target Hgb level of 10 g/dL. The study was terminated early due to an increased incidence of serious adverse events in the no-transfusion arm. Compared with no transfusion, those who received preoperative transfusion had fewer serious adverse events (3% vs. 30%) and fewer episodes of acute chest syndrome (3% vs. 27%).

6. **When should transfusion NOT be used in patients with SCD?**
   - Uncomplicated vaso-occlusive pain episode without symptomatic anemia (no evidence of benefit)

IRON OVERLOAD IN SCD

1. **Why are patients with SCD at risk for iron overload?**
   - For every 3 to 4 units of RBCs that a patient receives, 1 g of iron enters the body (adults normally have only 4–5 g iron in their body).
   - There is no physiologic means to remove excess iron as regulation of iron homeostasis normally occurs at the level of absorption through the hormone hepcidin, which inhibits the transport of gastrointestinal iron into the body. Because transfused blood represents iron that circumvents the normal pathways of iron regulation, this excess iron accumulates in tissues and can result in organ dysfunction.

2. **How is iron overload diagnosed?**
   - Serum ferritin
     - Level of >2,500 ng/mL had a sensitivity of 62.5% and specificity of 77.8% for identifying liver iron concentrations of 7 mg iron/g dry liver tissue or greater
   - Liver iron concentration by MRI

3. **List treatments for iron overload**
   - Deferiprone, deferoxamine, and deferasirox

ADVANCED THERAPIES IN SCD

1. **In whom would you consider a stem cell transplant for SCD?**
   - Patient with severe symptoms of SCD unresponsive to treatment with transfusions and hydroxyurea for whom there is a human leukocyte antigen (HLA)-matched sibling donor

QUESTIONS

1. You suspect sickle cell disease in a patient and order a hemoglobin electrophoresis. The following result is consistent with which diagnosis?

HbA	0%
HbS	87%–92%
HbC	0%
HbF	2%–15%
HbA2	>3.5%

A. Sickle cell disease (HbSS)
B. Sickle cell trait
C. Sickle beta(+) thalassemia
D. Sickle beta(0) thalassemia

2. Which lane on the following electrophoresis corresponds to a diagnosis of sickle cell trait?

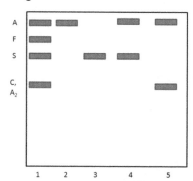

A. 1
B. 2
C. 3
D. 4
E. 5

3. A patient states he or she had a history of sickle cell. The smear shows an abundance of target cells. What type of sickle cell disease may you suspect?
A. SS
B. Sickle beta thalassemia
C. SC
D. Sickle cell trait

4. Which of the following is not recommended in children with sickle cell disease (SCD)?
A. Annual transcranial Doppler
B. Empiric iron chelation therapy at age 10 years

C. Annual eye exam
D. Daily penicillin prophylaxis

5. **A patient is undergoing a cholecystectomy. His hemoglobin is 8 g/dL. What is the appropriate perioperative transfusion strategy?**
   A. Patient does not need a transfusion
   B. Transfuse to a goal of 9 g/dL
   C. Transfuse to a goal of 10 g/dL
   D. Transfuse to a goal of 11 g/dL

6. **What level of ferritin would make you concerned your patient may be developing iron overload?**
   A. 250 ng/mL
   B. 500 ng/mL
   C. 750 ng/mL
   D. 2,500 ng/mL

7. **Which of the following is not part of the definition of acute chest syndrome?**
   A. Fever
   B. Chest pain
   C. Respiratory symptoms
   D. New infiltrate on chest x-ray (CXR)

8. **What mutation causes sickle cell disease?**
   A. Point mutation in the beta globin gene
   B. Frameshift mutation in the beta globin gene
   C. Deletion in the beta globin gene
   D. Insertion in the beta globin gene

9. **For a patient with sickle cell disease (SCD) at high risk for stroke, which is the appropriate treatment for primary prevention?**
   A. Hydroxyurea
   B. Chronic exchange transfusions to maintain hemoglobin S <30%
   C. L-glutamine
   D. Aspirin

10. **Which of the following does not play a role in the clinical manifestations and disease severity of sickle cell disease (SCD)?**
    A. Beta globin genotype
    B. Age at diagnosis
    C. Concentration of hemoglobin F
    D. Coexistence of alpha thalassemia

11. **Which of the following is recommended for infectious prophylaxis in children with sickle cell disease (SCD)?**
    A. Oral penicillin prophylaxis BID until age 3 years
    B. Oral penicillin prophylaxis BID until age 5 years
    C. Vaccinate against meningococcal B before age 3 years
    D. Vaccinate against *Haemophilus influenzae* at birth

ANSWERS

1. **D. Sickle beta(0) thalassemia.** This patient has ~90% HbS and no HbA or HbC; therefore the patient either has HbSS or sickle beta (0) thalassemia. The elevated HbA2 is consistent with the latter.

2. **D. 4.** Patients with sickle cell trait have HbA and HbS (+/− HbF but with no HbC) on hemoglobin electrophoresis.

3. **C. SC.** Abundance of target cells is a characteristic feature of hemoglobin SC disease.

4. **B. Empiric iron chelation therapy at age 10 years.** Empiric iron chelation is not routinely recommended in patients with SCD. Iron chelation should be done when there is evidence of iron overload.

5. **C. Transfuse to a goal of 10 g/dL.** Transfusion to a hemoglobin goal of 10 g/dL has been shown (in the Transfusion Alternatives Preoperatively in Sickle Cell Disease [TAPS] trial) to result in reduced incidence of adverse events and acute chest syndrome.

6. **D. 2,500 ng/mL.** A ferritin of 2,500 ng/mL or more has a sensitivity of 62.5% and specificity of 77.8% for identifying liver iron concentration of 7 mg iron/g dry liver tissue or greater.

7. **B. Chest pain.** Acute chest syndrome is defined as acute illness characterized by fever and/or respiratory symptoms, accompanied by a new pulmonary infiltrate on a chest X-ray.

8. **A. Point mutation in the beta globin gene.** Sickle cell disease is caused by a mutation resulting in valine to glutamic acid substitution at the sixth amino acid of beta globin.

9. **B. Chronic exchange transfusions to maintain hemoglobin S <30%.** According to the Stroke Prevention Trial in Sickle Cell Anemia (STOP), patients at high risk of stroke based on transcranial Doppler are treated with exchange transfusions to maintain HbS < 30%.

10. **B. Age at diagnosis.** Age at diagnosis does not play a role in the clinical manifestations or disease severity of SCD. Higher concentration of hemoglobin F is associated with reduced severity of clinical manifestations. Coexisting alpha thalassemia reduces the severity of some disease manifestations for select sickle cell haplotypes, and the beta globin genotype (AS, S-beta thal, SC, and SS) plays a significant role in clinical manifestations and disease severity.

11. **B. Oral penicillin prophylaxis BID until age 5 years.** Oral penicillin prophylaxis is recommended for children with SCD until age 5. Vaccination against *Streptococcus pneumoniae* is recommended. The other vaccinations are given as per the normal pediatric vaccination schedule.

White Blood Cell Disorders

5

Thomas Michniacki and Kelly Walkovich

Granulocyte Disorders

NEUTROPHIL OVERVIEW

1. **How are neutropenia and neutrophilia defined?**
   - Typically define neutropenia as absolute neutrophil count (ANC) below 1,500 cells/microL (1.5×10^9/L)
   - Mild neutropenia: ANC greater than 1,000 but less than 1,500 cells/microL
   - Moderate neutropenia: ANC greater than 500 but less than 1,000 cells/microL
   - Severe neutropenia: ANC less than 500 cells/microL
   - Very severe neutropenia: ANC less than 200 cells/microL
   - ANC = White blood cells/microL × (percent [polymorphonuclear cells + bands]/100)
   - Be aware of benign ethnic neutropenia with individuals of certain ethnic descent (especially African, West Indian, Sephardic Jews, and Yemenites) having lower baseline ANCs with values typically greater than 1,200 cells/microL (though they might be less than 1,000 cells/microL). Low ANC is correlated with a Duffy antigen/receptor null (FyA-/FyB-) phenotype in these individuals.
   - Neutrophilia leukocytosis is defined as a total white blood cell count greater than 11,000/microL along with an absolute neutrophil count greater than 7,700/microL in adults (more than two standard deviations above the mean)

2. **What is the maturation process and life cycle for neutrophils?**
   - Steps of maturation: myeloblast → promyelocyte → myelocyte → metamyelocyte → band → neutrophil
   - Neutrophils spend approximately 14 days within the bone marrow, including retention of mature cells within a large, non-mitotic storage pool that can be released into circulation rapidly if needed (e.g., secondary to infection)
   - The chemokine receptor, CXCR4, is an important regulator of neutrophil release from the marrow
   - Once released, neutrophils typically last 24 to 48 hours within the circulation
   - Neutrophils depart the circulation and move into inflamed/injured tissue via chemotaxis and ultimately diapedesis across or between endothelial cells. This process occurs via three main classes of proteins: selectins, integrins, and chemokines. Initial vessel adhesion and transient rolling across the endothelial wall by the neutrophil occurs through selectins. Further actions by integrins and chemokines ultimately lead to movement arrest and migration across the vessel wall into tissues

- Once within tissues, neutrophils are believed to not undergo phagocytosis by macrophages or apoptosis for another few days

3. How do neutrophils function?

- Assist in the recruitment and activation of additional cells of the immune system
- Have three direct antimicrobial functions: degranulation, phagocytosis, and creation of neutrophil extracellular traps (NETs)
- Degranulation results in the release of azurophilic, specific, and tertiary granules
- Phagocytosis ultimately generates reactive oxygen species (the "respiratory burst")
- The respiratory burst involves the activation of the enzyme nicotinamide adenine dinucleotide phosphate (NADPH) oxidase, which helps create superoxide. Superoxide is converted to hydrogen peroxide by superoxide dismutase with hydrogen peroxide next undergoing enzymatic reaction with myeloperoxidase to create the bactericidal hypochlorous acid
- NETs: Weblike extracellular structures, extruded by dying neutrophils, that consist of granule proteins and chromatin that can further facilitate microbe killing

ACQUIRED NEUTROPHIL DISORDERS

1. What are the acquired causes of neutropenia?

- Medications:
  - Usually begins within 3 months of starting the medication with the pathogenesis felt to be secondary to drug-dependent autoimmune destruction of neutrophils and/or their precursors
  - Numerous medications are implicated but the most commonly reported include clozapine, the thionamides (antithyroid medications), nonsteroidal anti-inflammatory drugs (NSAIDs), dapsone, antibiotics, sulfa-containing drugs, angiotensin-converting enzyme (ACE) inhibitors, histamine blockers, and ticlopidine
  - Be aware of levamisole-tainted cocaine and heroin causing neutropenia in illicit drug users
- Infections:
  - Bacterial infections commonly described include *Shigella* enteritis, typhoid fever, tuberculosis, brucellosis, and rickettsial pathogens
  - Malaria is a known cause as are numerous viral agents, most notably HIV, Epstein-Barr virus (EBV), cytomegalovirus (CMV), hepatitis viruses, human herpesvirus 6 (HHV-6), and varicella
- Nutritional deficiencies:
  - Deficiencies of vitamin B12, folate, and copper
  - Anorexia nervosa and/or severe malnutrition
- Autoimmune disorders:
  - Systemic lupus erythematosus and rheumatoid arthritis most commonly
  - Felty's syndrome is the combination of neutropenia, rheumatoid arthritis, and splenomegaly

- Chronic idiopathic neutropenia:
  - A benign chronic neutropenia with no obvious cause that may present in adulthood
  - ANC typically ranges from 500 to 1,000 cells/microL with an associated monocytosis
  - Patients usually do not suffer from increased infections; they may merely be monitored and do not often require granulocyte colony stimulating factor (G-CSF)
- Bone marrow disorders such as myelodysplastic syndromes
- Large granular lymphocyte (LGL) leukemia

2. **What are the acquired causes of neutrophilia?**
   - Neutrophilia can be secondary to increased production, reduced margination, enhanced release from marrow storage pool, and decreased removal from circulation
   - Increased production due to infection, autoimmune conditions, malignancy, myeloproliferative disease, chronic idiopathic neutrophilia, post-neutropenia recovery, and medications (lithium and quinidine)
   - Increased marrow storage pool release secondary to corticosteroids, stress, infection, endotoxin stimulation, and hypoxia
   - Reduced margination from stress, exercise, epinephrine, and infection
   - Decreased circulation clearance of neutrophils due to corticosteroids or splenectomy

3. **What are the acquired qualitative disorders of neutrophils?**
   - Numerous acquired conditions can affect the functional abilities of neutrophils
   - These include diabetes mellitus, trauma, severe burns, renal failure, liver disease, alcoholism, infections (most commonly HIV and influenza), and autoimmune conditions

INHERITED NEUTROPHIL DISORDERS

1. **What are the inherited causes of neutropenia?**
   - Benign ethnic neutropenia as noted earlier
   - Shwachman-Diamond syndrome:
     - Mutations in the *SBDS* gene that leads to bone marrow failure, exocrine pancreatic insufficiency, and skeletal abnormalities. Pancreatic and skeletal features may be mild and not clinically apparent. Neutropenia can progress to pancytopenia with bone marrow failure/leukemia
   - Cyclic neutropenia:
     - Recurrent neutropenia every 14 to 35 days but most patients exhibit a 21-day cycle period with 7 to 10 days of profound neutropenia
     - Often see a reciprocal monocytosis during times of neutropenia
     - Recurrent infections, fevers, and/or mouth ulcers during times of neutropenia with signs of chronic inflammation of the gingiva and oral mucosa
     - Patients are also at risk of *Clostridium septicum* infections

- Diagnosis requires monitoring neutrophil counts two to three times per week for 6 to 8 weeks
- Ninety percent of patients have mutations in the elastase gene (*ELA1*, *ELANE*) that leads to cyclic arrest in myelocyte maturation and selective apoptosis of neutrophil precursors
- Treatment involves recombinant granulocyte colony stimulating factor (G-CSF) and supportive care
- Severe congenital neutropenia:
  - Increased apoptosis of myeloid cells leading to severe neutropenia and risk of death from infection
  - Can be due to various mutations, including elastase/*ELANE* (autosomal dominant, 50%–60% of cases) and *HAX1* (formerly known as Kostmann syndrome, autosomal recessive)
  - At risk for malignant transformation into myelodysplastic syndrome (MDS) and acute myeloid leukemia (AML). Following 10 years of G-CSF therapy, the annual risk of MDS/AML appears to be 2.3%/year with a cumulative MDS/AML incidence after 15 years on G-CSF of 22%. Annual bone marrows are thus recommended for malignancy screening
  - Treatment with escalating doses of G-CSF until an ANC of 1,000 to 2,000 cells/microL is reached
  - Hematopoietic cell transplantation should be considered in those unable to tolerate G-CSF, with continued infections despite G-CSF usage or requiring high doses of G-CSF (greater than 8 mcg/kg/day)
- Neutropenia can also be associated with WHIM (warts, hypogammaglobulinemia, infections, and myelokathexis) syndrome and GATA2 deficiency

2. **What are the inherited functional disorders of neutrophils?**
   - Myeloperoxidase (MPO) deficiency:
     - The most common primary phagocyte disorder but may also be acquired
     - MPO catalyzes hydrogen peroxide into hypochlorous acid
     - Greater than 95% of patients are asymptomatic but may be unmasked in the setting of poorly controlled diabetes mellitus
     - Symptomatic individuals have an increased risk of *Candida* species infections and vasculitis
     - Diagnosis is obtained by histochemical staining for MPO
     - Treatment is supportive
   - Chronic granulomatous disease (CGD):
     - Caused by defects in NADPH oxidase, which leads to inability of phagocytes to kill certain microbes
     - Most mutations are X linked, although female carriers have increased autoimmune features and may have skewed lionization leading to infection susceptibility
     - Patients are particularly susceptible to catalase-positive organisms with the most common pathogens being *Staphylococcus aureus*, *Aspergillus*, *Burkholderia* (*Pseudomonas*), *Serratia*, and *Nocardia*

- ○ The lung, skin, lymph nodes, and liver are most frequently infected with recurrent abscesses common
- ○ Diagnosis is made via neutrophil function testing (nitroblue tetrazolium [NBT] or dihydrorhodamine [DHR] 123 tests) and confirmed via genetic studies
- ○ Treatment involves antimicrobial prophylaxis with trimethoprim-sulfamethoxazole and itraconazole with consideration for usage of interferon-gamma
- ○ Treat all acute infections aggressively
- ○ Corticosteroids may be used to control the inflammatory manifestations of CGD
- ○ Hematopoietic stem cell transplantation is curative
- Leukocyte adhesion deficiencies affect the ability of neutrophils to emigrate to sites of inflammation due to mutations in key integrins and selectins
- ○ May cause neutrophilia
- Neutrophil dysfunction is associated with numerous other syndromes including Chediak-Higashi syndrome, Griscelli syndrome, and STAT3 loss of function (autosomal dominant hyper-immunoglobulin E syndrome)

TREATMENT OF NEUTROPENIA

1. How are neutropenic conditions associated with an increased risk of infection treated?

- See preceding text for disease-specific recommendations, but most involve the usage of G-CSF and aggressive supportive therapy
- Granulocyte colony stimulating factor:
- ○ Initial dosing of G-CSF is 5 mcg/kg/d with escalation until appropriate ANC is reached (of note, patients with cyclic neutropenia typically respond to lower dosing of 2–3 mcg/kg)
- ○ May be associated with bone pain, neutrophilia, splenomegaly, and rarely splenic rupture
- Infection prophylaxis:
- ○ Trimethoprim-sulfamethoxazole, itraconazole, and interferon-gamma in chronic granulomatous disease (CGD) patients
- ○ Prophylactic antibiotics have not been found to be of value in most cases of non-chemotherapy-related neutropenia (this should be individualized)
- ○ Emphasize excellent hand and dental hygiene to reduce the risk of serious infections, including bacteremia

MONOCYTE OVERVIEW

1. What is the life cycle and function of monocytes?

- Following development from monoblasts within the marrow, monocytes move to the circulation for 1 to 3 days prior to moving to the tissue, where they differentiate into macrophages or dendritic cells
- Monocytes and their progeny serve three main functions within the immune system: phagocytosis, cytokine production, and antigen presentation

2. **What is the definition of monocytosis and monocytopenia?**
   - Monocytosis is defined as a total monocyte count of more than 500 cells/microL
   - Monocytopenia is a rare isolated finding and is usually associated with additional cytopenias

CAUSES OF MONOCYTOSIS AND MONOCYTOPENIA

1. **What are the major causes of monocytosis?**
   - Infectious causes: Subacute bacterial endocarditis, tuberculosis, syphilis, and protozoal and rickettsial infections (Rocky Mountain spotted fever and kala-azar)
   - Autoimmune conditions: Systemic lupus erythematosus, sarcoidosis, inflammatory bowel disease, and rheumatoid arthritis
   - Malignancy: Chronic myelomonocytic leukemia, chronic myeloid leukemia (CML), acute myeloid leukemia (AML), and lymphoma
   - Miscellaneous conditions: Post-neutropenia recovery, post-splenectomy, cyclic neutropenia (reciprocal monocytosis during times of neutropenia), corticosteroids, tetrachloroethane poisoning, and alcoholic liver disease

2. **What are the causes of monocytopenia?**
   - Typically found with other immune cytopenias but may be additionally observed with corticosteroid usage, infections with endotoxin production, stress, and GATA2 deficiency
   - Hairy cell leukemia (a monocyte count of 0 should raise the suspicion of this disorder in the right clinical setting)

EOSINOPHIL OVERVIEW

1. **What is an eosinophil?**
   - Eosinophils are granulocytes that play a vital role in combating viral and parasitic infections, along with mediating the body's response to allergens (in addition to mast cells and basophils)
   - Activated eosinophils may damage tissues through recruitment of other inflammatory cells, cytokine release, and toxic granule production

2. **What defines eosinophilia?**
   - Eosinophilia is defined as a total eosinophil count of greater than 500 cells/microL
   - Eosinophilia can be further classified as mild (500 to 1,500 cells/microL), moderate (1,500 to 5,000 cells/microL), or severe (>5,000 cells/microL)
   - Hypereosinophilia (HE) is defined as moderate-to-severe eosinophilia (greater than or equal to 1,500 cells/microL)
   - Keep in mind that the level of peripheral blood eosinophilia does not always predict the risk of organ damage

CAUSES OF EOSINOPHILIA AND EOSINOPENIA

1. **What are the major causes of eosinophilia?**
   - Allergic disorders: asthma, acute urticaria, atopic dermatitis, allergic bronchopulmonary aspergillosis, eosinophilic gastroenteritis, food allergy, and atopic rhinitis

- Parasites and infections: invasive helminths, EBV, malaria, toxoplasmosis, tuberculosis, amebiasis, cat scratch fever, coccidioidomycosis, fungal rhinosinusitis, and scabies
- Hereditary disorders: Hyper-immunoglobulin E syndrome, familial eosinophilia, and hereditary angioedema
- Drug reactions, including drug reaction with eosinophilia and systemic symptoms (DRESS)
- Miscellaneous: adrenal insufficiency, graft-versus-host disease (GVHD), and peritoneal/hemodialysis
- Rheumatological disorders: eosinophilic fasciitis, polyarteritis nodosa, sarcoidosis, and scleroderma
- Hypereosinophilic syndrome and clonal eosinophilia
  - Eosinophilia associated with *PDGFRA*, *PDGFRB*, *FGFR*, or *JAK2* rearrangements. These rearrangements could be tested for by fluorescence in situ hybridization (FISH), polymerase chain reaction (PCR), or bone marrow cytogenetics
  - If other cytogenetic abnormalities or excess blasts are present, the diagnosis could be chronic eosinophilic leukemia or other World Health Organization (WHO)-defined myeloid neoplasm
  - Lymphocyte variant eosinophilia (associated with abnormal or clonal lymphocytes)
  - In the absence of all the above clonal findings, the diagnosis could be idiopathic eosinophilia including hypereosinophilic syndrome. The latter two disorders do not have clonal findings
    - Hypereosinophilic syndrome is characterized by absolute eosinophil count of 1,500 cell/microL or greater for at least 6 months with evidence of organ damage from infiltrating eosinophils. In the absence of end-organ damage, the diagnosis of hypereosinophilic syndrome cannot be made
    - Patients with hypereosinophilic syndrome may present with fever, fatigue, weight loss, hepatosplenomegaly, pulmonary infiltrates, and skin manifestations
    - Cardiac damage is the leading cause of morbidity and mortality with Loeffler endocarditis as a possible complication
  - Treat the underlying condition if one can be found with consideration for corticosteroids in symptomatic patients
  - Imatinib therapy has been successfully used in those found to have *PDGFRA* rearrangements. If cardiac involvement is present, concomitant steroid therapy should be considered
  - In those severely affected with clonal eosinophilic disorder, consider hematopoietic stem cell transplantation
- Mastocytosis:
  - A clonal expansion of mast cells causing cutaneous (urticaria pigmentosa) or systemic multiorgan (bone marrow, spleen, liver, and lymph node) infiltration
  - Infiltrating mast cells typically express CD2 and/or CD25 in addition to normal mast cell markers

- ○ Patients often are found to have a mutation involving *c-KIT*
- ○ Patients may present with episodic signs/symptoms of mast cell activation, including hypotension, syncope, urticaria, flushing, fatigue, diarrhea, and musculoskeletal pain
- ○ Adults presenting with skin manifestations should be evaluated for presence of systemic disease
- ○ Cytopenias due to marrow infiltration; abnormal liver enzymes and elevated serum tryptase (persistently exceeds 20 ng/mL) are additionally found
- ○ Patients should have ready access to epinephrine injections given the risk of anaphylaxis
- ○ Treatment is aimed at preventing mast cell mediator release through the use of antihistamines, cromolyn sodium, and antileukotriene agents
- ○ Imatinib can be used if the systemic mastocytosis is not *c-KIT* mutated
- ○ Advanced systemic mastocytosis can be treated with midostaurin (regardless of *c-KIT* mutation status).
- ○ Severe cases may require cytoreductive therapies. Hematopoietic stem cell transplantation can be considered as part of a clinical trial (experimental)
- Many malignancies are associated with eosinophilia
  - ○ Eosinophilia is notably present in adenocarcinomas, primary (neoplastic) hypereosinophilic syndrome, Sezary syndrome, acute and chronic eosinophilic leukemia, chronic myeloid leukemia (CML), and myeloproliferative neoplasms

2. What are the causes of eosinopenia?
   - Eosinopenia may be secondary to conditions causing release of adrenal corticosteroids, prostaglandins, and epinephrine
   - Exposure to corticosteroids or epinephrine

BASOPHIL OVERVIEW

1. What is a basophil?
   - Basophils are the least common but the largest granulocyte
   - They assist in the formation of inflammatory reactions during immune and allergic responses
   - They are capable of phagocytosis and releasing heparin, serotonin, and histamine

CAUSES OF BASOPHILIA AND BASOPHILOPENIA

1. What are the major causes of basophilia?
   - Malignant disorders, most notably chronic myeloid leukemia (CML), AML, MDS, and myeloproliferative neoplasms
   - Hypersensitivity reactions to drugs and foods
   - Infections: Smallpox, tuberculosis, varicella, helminths, and influenza
   - Allergic syndromes
   - Mastocytosis

- Autoimmune conditions, most notably rheumatoid arthritis and ulcerative colitis
- Severe hypothyroidism and administration of estrogen

2. **What are the major cause of basophilopenia?**
   - Glucocorticoids
   - Thyrotoxicosis

Lymphocyte Disorders

CAUSES OF LYMPHOPENIA AND LYMPHOCYTOSIS

1. **What are the major acquired causes of lymphopenia?**
   - Infections:
     - Bacterial: tuberculosis, severe bacterial sepsis, brucellosis, and typhoid fever
     - Viral: HIV, measles, severe acute respiratory syndrome (SARS), and hepatitis
     - Severe fungal sepsis and histoplasmosis
     - Malaria
   - Autoimmune disorders, including systemic lupus erythematosus, Sjögren syndrome, and rheumatoid arthritis
   - Iatrogenic: corticosteroid usage, immunosuppressive therapy, and radiation
   - Miscellaneous: thoracic leak, protein-losing enteropathy, Cushing's syndrome, alcoholism, stress, trauma, zinc deficiency, malnutrition, and renal failure

2. **What are the major acquired causes of lymphocytosis?**
   - Numerous malignancies including chronic lymphocytic leukemia and other lymphoproliferative neoplasms, thymoma
   - Infections (notably viral), hypersensitivity reactions (including drug reactions), and autoimmune conditions
   - Miscellaneous: post-splenectomy, trauma, stress, cigarette smoking (persistent polyclonal B-cell lymphocytosis), and hyperthyroidism

QUESTIONS

1. **You are referred a 45-year-old African American for evaluation of persistent neutropenia. Over the past 3 months, he has had absolute neutrophil count (ANC) values of 1,250 cells/microL, 1,300 cells/microL, and 1,205 cells/microL. There is no reciprocal monocytosis with his neutropenia and he states that he has been told throughout his life that his neutrophils have always been slightly low. He denies any history of recurrent serious infections. What should be your next step in his care?**
   A. Perform a bone marrow evaluation
   B. Place him on prophylactic antibiotics
   C. No need for continued monitoring
   D. Prescribe daily granulocyte colony stimulating (G-CSF) factor injections

2. A woman is placed on a course of high-dose corticosteroids by her primary care physician for a case of severe atopic dermatitis. What complete blood count (CBC) abnormality would one likely find if a CBC was obtained on this patient while receiving her corticosteroids?
   A. Neutrophilia
   B. Anemia
   C. Eosinophilia
   D. Thrombocytopenia

3. You are taking over the care of a 25-year-old man from your pediatric hematology colleague. He has a history of recurrent liver abscesses and *Aspergillus* pulmonary infection in the past but is now doing well. He is currently receiving prophylaxis with itraconazole, trimethoprim-sulfamethoxazole, and interferon-gamma. What is the underlying inherited cause of his condition?
   A. Lack of myeloperoxidase (MPO)
   B. Mutations affecting the nicotinamide adenine dinucleotide phosphate (NADPH) oxidase complex
   C. SBDS gene mutation
   D. Duffy antigen/receptor null phenotype

4. You are the consulting hematologist for a patient found to have an absolute eosinophil count of 4.5×10^9/L along with urticarial rash, persistent cough with hypoxia, and a mild transaminitis. CT chest/abdomen shows pulmonary and hepatic infiltrates. Genetic testing reveals the presence of a FIP1L1-PDGFRA fusion within clonal marrow cells. Based on the patient's genetic analysis results, what medication should be included in the patient's treatment regimen?
   A. Imatinib
   B. Ipilimumab
   C. Ivermectin
   D. Trametinib

5. A 27-year-old Caucasian woman is seen in your clinic for an evaluation of neutropenia. Her past medical history is notable for a rheumatoid factor–positive rheumatoid arthritis diagnosis for which she was recently evaluated by a rheumatologist. She states she was prescribed a course of scheduled prednisone and naproxen as needed by her rheumatologist but has yet to begin the medications. A complete blood count (CBC) reveals an absolute neutrophil count (ANC) of 950 cells/microL, platelet count of 135,000/microL, and a microcytic anemia with a hemoglobin value of 10.5 g/dL. Eosinophil count is normal. Physical exam is notable for numerous swollen and painful joints and splenomegaly. What is your most likely diagnosis for this patient?
   A. Systemic mastocytosis
   B. Benign ethnic neutropenia
   C. Severe congenital neutropenia
   D. Felty's syndrome

6. A 24-year-old woman is receiving propylthiouracil treatment for her Graves' disease. What hematological lab abnormality is the patient at the highest risk of suffering from due to her medication history?
   A. Thrombocytosis
   B. Neutropenia
   C. Eosinophilia
   D. Anemia

7. You are evaluating a 22-year-old man who was referred to your clinic for workup of monomorphic urticaria pigmentosa and intermittent episodes of flushing, pruritus, abdominal pain, and diarrhea. His history is additionally notable for apparent episodes of anaphylaxis in association with alcohol ingestion or emotional stress. His workup thus far at other providers has not yielded a causative allergy. What laboratory study may be helpful in making a correct diagnosis for this patient?
   A. Dihydrorhodamine (DHR) 123 test
   B. Screening for mutations in the elastase gene
   C. Serum tryptase
   D. Serum lipase

8. A 32-year-old woman smokes two packs of cigarettes a day. She is currently relatively healthy despite her high tobacco usage. What benign proliferative hematological condition is this patient at risk for given her history of cigarette smoking?
   A. Persistent polyclonal B cell lymphocytosis
   B. Hemophagocytic lymphohistiocytosis (HLH)
   C. Autoimmune lymphoproliferative syndrome (ALPS)
   D. Primary myelofibrosis

9. A man is seen by an endocrinologist for hypertension, insulin resistance, and central obesity with prominent striae. Following a thorough evaluation, he is ultimately diagnosed with Cushing's syndrome. Given his new diagnosis, what value would one expect to find when a complete blood cell count is obtained on the patient?
   A. Absolute neutrophil value of 750 cells/microL
   B. Platelet count of 35,000 platelets/microL
   C. Absolute lymphocyte value of 0.8×10^9/L
   D. Hemoglobin of 9.0 g/dL

10. A 42-year-old woman is receiving treatment with pegylated interferon-alfa and ribavirin for a history of hepatitis C infection. Her treating physician has decided to begin treatment with granulocyte colony stimulating factor (G-CSF) to help lessen neutropenia associated with her antiviral regimen. What adverse reaction can commonly be seen with G-CSF administration?
    A. Hyperactivity
    B. Thrombocytosis
    C. Hirsutism
    D. Ostealgia

11. You have recently taken over the care of a 34-year-old woman with a diagnosis of systemic mastocytosis. Which genetic alteration is most often found associated with this disorder?
    A. *BCR-ABL*
    B. *c-KIT*
    C. *JAK2*
    D. *TET2*

12. A 25-year-old male with a history of cocaine usage is found to have significant neutropenia with an absolute neutrophil count of 100 cells/microL. Which substance now known to be frequently found as a contaminant in cocaine has strongly been associated with neutropenia?
    A. Levofloxacin
    B. Methylamphetamine
    C. Levamisole
    D. Mannitol

ANSWERS

1. **C. No need for continued monitoring.** This patient most likely has benign ethnic neutropenia and thus requires no further monitoring or treatment. There is no evidence of cyclic neutropenia with reciprocal monocytosis or episodes of severe infections. Chronic idiopathic neutropenia is a consideration but patients typically have ANC values ranging from 500 to 1,000 cells/microL with an associated monocytosis. Given his lack of recurrent severe infections, he does not require prophylactic antibiotics or G-CSF.

2. **A. Neutrophilia.** Patients placed on corticosteroids often manifest neutrophilia. Anemia and thrombocytopenia should not be seen. Additionally, corticosteroids often cause eosinopenia rather than eosinophilia.

3. **B. Mutations affecting the nicotinamide adenine dinucleotide phosphate (NADPH) oxidase complex.** This patient is suffering from chronic granulomatous disease (CGD), which is caused by various mutations leading to alterations of the NADPH oxidase protein complex. A lack of MPO is seen in myeloperoxidase deficiency with these patients typically being asymptomatic. SBDS mutations cause Shwachman-Diamond syndrome, and the Duffy antigen/receptor null phenotype is observed in those with benign ethnic neutropenia.

4. **A. Imatinib.** PDGFRA rearrangement is the diagnosis given the patient's eosinophilia and presence of FIP1L1-PDGFRA fusion. Such patients can be treated with Imatinib. Ipilimumab and trametinib are cytotoxic T-lymphocyte-associated antigen 4 (CTLA-4) and MEK inhibitors, respectively, and do not seem to play a role in this disease. Ivermectin is used to treat parasitic infections that may lead to eosinophilia.

5. **D. Felty's syndrome.** The triad of neutropenia, splenomegaly, and rheumatoid arthritis is classic for a diagnosis of Felty's syndrome. The patient additionally has anemia and mild thrombocytopenia, which can also be found with the syndrome. The patient's cytopenias may be partially explained by splenic sequestration, but with microcytic anemia a concurrent diagnosis of anemia of chronic disease should be considered. With Felty's syndrome, neutropenia cannot be explained by concurrent illnesses or medications and is often persistent. Benign ethnic neutropenia is characterized by lifelong mild neutropenia with normal hemoglobin and platelet counts. Severe congenital neutropenia typically presents in early childhood with ANC values of less than 200 cells/microL and requires granulocyte colony stimulating factor injections to help prevent serious infections.

6. **B. Neutropenia.** Thionamides, such as methimazole, carbimazole, and propylthiouracil (PTU), are used in the treatment of Graves' hyperthyroidism but may cause agranulocytosis. PTU appears to more likely cause the condition compared to methimazole. Neutropenia often occurs within the first 1 to 3 months of treatment and is dose dependent with methimazole usage. The thionamides may be associated with aplastic anemia but this complication is less common than agranulocytosis.

7. **C. Serum tryptase.** The patient's history is concerning systemic mastocytosis, which can be associated with an elevation of serum tryptase (>20 ng/mL). Serum tryptase should be measured when the patient is at baseline state and not during or immediately following an apparent mast cell mediator release episode. Values obtained following a symptomatic incident indicate mast cell activation but cannot distinguish between mastocytosis and anaphylaxis secondary to another cause. DHR 123 testing is used for diagnostic evaluation of chronic granulomatous disease. Elastase gene mutations may be found in cyclic neutropenia and severe congenital neutropenia but have no apparent association with mastocytosis. Patients with systemic mastocytosis can present with pancreatitis and thus serum lipase may be elevated but serum tryptase is more specific for mastocytosis.

8. **A. Persistent polyclonal B cell lymphocytosis.** Persistent polyclonal B-cell lymphocytosis is significantly associated with cigarette smoking and is characterized by a persistent elevation in peripheral blood polyclonal binucleated atypical-appearing lymphocytes. Serum IgM is often elevated and there appears to be an association with the HLA-DR7 allele. Women are more at risk for the condition than men. ALPS is more commonly seen in pediatric patients and does not appear to be associated with cigarette smoking. HLH and primary myelofibrosis additionally do not have a clear association with tobacco exposure.

9. **C. Absolute lymphocyte value of 0.8 × 10⁹/L.** Lymphocytopenia often accompanies Cushing's syndrome. Polycythemia has been associated with Cushing's syndrome rather than anemia. There is additionally no association of thrombocytopenia with the condition.

10. **D. Ostealgia.** Musculoskeletal discomfort is a frequent finding following G-CSF administration. Alopecia, thrombocytopenia (possibly due to splenomegaly, a rare side effect of G-CSF), and fatigue have been reported rather than hirsutism, thrombocytosis, and hyperactivity.

11. **B. *c-KIT.*** The majority of systemic mastocytosis patients possess a gain-of-function mutation in the tyrosine kinase receptor, KIT. *JAK2* and *TET2* mutations may be found in those with systemic mastocytosis but are much less common than KIT alterations. *BCR-ABL* gene fusions are most often associated with chronic myelogenous and acute lymphoblastic leukemias.

12. **C. Levamisole.** Numerous reports have now noted cocaine laced with levamisole, an agent historically used to treat malignancies and parasitic infections, as a cause of neutropenia in illicit drug users. Mannitol and methylamphetamine are additional substances that may be found in altered cocaine but are not associated with reports of significant agranulocytosis. Levofloxacin has not reportedly been associated with cocaine manufacturing or with neutropenia.

Bone Marrow Failure/Aplastic Anemia

6

Austin Poole and Michael W. Deininger

Bone Marrow Failure/Aplastic Anemia

DEFINITION

- Pancytopenia resulting from stem cell injury with subsequent deficient hematopoiesis

EPIDEMIOLOGY

- Varied but usually biphasic age distribution: teens to 20s (inherited/constitutional) and elderly (acquired). Men and women are equally affected.
- Incidence: ~ 2 persons per million, higher in East Asia ~4 persons per million

DIAGNOSTIC CRITERIA

1. **What are the two main categories of bone marrow failure?**
   - Acquired
   - Inherited/constitutional

2. **What are major clinical manifestations?**
   - Typically cytopenia related
     - Anemia: fatigue and dyspnea
     - Leukopenia: infection
     - Thrombocytopenia: mucosal bleeding (menorrhagia, epistaxis, easy bruising)

3. **Major peripheral blood morphologic findings**
   - Pancytopenia with normocytic-to-macrocytic red blood cells
   - Reticulocytopenia

4. **What are typically bone marrow biopsy findings?**
   - Paucity of hematopoietic cells (hypocellular)
     - <25 cellularity in severe aplastic anemia *or*
     - <50% with less than 30% hematopoietic cells
       - Preponderance of adipocytes
       - Usually normal karyotype—as opposed to hypoplastic myelodysplastic syndrome (MDS)
       - Low frequency of somatic mutations in *BCOR/BCORL1, DNMT3A, ASXL1*

STAGING

1. **What historical findings are indicative of an inherited/constitutional process (i.e., not acquired)?**

   - Inherited/constitutional
     - Young age at onset, abrupt onset of manifestations
     - Lack of symptoms unrelated to cytopenias (no symptoms suggestive of rheumatologic disease such as arthritis/serositis/rash *or* malignancy/infection/granulomatous disease i.e., constitutional symptoms)
     - Lack of known exposures to insults such as chemotherapy/radiation, drugs (nonsteroidal anti-inflammatory drugs [NSAIDs], sulfonamides, antihistamines, anticonvulsants), and alcohol

SIGNS AND SYMPTOMS

1. **What physical exam/clinical elements may be indicative of an inherited/constitutional process (i.e., not acquired)?**

   - Inherited/constitutional:
     - Physical features (not always present)
       - Fanconi anemia: short stature, anomalies involving radius/thumb, café au lait spots, microcephaly
       - Dyskeratosis congenita: mucous membrane leukoplakia, dystrophic nails, and reticular hyperpigmentation
       - Shwachman-Diamond syndrome: short stature, cognitive impairment
       - Telomeropathies: early graying of the hair
     - Other clinical manifestations:
       - Fanconi anemia: malformed/absent kidneys, gastrointestinal (GI) and heart defects, infertility; 10% to 30% increased risk of malignancy
       - Dyskeratosis congenita: lacrimal duct atresia, pulmonary fibrosis
       - Phenotypic variants of dyskeratosis congenita
         - Hoyeraal-Hreidarsson syndrome: hypoplastic cerebellum, immunodeficiency, intrauterine growth restriction
         - Revesz syndrome: exudative retinopathy, intracranial calcifications, hypoplastic cerebellum
       - Shwachman-Diamond syndrome: exocrine pancreatic insufficiency with malabsorption
       - Telomeropathies: spectrum disease with dyskeratosis congenita as most severe childhood variant, with some adults being diagnosed with bone marrow failure in absence of other stigmata of disease. Associated with hepatic cirrhosis and pulmonary fibrosis

2. **What are some of the genetic aberrations present in inherited/constitutional bone marrow failure syndrome?**

   - Fanconi anemia
     - Autosomal recessive, 15 identified genes involved in Fanconi anemia (FA) pathway

- ○ Eighty-ninety percent of affected individuals with aberrations in *FANCA, FANCC, FANCG*
- ○ Pathway activates FANCD2 and FANCI proteins in response to DNA damage, in particular, interstrand cross-links (ICLs). These proteins bring DNA repair proteins to the area of ICLs
- ○ Diagnosed by demonstrating chromosomal breakage of peripheral blood lymphocytes when exposed to mitomycin C or diepoxybutane
- ○ Ten percent demonstrate hematopoietic somatic mosaicism; therefore skin biopsy required
- Dyskeratosis congenita
  - ○ Mutations in the telomerase complex, which maintains telomere length and thus genetic stability
  - ○ X-linked mutation in gene *DKC1* (dyskerin) causes destabilization of the telomerase repair complex
  - ○ Autosomal dominant (less common) mutation in *TERC* and *TERT*, responsible for the RNA template in the telomerase complex and catalytic reverse transcriptase, respectively
  - ○ Hoyeraal-Hreidarsson syndrome: X-linked recessive, *DCK1* gene (Xq28)
  - ○ Revesz syndrome: Autosomal dominant, *TINF2* (14q12) encoding a component of the shelterin complex that protects telomeres
  - ○ Diagnosed via blood leukocyte telomere length and identification of aforementioned genetic mutations
- Shwachman-Diamond syndrome
  - ○ Autosomal recessive aberration in *SBD2* on 7q11. *SBD2* may have role in ribosomal assembly and function but exact function is unknown
  - ○ Clinical diagnosis with *SBDS* gene sequencing as confirmatory (despite roughly 10% of these patients lacking said mutation)
- Telomeropathies
  - ○ Mutations in *TERT* and *TERC*
  - ○ Diagnosed via blood leukocyte telomere length analysis

3. **What are some acquired causes of aplastic anemia/bone marrow failure?**
- **Paroxysmal nocturnal hemoglobinuria**
  - ○ Present in roughly 50% of patients with aplastic anemia
  - ○ Acquired mutation in *PIG-A* gene, which encodes the enzyme that anchors lipids on cell membranes, which prevents complement-mediated destruction
  - ○ X-linked somatic mutation that affects men and women equally
  - ○ Disease of adulthood
  - ○ Characterized by complement-mediated hemolysis due to absence of glycosylphosphatidylinositol (GPI)-anchored proteins
  - ○ Associated with aplastic anemia, thrombosis, smooth muscle dysfunction (erectile dysfunction/pulmonary hypertension)

○ Diagnosed by flow cytometry evaluating for a variety of GPI-anchored proteins (CD55 and CD59) bound by bacterial toxin aerolysin (FLAER—fluorescent aerolysin—assay)

○ Associated with improved responses to immune suppression

- **Toxins**
  - ○ Benzene: solvent in rubber and leather goods
    - Highly regulated in the United States
  - ○ Organophosphates/organochlorine pesticides
- **Drug: extremely rare, difficult to prove causality**
  - ○ Chloramphenicol (strongest evidence as drug precipitant of aplastic anemia)
  - ○ Cimetidine
  - ○ Nonsteroidal anti-inflammatory drugs (NSAIDs)
  - ○ Sulfa drugs including thiazide diuretics
  - ○ Antimalarials
  - ○ Chemotherapy
- **Infections**
  - ○ Viral hepatitis
    - Classically bone marrow failure occurs weeks to months after resolution of hepatitis
    - Typically occurs in young men
  - ○ Epstein-Barr virus (EBV)
    - Again, classically occurs weeks after infection, which can be subclinical
  - ○ HIV
    - Typically, HIV does not cause hypocellular marrow but case reports of subsequent aplastic anemia
- **Rheumatologic/autoimmune**
  - ○ Eosinophilic fasciitis: inflammation of the fascia with resulting skin changes and swelling, typically asymmetric, in the limbs with peripheral blood eosinophilia. Skin changes are often described as "peau d' orange"
  - ○ Rheumatoid arthritis (RA)
  - ○ Systemic lupus erythematosus (SLE)/lupus
    - Difficult to delineate whether disease or treatment in SLE/RA responsible for association with aplastic anemia
- **Radiation therapy**
- **Pregnancy**
  - ○ Occasionally resolves with delivery or termination
  - ○ Case reports of recurrence with subsequent pregnancy

PROGNOSTIC FACTORS

1. **How is severity of aplastic anemia determined?**
   - **Severe aplastic anemia**

- ○ Bone marrow biopsy <25% or <30% (used in NIH trials) normal cellularity or biopsy with <50% normal cellularity in which 30% of the cells are hematopoietic

  and at least two or three of the following:

- ○ Absolute reticulocyte count <40,000/microL or <60,000/microL (used in NIH trials)
- ○ Neutrophil count <500/microL
- ○ Platelets <20,000/microL
- **Very severe**
  - ○ Blood counts meeting severe criteria

    and
  - ○ Neutrophil count <200/microL
- **Moderately severe aplastic anemia**
  - ○ Bone marrow cellularity <30%
  - ○ Absence of severe pancytopenia
  - ○ Blood counts of at least two or three blood elements below normal

TREATMENT

1. What is the treatment for aplastic anemia?

- **General principles of treatment:**
  - ○ Acquired cases of bone marrow failure rarely respond to erythropoietin stimulating agents/colony-stimulating factors or androgens
  - ○ Inherited cases rarely respond to immunosuppression
- **Criteria for response**
  - ○ Hematologic response
    - Two of the following on two separate blood tests measured at least 1 week apart
  - ○ Absolute neutrophil count >500/microL; platelet count >20,000/microL; reticulocyte count >60,000/microL
- **Removal of offending drug if one identified**
- Histocompatibility testing of patient/siblings in anticipation of possible allogeneic stem cell transplant
- **Supportive measures**
  - ○ Judicious transfusion of blood products to prevent alloimmunization
    - Cytomegalovirus (CMV)-negative, leukoreduced product
  - ○ Aggressive treatment of potential infection(s)
  - ○ Aggressive treatment of iron overload/secondary hemochromatosis, if present
- **Allogeneic hematopoietic stem cell transplantation (SCT)**
  - ○ Young patients (<40 years of age, acquired or inherited) with human leukocyte antigen (HLA)-matched sibling donor
    - In patients 20 years of age, 80% to 90% survival versus ~50% in those > 40 years of age

- Chronic graft-versus-host disease (GVHD) can complicate up to 40% of those treated with SCT
- Recommended source of stem cells is bone marrow as opposed to peripheral blood
- **Antithymocyte globulin (ATG) and cyclosporine +/− eltrombopag**
  - Older patients (>40 years of age) or those without HLA-matched sibling donor
  - Equine ATG (h-ATG) has demonstrated superior response rates compared to rabbit
  - Hematologic response at 6 months in ~70% of patients (>95% with addition of eltrombopag)
  - Survival roughly >90% at 3 years in all comers treated with combined immunosuppressive therapy (>95% with addition of eltrombopag at 2 years)
  - Immune suppression is associated with increased risk of subsequent hematologic malignancy
  - Equine ATG/cyclosporine +/- eltrombopag typically administered frontline with consideration of reinduction with rabbit-ATG/cyclosporine if no response at 6 months and no HLA-matched sibling *or* not suitable for nonsibling HLA-matched donor
    - Sample regimen
      - h-ATG 40 mg/kg per day, day 1 to 4
      - Cyclosporine 6 mg/kg per day in two divided doses with goal trough level of 200–400 ng/mL
      - Eltrombopag 150 mg daily for 6 months (adult dose)
    - Toxicities
      - h-ATG
        - Serum sickness: Type III hypersensitivity reaction characterized by rash, arthralgias, and fevers. Occurs ~7 days after exposure
      - Cyclosporine
        - Nephrotoxicity, hepatotoxicity, hypertension, PRES, osteopenia
      - Eltrombopag
        - Hepatotoxicity
  - 1/3 will be cured, ~ 1/3 will remain dependent on cyclosporine, ~1/3 will relapse or develop clonal hematologic disorder
  - Retreatment after relapse may salvage ~50% of patients
- **Alternatives/adjuncts**
  - Eltrombopag monotherapy (50–150 mg PO daily)
  - Androgens (danazol PO 400 mg twice daily)
  - Erythropoietin stimulating agents/granulocyte colony-stimulating factors
  - Other immunosuppressive therapies:
    - High-dose cyclophosphamide (50 mg/kg of ideal body weight intravenous [IV] for 4 days)
    - Alemtuzumab (10 mg per day IV for 10 days)

○ Other bone marrow transplant (BMT) strategies: haploidentical transplant, mismatched unrelated transplant

○ Rituximab for Epstein-Barr virus (EBV)-related lymphoproliferative disorders

QUESTIONS

1. Patient is a 9-month-old boy, who is seen by his pediatrician for failure to thrive and diarrhea. The patient's parents have changed formula from milk-based formula to a soy-based formula without improvement. He is currently on an elemental formula without improvement in greasy foul-smelling stools and with little appreciable weight gain. The child is in less than the fifth percentile for height and weight. Physical examination is remarkable for short stature and abdominal distension without peritoneal signs.

Laboratory testing is as follows:

Laboratory test	Patient's result	Reference range
Hematocrit	30.9%	33.0%–39.0%
Hemoglobin	10 g/dL	11.0–13.0 g/dL
Mean corpuscular volume	100.5 fL	76–90 fL
White blood cell count	4.17×10^9/L	4×10^9–10×10^9/L
Differential		
Segmented neutrophils	9%	20%–45%
Lymphocytes	80.3%	40%–65%
Monocytes	10.2%	1%–3%
Platelet count	402×10^9/L	150×10^9–450×10^9/L

Fecal elastase is undetectable.

Which of the following diagnostic tests should be ordered next?
A. Chromosome breakage analysis
B. High-resolution karyotyping
C. *SBDS* gene sequencing
D. Bone marrow biopsy/aspirate
E. Telomere length analysis

2. Patient is a 17-year-old man who presents to the emergency room (ER) with 1 week of fevers at home >39° C. Examination demonstrates short stature, conjunctival pallor, and polydactyly of the thumb on the right hand. No other abnormalities on physical examination were noted.

Laboratory test	Patient's result	Reference range
Hemoglobin	6.4 g/dL	14.6–17.8 g/dL
Mean corpuscular volume	100 fL	78–94 fL
White blood cell count	1.9×10^9/L	3.2×10^9–10.6×10^9/L

(continued)

Laboratory test	Patient's result	Reference range
Absolute neutrophil count	0.3×10^9/L	1.4×10^9–7.5×10^9/L
Absolute reticulocyte count	10×10^9/L	20×10^9–80×10^9/L
Platelet count	8×10^9/L	177×10^9–406×10^9/L

Patient is started on broad-spectrum antibiotics and transfused appropriately with packed red blood cells and platelets. Bone marrow evaluation was hypocellular at <10%. Bone marrow cytogenetics revealed 46, XY.

What is the most appropriate likely next step in the management of this patient?
A. Horse antithymocyte globulin (ATG) plus cyclosporine
B. Rabbit ATG plus cyclosporine
C. Alemtuzumab
D. Human leukocyte antigen (HLA) typing of older sibling for possible matched related hematopoietic stem cell transplantation
E. Matched unrelated hematopoietic stem cell transplantation
F. Single agent eltrombopag

What would be the best test to confirm the diagnosis of the underlying condition?
A. Chromosome breakage analysis
B. High-resolution karyotyping
C. *SBDS* gene sequencing
D. Erythrocyte adenosine deaminase level
E. Telomere length analysis

3. Patient is a 45-year-old female with a history of obesity and hypothyroidism who presented to her endocrinologist's office with fatigue and dyspnea on exertion. She was started on topiramate roughly 2 weeks prior for weight loss. Vital signs are significant for a BP 104/70 mmHg I Pulse 104 I Temp (Src) 36.8°C (98.2°F) (Temporal) I Resp 16 I SpO$_2$ 97% on room air. Physical exam is remarkable for pallor and tachycardia. She takes no other medications other than omeprazole for gastroesophageal reflux disease (GERD).

Laboratory studies are as follow:

Laboratory test	Patient's result	Reference range
Hemoglobin	3.8 g/dL	12.6–15.9 g/dL
Mean corpuscular volume	76.8 fL	81.9–101 fL
White blood cell count	3.25×10^9/L	4.3×10^9–11.3×10^9/L
Absolute neutrophil count	0.4×10^9/L	2.0×10^9–7.4×10^9/L
Platelet count	63×10^9/L	159×10^9–439×10^9/L
Absolute reticulocyte count	30×10^9/L	20×10^9–80×10^9/L

Bone marrow biopsy demonstrates hypocellular marrow with trilineage hematopoiesis. Chromosome analysis is 46, XX. Topiramate is subsequently discontinued.

What is the most appropriate likely next step in the management of this patient?

A. Horse antithymocyte globulin (ATG), cyclosporine
B. Rabbit ATG, cyclosporine plus eltrombopag
C. Alemtuzumab
D. Human leukocyte antigen (HLA) typing of older sibling for possible matched related hematopoietic stem cell transplantation
E. Single agent eltrombopag

4. A 22-year-old man presented to urgent care with a 5-day history of sore throat and malaise. He reports no medical history other than "nail fungus," which is a cosmetic concern but he has never been evaluated. He has no allergies and takes no medications. On physical examination, whitish plaques were noted on his tongue, which could not be scraped off with a tongue blade. The nails on the hands demonstrate atrophy and splitting. His skin seems spotted with pigmentation on the anterior chest and neck. Patient reported family history of leukemia and "lung problems." His rapid strep test was negative; however, his complete blood count demonstrated anemia and thrombocytopenia.

Which of the following diagnostic tests should be ordered next/would confirm diagnosis?

A. Chromosome breakage analysis
B. High-resolution karyotyping
C. *SBDS* gene sequencing
D. Telomere length analysis
E. Soluble IL-2 receptor level

5. Patient is an 89-year-old female with multiple medical comorbidities and a long-standing history of severe aplastic anemia, who relapsed after ATG and cyclosporine in the past. She remains transfusion dependent, requiring packed red blood cell (PRBC) transfusion every 1 to 2 months for symptomatic anemia. Her last transfusion was 2 weeks ago. She presents for further management.

Physical exam reveals a frail, chronically ill–appearing female in no acute distress with conjunctival pallor. No hepatosplenomegaly was appreciated.

Laboratory studies are as follows:

Laboratory test	Patient's result	Reference range
Hemoglobin	10.8 g/dL	12.6–15.9 g/dL
Mean corpuscular volume	101.8 fL	81.9–101 fL
White blood cell count	5.25×10^9/L	$4.3 \times 10^9 - 11.3 \times 10^9$/L
Absolute neutrophil count	1.25×10^9/L	$2.0 \times 10^9 - 7.4 \times 10^9$/L
Platelet count	23×10^9/L	$159 \times 10^9 - 439 \times 10^9$/L

Serum creatinine is 2.25 mg/dL. Ferritin is 1,300 ng/mL. Liver iron quantification is calculated at 10 mg/g.

What is the most appropriate likely next step in the management of this patient?

A. Rabbit antithymocyte globulin, cyclosporine
B. Alemtuzumab
C. Evaluation for matched related hematopoietic stem cell transplantation
D. High-dose cyclophosphamide
E. Single agent eltrombopag

6. Patient is a 68-year-old Caucasian male who was referred to hematology for pancytopenia with a white blood cell count of 2,200, hemoglobin of 11.3 g/dL, and platelets of 105,000. Reticulocyte percentage was 5.4%; absolute neutrophil count (ANC) 900; lymphs 800. Coombs test was negative. Nutritional studies were performed: B12 level and folate were within reference range, ferritin was 295 ng/mL, and transferrin saturation was 55%. His indirect bilirubin was 1.2 mg/dL (upper limit of normal [ULN] 1.1 mg/dL). Lactate dehydrogenase (LDH) was >932 IU/L and haptoglobin was low at 2.0 mg/dL (lower limit of normal [LLN] 30 mg/dL). He was started on folic acid and paroxysmal nocturnal hemoglobinuria (PNH) flow cytometry was sent, which demonstrated 17.63% glycophosphatidylinositol (GPI)-deficient granulocytes, 66.79% deficient monocytes, 1.56% type II red blood cells (RBCs), 17.25% type III RBCs. He was started on eculizumab. He has two siblings: a sister and a brother.

He is referred for a second opinion. Labs after four doses of eculizumab are provided below:

Laboratory test	Patient's result	Reference range
Hemoglobin	8.5 g/dL	14.8–17.8 g/dL
Mean corpuscular volume	110.1 fL	81.9–101 fL
White blood cell count	2.32×10^9/L	4.3×10^9–11.3×10^9/L
Absolute neutrophil count	1.08×10^9/L	2.0×10^9–7.4×10^9/L
Platelet count	82×10^9/L	159×10^9–439×10^9/L
Absolute reticulocyte count	98.5×10^9/L	47×10^9–152×10^9/L
Lactate dehydrogenase	367 U/L	100 U/L – 253 U/L

Peripheral blood smear: Red blood cells with 1+ anisocytosis, 2+ poikilocytosis with a few tear drops and paucity of polychromatophilic cells. Neutropenia is present with a few of the neutrophils with segmentation abnormalities (hyposegmented). No large granular lymphocytes were appreciated. No left shift, basophilia, eosinophilia, or blasts seen. Platelet count is decreased and morphologically normal.

What is the next best step in therapy/evaluation?
A. Discontinue eculizumab and recheck PNH panel
B. Add horse antithymocyte globulin and cyclosporine to eculizumab
C. Bone marrow biopsy and aspirate
D. HLA typing of siblings for possible matched related hematopoietic stem cell transplantation
E. Telomere length analysis

7. Patient is a 38-year-old male who presents to the emergency department with a rash on bilateral lower extremities. The emergency room physician identified the rash as petechiae and a complete blood count was obtained and is noted as follows:

Laboratory test	Patient's result	Reference range
Hemoglobin	11.6 g/dL	14.8–17.8 g/dL
Mean corpuscular volume	88.2 fL	81.9–101 fL
White blood cell count	3.22×10^9/L	4.3×10^9–11.3×10^9/L
Absolute neutrophil count	0.44×10^9/L	2.0×10^9–7.4×10^9/L
Platelet count	$<6 \times 10^9$/L	159×10^9–439×10^9/L
Absolute reticulocyte count	27.4×10^9/L	47×10^9–152×10^9/L
Lactate dehydrogenase	173 U/L	100 U/L – 253 U/L

Paroxysmal nocturnal hemoglobinuria (PNH) flow cytometry was sent, which demonstrated 2.7% glycophosphatidylinositol (GPI)-deficient monocytes, 2.6% deficient neutrophils, and 0.041% deficient red blood cells (RBCs).

A bone marrow biopsy was performed, which demonstrated variably cellular marrow (overall hypocellular) with decreased trilineage hematopoiesis. No dysplasia was identified. Karyotype was normal male, XY. The patient has one sibling who is not a human leukocyte antigen (HLA) match.

What is the most appropriate likely next step in the management of this patient?
A. Matched unrelated hematopoietic stem cell transplantation
B. Rabbit antithymocyte globulin (ATG), cyclosporine, and eltrombopag
C. Haploidentical hematopoietic stem cell transplantation
D. Horse ATG plus cyclosporine
E. High-dose cyclophosphamide (50 mg/kg of ideal body weight intravenous [IV] for 4 days)

Which of the following clinical/laboratory features would be predictive of a better response to immune suppressive therapy in this patient?
A. Age of the patient
B. Pretreatment neutrophil count
C. Pretreatment reticulocyte count
D. Presence of a PNH clone

ANSWERS

1. **C. *SBDS* gene sequencing.** Patient has pancreatic insufficiency and severe aplastic anemia, which goes along with Shwachman-Diamond syndrome. Shwachman-Diamond syndrome is the second leading cause of exocrine pancreatic insufficiency. Patients typically present early in life with failure to thrive and signs and symptoms of exocrine pancreatic insufficiency. The test of choice is sequencing the *SBDS* gene, which is abnormal in roughly 90% of cases. Karyotyping would not identify this genetic anomaly. Bone marrow aspirate and biopsy would likely demonstrate a hypoplastic bone marrow but this would be a nonspecific finding. Telomere length analysis would be helpful if there was concern for dyskeratosis congenita; however, this patient does not have stigmata that would raise suspicion for the disease (oral leukoplakia, skin hyperpigmentation, and dystrophic nails).

2. **D. Human leukocyte antigen (HLA) typing of older sibling for possible matched related hematopoietic stem cell transplantation; A. Chromosome breakage analysis.** Current standard of care for younger patients (<40 years) is to proceed directly to allogeneic stem cell transplantation with a matched related donor (*Blood* 2006 Oct 15; 108(8):2509–2519). Horse ATG cyclosporine would be reasonable should the patient have comorbidities or geographic and donor constraints that would make transplantation not feasible. Horse and rabbit ATG were compared head-to-head with superior response rates and overall survival in the horse ATG arm (*N Engl J Med* 2011; 365:430–438). While alemtuzumab has activity in aplastic anemia, it is more in the relapsed refractory setting and is not recommended for up-front treatment outside of a clinical trial (*Blood* 2012; 119:345–354). Single agent eltrombopag is not curative therapy and should not be used in otherwise healthy individuals fit for transplant or intensive immune suppression. Patient has stigmata of Fanconi anemia with abnormalities at the thumb, short stature, and severe aplastic anemia. The test of choice for diagnosis would be chromosome breakage analysis. *SBDS* gene sequencing would be useful in Shwachman-Diamond syndrome, which is characterized by pancreatic insufficiency, short stature, and skeletal dysostosis. Erythrocyte adenosine deaminase levels can be elevated in Diamond-Blackfan anemia but not Fanconi anemia. Telomere length analysis would be helpful in dyskeratosis congenita, which is characterized by oral leukoplakia, hyperpigmented skin, nail dystrophy, and aplastic anemia.

3. **A. Horse antithymocyte globulin (ATG), cyclosporine.** This case underscores the importance of recognizing the possibility for drug-induced aplastic anemia (in this case, topiramate). Current standard of care for older patients (>40 years) with severe aplastic anemia is horse ATG and cyclosporine plus or minus the addition of eltrombopag. Horse and rabbit ATG were compared head-to-head with superior response rates and overall survival in the horse ATG arm (*N Engl J Med* 2011; 365:430–438). While the addition of eltrombopag has demonstrated improved response

rates against historical cohorts, this has not been demonstrated with rabbit ATG and is thus the wrong answer (*N Engl J Med* 2017; 376:1540–1550). While alemtuzumab has activity in aplastic anemia, it is more in the relapsed refractory setting and is not recommended for up-front treatment outside of a clinical trial (*Blood* 2012; 119:345–354). While allogeneic stem cell transplant is not the wrong answer, it is generally reserved for up-front treatment in younger patients (*Blood* 2012 Aug 9; 120(6): 1185–1196), and ATG/cyclosporine is the more correct answer. Single agent eltrombopag is not definitive therapy and therefore cannot be a recommended first-line therapy in this otherwise healthy individual.

4. **D. Telomere length analysis.** Patient has stigmata of dyskeratosis congenita with oral leukoplakia, dystrophic nails, hyperpigmented skin, and cytopenias. The family history of leukemia and pulmonary disease underscore the spectrum of disease manifestations of telomeropathies, with dyskeratosis congenita being one of the more severe manifestations. Telomere length analysis, usually of peripheral blood leukocytes, will confirm the diagnosis. High-resolution karyotyping will not give information on telomere length. *SBDS* gene sequencing would be appropriate if there was suspicion for Shwachman-Diamond syndrome. Patient does not have stigmata of Schwachman-Diamond syndrome—short stature and pancreatic insufficiency. Soluble IL-2 receptor is usually elevated in hemophagocytic lymphohistiocytosis (HLH). It would be unlikely for a stable outpatient to present with HLH.

5. **E. Single agent eltrombopag.** Patient is an elderly infirm female with symptomatic anemia related to aplastic anemia and secondary hemochromatosis with significant liver iron deposition by liver MRI. Given her general state of health, of all the options mentioned, single agent eltrombopag would likely be the best option. Hematologic response rates were 44% with single agent eltrombopag, with 3 of 25 patients becoming transfusion independent (*N Engl J Med* 2012; 367:11–19). While response rates with rabbit ATG and cyclosporine after horse ATG and cyclosporine are around 65%, given the patient's age and comorbidities (in particular, renal insufficiency), she would be unlikely to tolerate a reinduction with intensive immunosuppression (*Br J Haematol* 2006 Jun;133(6):622–627). The same argument can be made for high-dose cyclophosphamide, stem cell transplant, and single agent alemtuzumab.

6. **C. Bone marrow biopsy and aspirate.** PNH can be thought of as a spectrum disorder with classical PNH on one end of the spectrum, with high PNH clone burdens and brisk intravascular hemolysis, and bone marrow failure on the other end, with relatively smaller PNH clones and limited to absent intravascular hemolysis. This case clearly demonstrates a case of an overlap between classical PNH and bone marrow failure (*Blood* 2006; 108(8):2509–2519). In particular, while the patient has evidence of classical PNH with evidence of intravascular hemolysis (elevated LDH, indirect bilirubin, reticulocyte count, and decreased haptoglobin), he also has evidence of concomitant bone marrow failure with significant cytopenias

not confined to the red cell lineage. His inappropriately normal reticulocyte response and dysplasia on peripheral blood smear are most concerning for myelodysplastic syndrome (MDS) underlying his bone marrow
failure. While these aforementioned features are suggestive, they are not
diagnostic of MDS and a bone marrow biopsy and aspirate should be
performed next. While a PNH clone is present in ~15% of patients with
MDS, these clones are usually small and are not associated with features
of classical PNH (*Ann Hematol* 2008; 87: 257). The identification of a PNH
clone in the setting of a diagnosis MDS, in particular those with a trisomy
8 cytogenetic abnormality, may suggest a more immunologic phenomenon underlying the marrow failure and thus predict a response to immunosuppression (*Blood* 2006; 107, 1308–1314) (*Blood* 2005; 106:841–851).
A diagnosis, however, via a bone marrow biopsy and aspirate would
be required before proceeding with immune suppression. In regard to
stopping eculizumab and rechecking PNH studies, this therapy is clearly
improving his markers of intravascular hemolysis (decreased LDH) and
thus should continue. Telomere length would be helpful in a younger
patient with aplastic anemia for which there was a concern for a telom-
eropathy.

7. **D. Horse ATG plus cyclosporine; B. Pretreatment neutrophil count
and D. Presence of a PNH clone.** Current standard of care for younger
patients (<40 years of age) is to proceed directly to allogeneic stem
cell transplantation with a matched related donor. A matched sibling
donor is only available, however, in 20% to 30% of cases (*Blood* 2006;
108(8):2509–2519.). If the patient does not have a matched related
donor, as in this scenario, the next best answer would be horse ATG plus
cyclosporine. Horse and rabbit ATG were compared head-to-head with
superior response rates and overall survival in the horse ATG arm (*N Engl
J Med* 2011; 365:430–438). While in a prospective, nonrandomized
trial, the addition of eltrombopag to ATG and cyclosporine improved
response rates in patients with aplastic anemia, this therapy was added
to horse ATG and not rabbit and therefore is the incorrect answer for
first-line treatment (*N Engl J Med* 2017; 376:1540–1550). While high-dose
cyclophosphamide had a response rate of 77% in both refractory and
treatment-naïve patients with severe aplastic anemia, the trial was discontinued early due to three deaths in the cyclophosphamide group and is
not considered a first-line therapy option (*Lancet* 2000; 356(9241):1554–
1559). Matched unrelated donor transplant has roughly twice the mortality rates as a matched sibling donor with 5-year survival estimated
to be around 39% and is also not preferred front-line therapy (*Blood*
2006; 108(8):2509–2519). Although haploidentical transplantation may
hold promise in the future as a front-line therapy for young patients with
severe aplastic anemia without a matched sibling, it is associated with an
increased incidence of chronic graft-versus-host-disease when compared
with matched sibling donors and would not be considered a first-line
therapy (*Blood* 2015; 126:3227). In an analysis performed in 97 patients
with severe aplastic anemia treated with immune suppressive therapy,

the presence of an absolute neutrophil count (ANC) > 2,000 and a PNH clone at diagnosis predicted a better response to immune suppression (*Ann Hematol* 2015; 94(7):1105–1110). While age is important in regard to transplantation-related complications, it has not been associated with responses to immune suppressive therapy. In the aforementioned trial, pretreatment reticulocyte count was not associated with improved responses with immunosuppressive therapy.

Platelet and Megakaryocyte Disorders

7

Maryann Shango and Asra Ahmed

MEGAKARYOCYTE AND PLATELET OVERVIEW

1. **What are the features of megakaryocytes?**
   - Megakaryocytes are large polypoid cells derived from megakaryocyte colony–forming cells (Meg-CFCs) and are responsible for the formation of platelets.
   - The average diameter of a megakaryocyte is 20 to 25 microns (2–3 × the size of a mature erythrocyte).
   - Megakaryocytes make up approximately 0.05% to 1% of all nucleated cells in the bone marrow.
   - Surface markers and granules associated with megakaryocytes are identical to those present on mature platelets.

2. **Describe the process of megakaryocyte maturation.**
   - Megakaryocytes initially undergo endomitosis, in which there is DNA replication without division of the nucleus, followed by progressive expansion and maturation of the cytoplasm. Once mature, anucleate cytoplasmic fragments bud off the megakaryocyte pseudopods, resulting in the formation of platelets. The entire process occurs over 5 to 7 days within the bone marrow.
   - A single megakaryocyte is responsible for the formation of 1,000 to 3,000 individual platelets.

3. **How is megakaryocytopoiesis regulated under physiological circumstances?**
   - Thrombopoietin (TPO) is a glycoprotein hormone consisting of 332 amino acids and is responsible for megakaryocytic differentiation, maturation, and proliferation. The N-terminal end has 144 amino acid homology with erythropoietin. The TPO gene is located on the long arm of chromosome 3 (q 26.3-27).
   - TPO is primarily produced in the liver sinusoidal cells, and to a lesser extent in bone marrow stroma and the proximal convoluted cells of the kidney. TPO production is regulated by circulating platelet mass.
   - The receptor for TPO is c-mpl.
   - TPO secreted by the liver is quickly taken up by circulating platelets (via c-mpl receptors) with residual levels providing basal stimulation for megakaryocytes. TPO binds receptors on megakaryocytes, resulting in the stimulation of megakaryocytic growth and endomitosis (ploidy).
   - The TPO levels in the blood are inversely related to megakaryocyte mass. A decline in circulating platelets will signal liver sinusoidal cells to produce and secrete more TPO, resulting in enhanced platelet production, and thus maintenance of platelet mass.

- IL-3 and IL-11 promote megakaryocyte colony–forming cell (Meg-CFC) growth, but have little impact on megakaryocyte endomitosis.

4. **What are the features of platelets?**
   - Platelets are anucleate cells made up of cytoplasmic fragments
   - The diameter of a platelet is 2 to 3 microns
   - When activated, platelets transform from a flattened disc to a sphere with multiple projecting pseudopods
   - Transmembrane receptors play a crucial role in platelet function
     - GPIb/IX/V, GPIa/IIa, integrin $\alpha_{IIb}\beta_3$ $\alpha_{IIb}\beta_3$ (formally known as GPIIb/IIIa)
   - The storage granules within platelets contain vital mediators of hemostasis
     - **Alpha granules** contain von Willebrand factor (vWF), platelet factor 4 (PF4), thrombospondin, fibrinogen, beta-thromboglobulin, platelet-derived growth factor (PDGF)
     - **Dense granules** contain adenosine diphosphate (ADP) and serotonin

5. **What are the key function of platelets?**
   - Platelets are an integral component of the hemostatic system and are responsible for primary hemostasis at the time of endothelial injury. Platelets are also involved in modulating systemic inflammatory responses.
   - Under physiological circumstances, platelets circulate in inactive form. Once exposed to subendothelial tissue, as a result of injury, platelets undergo a series of conformational and biochemical changes, which culminate with the formation of a platelet plug (i.e., primary hemostasis). For more details, please refer to Chapter 8.

6. **What is the life cycle of a platelet?**
   - The life span of a platelet is approximately 9 days. Platelet counts remain stable throughout life unless disturbed by physiologic or pathologic processes.
   - Once released into systemic circulation, the platelets will enter the spleen. Approximately, two thirds of the platelets will enter the general circulation and one third will remain in the spleen.
     - Platelets sequestered in the spleen contribute to the total platelet mass and can be demarginated via splenic contraction, when the need for additional platelets arise.
   - Old platelets are phagocytosed by the splenic macrophages, liver Kupffer cells, and other components of the reticuloendothelial system.
   - Cytokines IL-6 and IL-11 stimulate platelet production independently of thrombopoietin (TPO). This typically occurs in inflammatory conditions.

LABORATORY EVALUATION OF PLATELETS

How are platelets evaluated?

1. **Complete blood count (CBC):** Platelets are quantified via an automated analyzer
   - **Normal platelet count: 150,000 to 450,000/microL**
     - **Thrombocytopenia:** platelet <150,000/microL

- Mild: 100 to 150,000/microL
- Moderate: 50 to 99,000/microL
- Severe: <50,000/mircoL
  - ○ **Thrombocytosis:** platelet >450,000/microL

2. **Peripheral blood smear:** provides morphological information about systemic processes, as well as clues about disorders limited to platelets
   - Large platelets: could reflect accelerated platelet turnover
   - Small platelets: are generally found in some congenital platelet disorders
   - Gray platelets: hypogranulated platelets due to storage granule defects
   - Schistocytes: presence indicates an underlying thrombotic mircoangiopathy

3. **Platelet aggregation assays:** laboratory evaluation used to measure specific platelet function defects. Differentiates between disorders of platelet adhesion, activation, or aggregation, based on platelet response to agonists such as adenosine diphosphate (ADP), arachidonic acid, thrombin, ristocetin, epinephrine, and collagen (see Chapter 8)

4. **Bleeding time (BT):** provides an assessment of general platelet function. It is being used less commonly due to inconsistencies in testing

5. **Rotational thromboelastometry (ROTEM):** provides information on the clotting time, clot formation, clot stability, and clot lysis for a comprehensive picture of whole blood hemostasis (see Chapter 8)

6. **Bone marrow biopsy:** provides information about bone marrow disorders affecting megakaryocyte production

PLATELET DISORDERS
Quantitative Platelet Disorders

Thrombocytopenia
1. **What are the symptoms of thrombocytopenia?**
   - The risk and severity of bleeding depends on the degree of thrombocytopenia and the presence of a concomitant qualitative platelet disorder and/or coagulopathy.
   - The clinical presentations are variable. Patients present with a range of symptoms from mild bruising and petechiae, to mucosal bleeding, including epistaxis, menorrhagia, and gastrointestinal (GI) hemorrhage.

2. **What are mechanisms of thrombocytopenia and corresponding disease manifestations?**
   A. **Pseudothrombocytopenia (or factitious thrombocytopenia):**
   - Idiosyncratic ex vivo agglutination of platelets due to presence of nonpathologic agglutinating immunoglobulins in the presence of EDTA.
   - Platelet clumps can be identified on the peripheral blood smear.
   - Incidence is estimated to be 0.1% to 0.2% of the hospitalized population.
   - Patients are asymptomatic and do not have an increased risk of bleeding.
   - Accurate platelet counts can be obtained by collecting blood in collection tubes using sodium citrate as the reagent instead of EDTA.

B. Thrombocytopenia due to synthetic defects

1. **Nutritional deficiencies**
   - Nutritional deficiencies will affect the bone marrow proliferative capacity of all the cell lines (myeloid, erythroid, and megakaryocytic).
   - Deficiencies of vitamin B12 and folic acid result in the formation of megakaryocytes with diminished ploidy and subsequent reduced platelet production.
   - Copper deficiency has also been associated with thrombocytopenia.

2. **Viral infection**
   - Viral particles directly suppress megakaryocytic development. The most common viruses implicated are HIV, *Epstein-Barr virus* (EBV), *hepatitis C virus* (HCV), cytomegalovirus (CMV), and Haanta virus. Of note, viruses can also cause immune-mediated thrombocytopenia (see section on immune-mediated consumptive thrombocytopenia).

3. **Marrow disease**
   - Infiltration of the bone marrow will result in multilineage hematopoietic defects.
   - Common causes include malignancy, infectious diseases, sarcoidosis, and storage diseases (e.g., Gaucher's disease).
   - Stem cell disorders such as MDS and aplastic anemia will also present with pancytopenia due to dyshematopoiesis and/or marrow aplasia.

4. **Drug- and toxin-induced thrombocytopenia**
   - Drug-induced thrombocytopenia results from direct bone marrow and or megakaryocyte toxicity. Chemotherapeutic agents, alcohol, gold, and thiazides are common causes.

5. **Liver disease**
   - In patients with chronic liver disease and/or cirrhosis, the liver's ability to produce tTPO is compromised, thus affecting platelet production. Patients with liver disease often have portal hypertension resulting in splenomegaly, which can also contribute to thrombocytopenia.

C. Thrombocytopenia due to accelerated consumption

Immune-mediated consumptive thrombocytopenia

- Heterogeneous group of diseases are characterized by immune-mediated destruction of platelets.
- The CBC will reveal evidence of isolated thrombocytopenia. The platelets tend to be large and well granulated, reflective of their young age due to compensatory accelerated platelet production.
- On bone marrow examination, there are an increased number of morphologically normal megakaryocytes and otherwise normal erythropoiesis and myelopoiesis.

1. **Immune thrombocytopenia (ITP)**

   What is ITP?

   - Thrombocytopenia caused by autoantibodies directed against the platelet membrane receptors, most commonly the GpIb/IX and GPIIb/IIIa receptors, resulting in accelerated platelet–antibody clearance mainly via the splenic macrophages but can also occur in other parts of the reticuloendothelial system.

   What are the clinical features of ITP?

   - ITP is seen in all age groups.
   - The of rate of spontaneous remission in adults is low (<20%) but is greater than 80% in children.

   What is the etiology of ITP?

   - An inciting event is not identified in the majority of cases.
   - Infections
     - Viral infections (HCV, CMV, EBV, and HIV) have been implicated. It is postulated that viral antigens stimulate production of antibodies that cross-react with platelet surface receptors.
     - *Helicobacter pylori* can provoke a molecular mimicry response with resultant autoimmune thrombocytopenia. This is particularly true of the strains found in East Asia.
   - Autoimmune diseases (systemic lupus erythematosus, rheumatoid arthritis and antiphospholipid antibody syndrome, common variable immune deficiency, Hashimoto's thyroiditis) are associated with ITP.
   - Chronic lymphocytic leukemia (CLL)
     - One percent of patients will develop ITP. ITP seen in CLL needs to be differentiated from bone marrow infiltration and splenomegaly.
   - Evan's syndrome
     - A disorder characterized by concomitant Coombs positive autoimmune hemolytic anemia and autoimmune thrombocytopenia and is often associated with other autoimmune diseases

   What are the symptoms of ITP?

   - Symptoms of ITP are variable and depend on degree of thrombocytopenia. Most patients are asymptomatic and have a low risk of spontaneous bleeding even with severe thrombocytopenia due to the presence of well-granulated functionally intact platelets.
   - The risk of spontaneous bleeding increases significantly when the platelets are <10,000 to 20,000/microL.

   How is ITP diagnosed?

   - There is no specific testing for ITP; a diagnosis is obtained by ruling out other identifiable causes of thrombocytopenia.
   - In patients >50 years (or >60 years), a bone marrow biopsy might be helpful to rule out underlying marrow disease.

What is the approach to the treatment of ITP?

- Most patients will not require treatment if asymptomatic and platelets are >30,000/microL.
- In children, observation is favored due to the high rate of spontaneous remission within 3 months of diagnosis.
- Treatment is recommended for the following situations:
  - Platelets <10,000/microL
  - Platelets between 10,000 and 30,000/microL with risk factors for bleeding
- The cornerstone of therapy is **immunosuppression**.
  - **Corticosteroids** are the standard first-line treatment. Corticosteroids suppress overall immune function and specifically impair the clearance of opsonized platelets by the reticuloendothelial system. Corticosteroids will also suppress both B and T lymphocytes, which are mediators of autoimmune processes.
  - The overall response rate of corticosteroids is 60% to 70%, with most patients responding within 5 days of treatment. The duration of therapy is dependent on patient response and side effects; however, the goal is to minimize the duration of therapy. Thirty percent of patients will relapse within 2 years.
  - **Intravenous immunoglobulin (IVIG):** It is thought that IVIG blocks the Fc receptors on reticuloendothelial cells and thereby prevent platelet binding and subsequent phagocytosis.
    - IVIG is administered when there is an immediate need to raise the platelet count as it raises platelet count within 1 to 2 days.
    - The overall response rate is 70% to 90% with peak platelet levels achieved within 1 week of treatment. The response is often temporary.
  - **Anti-Rh(D)** is an alternative to IVIG for patients with Rh(D)-positive RBCs and works by saturating Fc receptor similarly to IVIG, thereby raising platelet count. Mild-to-moderate hemolysis is expected, so it should be avoided in patients prone to hemolysis.
  - Splenectomy is considered a second-line therapy in patients who fail primary therapies. Removal of the spleen eliminates a major site of platelet destruction as well as the primary site of autoantibody production.
    - The 10-year remission rate is 60% to 65%.
    - Patients who undergo splenectomy have a lifelong risk of infection. They are particularly prone to overwhelming sepsis with encapsulated organisms and require immunization against *Streptococcus pneumoniae*, *Haemophilus influenzae*, and *Neisseria meningitides* prior to splenectomy.
  - **Rituximab** is a monoclonal antibody used in the treatment of B-cell lymphomas directed against the CD20 antigen on B lymphocytes. The exact mechanism of action in ITP is not clearly understood but it is

postulated that depletion of the CD20-positive lymphocytes mitigates platelet autoantibody production.

- Rituximab may be used in ITP as second-line therapy in patients who fail corticosteroids, especially if the patient is not a candidate for splenectomy.
- The overall response rate is 40% to 60%.

○ **Other immunosuppressant agents:** generally used in relapsed/refractory ITP patients who failed first- and second-line options and have symptomatic disease

- **Cyclophosphamide**
- **Vincristine**
- **Cyclosporine**
- **Danazol**

○ **Thrombomimetic agents:** Romiplostim and eltrombopag are thrombopoietin analogues that stimulate different portions of the thrombopoietin receptors present on megakaryocytes. They stimulate and promote megakaryopoiesis and thus platelet production. The thrombomimetic agents do not impact platelet clearance. Initial experience suggests sustained long-term remission. Patients who have undergone splenectomy appear to have superior responses. Risks of thrombomimetic agents include thrombocytosis, thrombosis, and increased bone marrow reticulin fibrosis. Increased liver enzymes have been seen with eltrombopag.

○ **Platelet transfusions** are recommended only if there is clinically significant bleeding.

2. **Drug-induced thrombocytopenia**

- In addition to direct bone marrow suppression, drug-dependent antibodies can develop that cross-react with platelets.
- Thrombocytopenia generally develops within 2 weeks of drug exposure and will usually resolve within 1 to 2 weeks of drug cessation.
- Common causes include beta-lactam antibiotics, vancomycin, quinine, and antiepileptic drugs.

What is heparin-induced thrombocytopenia (HIT)?

- **Type 1:** *nonimmune-mediated* drop in platelets in response to direct effect of heparin on platelet activation. Mild thrombocytopenia usually occurs within first 2 days of heparin exposure

  ○ No clinical effects and not associated with thrombosis

- Type 2: immun*e mediated*—HIT is a clinicopathological syndrome associated with exposure to heparin or heparin derivatives.

  ○ Less than 5% of patients exposed to heparin or heparin derivatives will develop immunoglobulin G (IgG) antibodies specifically to the heparin/platelet factor 4 (PF4) epitope complex paradoxically leading platelet activation and thrombosis. If there is associated thrombosis, the condition is referred to as heparin-induced thrombocytopenia thrombosis syndrome (HITTS)

○ Disease characteristics
   ■ At least 50% drop in platelet count within 7% to 10 days of first heparin exposure and within 1 to 3 days of subsequent heparin exposure
   ■ Patients are at risk of developing life- and/or limb-threatening venous and arterial thrombosis

How is HIT/HITTS diagnosed?
● Clinical suspicion is based on the 4Ts score, which assigns points based on the following:
   1. Degree of Thrombocytopenia → 50% drop from baseline, but usually not less than 20,000/ microL
   2. Timing of platelet drop → within 7 to 10 days of heparin exposure
   3. Thrombotic events → venous more common than arterial
   4. Alternative cause of Thrombocytopenia
● If the 4Ts score is intermediate or high risk, initiate empiric therapy for HIT and pursue HIT antibody testing
   ○ Screen with immunoassay for anti-heparin/platelet factor 4 (PF4) complex, which is an enzyme-linked immunosorbent assay (ELISA) test that detects circulating antibodies. If positive, confirm with a functional assay, such as the serotonin release assay (SRA).
   ○ SRA measures release of radiolabeled serotonin from donor platelets after exposure to heparin and patient's serum if heparin-induced antibody is present.

How is HIT/HITTS treated?
● Discontinue all heparin products and start an alternative anticoagulation such as parenteral direct thrombin inhibitor (DTI), either argatroban or bivalirudin. The DTI should be continued until the platelet count is greater than 150,000/microL. If a thrombosis is identified, then patient should undergo anticoagulation with warfarin for at least 3 months or longer depending on the severity of the thrombosis. If no thrombosis is identified, anticoagulation with warfarin should be administered for 1 month. Warfarin should only be initiated after resolution of acute HIT as indicated by normalization of the platelet count due to risk of thrombosis from depletion of protein C.
● Immunoassays can remain positive for several months after discontinuation of heparin. Care should be taken to avoid all future exposure to heparin products.

3. **Post-transfusion purpura (PTP)**
   ● Severe thrombocytopenia develops 1 to 2 weeks after transfusion of a blood product
   ● Develops as a result of platelet alloantibodies (usually to HPA-1a antigen) that cross-react with autologous platelets
   ● Patients become sensitized to HPA-1a antigen from a previous pregnancy or from a previous transfusion
   ● Diagnosis is made by detection of the presence of the HPA-1a antigen

- Treatment: Most patients respond to treatment with intravenous immunoglobulin (IVIG), and less commonly plasma exchange is required. Platelet recovery occurs within 4 to 5 days of receiving IVIG
- Future blood products should be screened for HPA-1a–positive antigen

4. **Antiphospholipid antibody syndrome** (please also refer to Chapter 9)

What is antiphospholipid antibody syndrome (APAS)?

- APAS is a thrombotic syndrome that is caused by antiphospholipid antibodies that activate the coagulation pathway, resulting in both arterial and venous thrombosis and recurrent first trimester miscarriages

How is APAS diagnosed? (See Chapter 9 for further details.)

- At least one thrombotic event or pregnancy morbidity occurring in the presence of persistent antiphospholipid antibodies (confirmed on two separate occasions at least 12 weeks apart):
  - Immunoglobulin G (IgG) and/or IgM anti-cardiolipin antibodies (ACAs) **OR** beta-2 glycoprotein I (B2GP1)

    OR
  - The presence of a lupus anticoagulant (LA; i.e., prolonged dilute Russell's viper venom time); presence of LA is the strongest predictor of recurrent venous thromboembolism (VTE)

How is APAS treated?

- Treatment of APAS mandates long-term anticoagulation. Patients who develop catastrophic antiphospholipid antibody syndrome (CAPS), characterized by widespread thrombosis, should undergo plasmapheresis followed by immunosuppression.

Nonimmune-mediated consumptive thrombocytopenias

What are the nonimmune-mediated causes of consumptive thrombocytopenias?

1. **Thrombotic microangiopathies**

   - Fulminant disorders consisting of microangiopathic hemolytic anemia (MAHA), thrombocytopenia, and microthrombi deposition in the capillaries and arterioles due to endothelial injury

Thrombocytopenic purpura (TTP)

What is TTP?

- TTP is a clinical condition that results from a congenital or acquired deficiency of ADAMTS-13 protease. This metalloprotease is responsible for cleavage of large von Willebrand factor (vWF) multimers. In the absence of the protease, there is an accumulation of vWF multimers, which leads to the formation of small-vessel platelet-rich thrombi.
- Potentially fatal multiorgan dysfunction develops as a result of platelet aggregates that are deposited in the microcirculation. The microthrombi create a shear force for red blood cells producing pronounced microangiopathic hemolytic anemia.

- Typically, the deficiency of the protease is due to an immunoglobulin G (IgG) autoimmune inhibitor directed against the protease, but can also be due to mutations in *ADAMTS13* (resulting in congenital/familial TTP).
- Certain drugs (such as ticlopidine, clopidogrel, mitomycin-c, tacrolimus) can also cause TTP.

How do patients with TTP present?

- Patients typically present with a pentad of clinical findings including fever, microangiopathic hemolytic anemia (MAHA), thrombocytopenia, renal dysfunction, and mental status changes. The cornerstone of diagnosis of TTP requires the presence of MAHA and thrombocytopenia. Other components of the pentad can occur with varying frequency.
- If diagnosis and/or treatment is delayed, the disease can be rapidly fatal.

How is TTP diagnosed?

- The diagnosis requires a strong clinical suspicion in anyone who presents with microangiopathic hemolytic anemia (MAHA) and thrombocytopenia.
- ADAMTS-13 level of <10% is usually diagnostic.
- In the autoimmune variant, the ADAMTS-13 inhibitor will be elevated.

How is TTP treated?

- Plasma exchange should be instituted as soon as the condition is suspected without waiting for confirmatory serology.
- If plasma exchange is not available, then patient can be transfused with fresh frozen plasma, which contains some ADAMTS-13, and transferred to a facility that can perform plasma exchange. Platelet transfusion is generally felt to be contraindicated in TTP.
  - ○ In some patients, additional immunosuppression may be required. Corticosteroids and rituximab are used most commonly.
    - ■ In drug-induced TTP, the drug should be stopped; this subtype of TTP does not typically respond well to plasma exchange.

Disseminated intravascular coagulation (DIC)

What is DIC? (See chapter 8.)

- Acquired systemic activation of intravascular coagulation resulting in microvascular thrombi complicated by end-organ damage, increased risk of venous thrombosis, and consumption of platelet and coagulation proteins with risk of bleeding and thrombocytopenia. Dysfunctional fibrinolysis may be present.

How is DIC diagnosed?

The diagnosis of DIC is made clinically. Laboratory evaluation shows thrombocytopenia, prolonged prothrombin time (PT) and partial thromboplastin time (PTT), elevated d-dimer, and low fibrinogen.

How is DIC treated?

- Manage the underlying cause (i.e., sepsis, pancreatitis, malignancy, trauma, etc.) and aggressive supportive care. Treatment of patients with DIC is complex and should be individualized. Patients should undergo transfusion of blood products for bleeding and coagulopathy. In the setting of a thrombotic event, consideration of anticoagulation should be made.

2. **Thrombocytopenia with massive transfusion**
   - Dilutional thrombocytopenia from extensive blood products transfusion
   - Treatment:
     - Replete coagulation proteins and platelets with massive RBC transfusions, in addition to aggressive supportive care
     - Most blood banks have massive transfusion protocol that takes into account the dilutional effect when dispensing blood products

D. Thrombocytopenia due to platelet sequestration

What are conditions that lead to platelet sequestration?

Splenomegaly

- In a patient with splenomegaly, up to 90% of total body platelet mass can be sequestered in the spleen (normal spleen sequesters 1/3 of total body platelets).
- The most common cause for splenomegaly is passive congestion due to portal hypertension
- Other causes of splenomegaly
  - Chronic extravascular hemolysis—due to thalassemia, hereditary RBC cytoskeletal defects, pyruvate kinase deficiency, and so forth
  - Hematologic neoplasms including lymphomas and myeloproliferative disorders
  - Infections such as mononucleosis
  - Storage diseases

How is splenomegaly managed?

- Even in the setting of massive splenomegaly, the platelet count is rarely less than 30,000/microL. Therefore, if the platelet count is lower, it should prompt a search for other causes of thrombocytopenia.
- In most patients, the splenomegaly is chronic and progressive.
- If feasible, treat the underlying condition.
- In patients with cirrhosis who undergo liver transplant, the splenomegaly does improve with consequential improvement of the platelet count.

Thrombocytosis

WHAT IS THROMBOCYTOSIS?

Thrombocytosis (or thrombocythemia) refers to a platelet count of >450,000/microL

What are the causes of thrombocytosis?

1. Reactive or secondary thrombocytosis

- Inflammation (inflammatory bowel disease, rheumatoid arthritis, infection) is the most common cause of thrombocytosis, resulting from IL-6 and IFN-gamma–mediated megakaryocytopoiesis
- Iron deficiency can be associated with thrombocytosis
- Rebound from thrombocytopenia (i.e., chemotherapy-induced thrombocytopenia)
- Asplenic state resulting in decreased physiologic clearance by phagocytes
- Treatment is directed at underlying cause

2. Clonal thrombocytosis

- Seen in several clonal hematopoietic disorders such as essential thrombocytosis, polycythemia vera, primary myelofibrosis, chronic myeloid leukemia (refer to Chapter 10), and in a subset of patients with myelodysplastic syndromes (Chapter 12)

Disorders of Platelet Function (refer to hemostasis chapter)

Congenital Disorders of Platelet Function

What are the most common congenital disorders of platelet function?

Disorders of adhesion

1. von Willebrand Disease (see Chapter 8)

What is von Willebrand disease (vWD)?

- Most common congenital bleeding disorders with an incidence of 1 in 10,000
- It is characterized by deficiency or dysfunction of vWF causing impaired platelet adhesion to the subendothelium and reduced stability of factor VIII
- Patients present with variable symptoms including easy bruising, mucosal bleeding such as epistaxis and menorrhagia, and postoperative hemorrhage

What are the different categories of von Willebrand Disease?

- Type 1: quantitative deficiency of vWF. Most common. Autosomal dominant
- Type 2: qualitative defect of vWF
  - Type 2A: autosomal dominant. Decreased intermediate and large vWF multimers due to defective protein synthesis or increased susceptibility to ADAMTS13 proteolysis. Reduced ristocetin-induced platelet aggregation (RIPA) and ristocetin cofactor activity compared to vWF antigen. Multimer electrophoresis with decreased intermediate and high-molecular-weight multimers
  - Type 2B: autosomal dominant. Mutation of the large vWF multimer results in high affinity of vWF to GP1b receptor on platelets. There is spontaneous binding of vWF to platelets, which results in rapid clearance of the platelet–vWF complex. Patients will have decreased large vWF multimers and thrombocytopenia. RIPA with hyperactive agglutination. Low-dose RIPA: increased platelet aggregation, which is only seen in type 2B vWD and in platelet-type vWD (see the following text)

- ○ 2M: usually autosomal dominant. Decreased affinity for platelet binding, resulting in hypoactive agglutination with ristocetin cofactor assay and RIPA, and normal multimer electrophoresis.
- ○ 2N: autosomal recessive. Defective factor 8 binding site on vWF, resulting in clinical picture similar to hemophilia A. Normal vWF activity, RIPA, and multimer electrophoresis, but factor 8 level is low (typically <15%)
- Type 3: complete deficiency of vWF. Autosomal recessive
- ○ Platelet-type vWD: "gain-of-function" mutation of GP 1b, resulting in similar phenotype to vWD type 2B. If the addition of normal vWF to the patient's platelets does not correct the increased platelet aggregation seen with low-dose RIPA, then the diagnosis is consistent with platelet-type vWD, rather than type 2B vWD. Bleeding in the setting of platelet-type vWD can be treated with platelet transfusion

Disorders of platelet activation and secretion (including storage pool defects)

1. What is Wiskott-Aldrich syndrome?

- X-linked recessive disorder characterized by a mutated WASp gene, which is responsible for actin cytoskeleton in hematopoietic stem cells.
- Manifests as storage pool–like disorder with platelets that cannot aggregate and microthrombocytopenia with a platelet count of less than 70,000/microL.
- Patients present with immunodeficiency with recurrent sinopulmonary infection, eczema, and lymphoproliferative disorders.

2. What is Chediak-Higashi syndrome?

- Autosomal recessive disorder characterized by abnormal microtubule function and the absence of dense granules from platelets
- The second wave of platelet aggregation is impaired due to decreased serotonin uptake
- Patients present with recurrent gram-positive infections due to defective degranulation and chemotaxis
- Oculocutaneous albinism is a prominent feature

3. What are the MYH9-related disorders?

- MYH9-related disorders are a group of platelet storage pool diseases characterized by mutations of *MYH9* gene on chromosome 22, encoding nonmuscle myosin heavy chain.
- This group of disorders include the following symptoms
  - ○ Patients present with mild bleeding diasthesis, macrothrombocytopenia, and leukocyte inclusions from myosin aggregates (Döhle-like inclusions).
  - ○ Some patients might have nephritis, hearing loss, and cataracts.

4. What is gray platelet syndrome?

- Condition characterized by defective alpha granules resulting in impaired release of von Willebrand factor (vWF), fibrinogen, platelet factor 4 (PF4), and platelet-derived growth factor (PDGF)

- Laboratory evaluation reveals normal platelet aggregation
- The constitutive secretion of PDGF results in splenomegaly and marrow fibrosis
- Patients present with mucocutaneous bleeding with trauma and thrombocytopenia with platelet count ~50,000/microL
- Platelets appear large and pale ("gray")

Disorders of platelet surface glycoproteins

1. What is Glanzmann's thrombasthenia?

- Autosomal recessive disorder characterized by abnormal integrin $\alpha_{IIb}\beta_3$ (also known as the fibrinogen receptor) resulting in defective platelet aggregation
- Patient will have a normal platelet count but will present with varying degrees of mucocutaneous bleeding with prolonged bleeding time
- Platelet aggregation is normal with ristocetin but defective with agonists like thrombin, collagen, or adenosine diphosphate (ADP)
- Treatment: platelet transfusions

2. What is Bernard-Soulier syndrome?

- Autosomal recessive disorder characterized by defective GP1b/IX/V receptors (von Willebrand factor receptor) resulting in defective platelet adhesion
- Platelets tend to be large (increased mean platelet volume [MPV]) but decreased in number
- Patients present with bleeding out of proportion to thrombocytopenia
- Diagnosis may be confirmed with absent GP1b/IX/V receptor on flow cytometry and absent aggregation with ristocetin, which does not correct with addition of normal plasma, thereby differentiating it from von Willebrand disease (vWD). Hypoactive agglutination with ristocetin-induced platelet aggregation (RIPA) and normal agglutination with ristocetin cofactor assay.
- Treatment: platelet transfusion

Acquired Functional Disorders of Platelets

What are the common causes of acquired functional disorders of platelets?

1. Antiplatelet drugs

a. Cyclooxygenase (COX) Inhibitors

- Inhibition of COX leads to impaired thromboxane formation, which results in defective intracellular signaling and ultimately platelet aggregation.
- Aspirin is an irreversible inhibition of COX 1 in platelets in doses as low as 50 to 100 mg daily.
- Nonsteroidal anti-inflammatory drugs (NSAIDs) are reversible inhibitors of the COX enzymes.

b. P2Y12 Inhibitors (adenosine diphosphate [ADP] receptor agonists)

- Inhibit platelet activation
- Examples include clopidogrel and ticlopidine

c. **Integrin αIIbβ3 inhibitors**
- Inhibit platelet aggregation
- Examples include abciximab, tirofiban, and eptifibatide

2. **Other drugs: Fibrinolytics**

3. **Hematologic diseases**
- Myeloid neoplasms are associated with dysmegakaryopoiesis resulting in dysfunctional platelets.

4. **Uremia**
- Retention of uremic toxins can inhibit all aspects of platelet function.
- Dialysis will partially mitigate the bleeding risk.

Platelet Disorders in Pregnancy

What are the common platelet disorders associated with pregnancy?

Thrombocytopenia

1. **Gestational thrombocytopenia**

What is gestational thrombocytopenia?
- Most common cause of thrombocytopenia in pregnancy
- This is a diagnosis of exclusion
- Commonly presents in the third trimester (but could occur as early as in the mid-second trimester)
- Pathogenesis unknown, platelets are typically >80,000/microL
- Patients are asymptomatic and the platelet count will normalize within 1 to 2 months of delivery
- Fetus/newborn does not have thrombocytopenia
- Recurrence in subsequent pregnancies is common
- Difficult to distinguish from immune thrombocytopenia (ITP), the latter more likely if thrombocytopenia is severe and occurring in first trimester
- Treatment is usually not required

2. **Immune thrombocytopenia**

How does immune thrombocytopenia (ITP) manifest in pregnancy?
- ITP in pregnancy accounts for 4% to 5% of all pregnancy-associated thrombocytopenia.
- Patients will often have a prior history of ITP.
- ITP in pregnancy can be difficult to distinguish from gestational thrombocytopenia.
  - In ITP, the platelet count drops early in pregnancy (typically below 70) and will progressively decline throughout pregnancy.
  - The platelet may recover, but does not typically normalize after pregnancy.
- Antiplatelet antibodies cross the placenta causing neonatal thrombocytopenia.

○ There is potential for newborn fetal hemorrhage, especially with vaginal birth due to neonatal thrombocytopenia. There are no methods currently to predict fetal platelet count at the time of delivery.

○ The mode of delivery should be determined by the obstetricians.

Treatment of ITP during pregnancy
When to treat?

- The cutoff platelet count to treat and timing of treatment should be discussed with the obstetrician. The platelet cutoff for epidural anesthesia should be discussed with the anesthesiologists (some consider a platelet count of >80,000 to be adequate for epidural anesthesia).

How to treat? What are the treatment options?

- Glucocorticoids
- IVIG
  ○ Can be used throughout pregnancy
  ○ Need to be cognizant of fluid overload issues
- Splenectomy
  ○ Laparoscopic splenectomy can be performed in the second trimester if there is failure to respond to IVIG and steroids
- Aniti-(Rh)D can cause maternal and fetal hemolysis, and is relatively contraindicated
- Rituximab and TPO mimetics are generally not recommended. Rituximab has been reported in the second trimester and beyond with risk of lymphopenia in the newborn for several months
- Newborn thrombocytopenia
  ○ Platelet count should be determined in neonates of mothers with immune thrombocytopenia (ITP) and further monitoring/management should be done in consultation with neonatology

Microangiopathic disorders
1. **Preeclampsia/eclampsia:** affects 5% to 8% of all pregnancies. Defined as new hypertension after 20 weeks gestation with proteinuria, or if without proteinuria, presence of one of the following:
   - Thrombocytopenia (platelet count <100,000/microL)
   - Abnormal liver function tests (LFTs)
   - Acute kidney Injury
   - Pulmonary edema
   - Cerebral/visual disturbances
   - If epileptic seizures are present => **eclampsia**

2. **HELLP (hemolysis, elevated liver enzymes, low platelets) syndrome**
   - This can occur in the setting of preeclampsia in 70% to 80% of patients, and usually in the peripartum period. Similar presentation as thrombocytopenic purpura (TTP), but abnormal LFTs more common

3. Acute fatty liver of pregnancy (ALFP)
   - A rare condition characterized by microvascular fatty infiltration of liver with subsequent liver failure and encephalopathy
   - Platelet count may be low with or without other signs of DIC
   - Usually diagnosed in third trimester

Treatment: Management of these disorders should be performed in discussion with the obstetricians.

QUESTIONS

1. An 18-year-old girl with no known past medical history presents with a mild splenic laceration from a motor vehicle accident while visiting her aunt. Complete blood count shows hemoglobin (Hgb) 7g/dL, white blood cells (WBCs) of 15, and platelets of 103,000. Prothrombin time (PT)/partial thromboplastin time (PTT) is within normal limits. She continues to require 2 to 3 units of packed red blood cells (PRBCs) per day. You are consulted for consideration of a bleeding disorder, and recommend platelet aggregation studies, which show normal ristocetin activity, but no aggregation in response to agonists such as adenosine diphosphate (ADP), epinephrine, or collagen. You recommend which of the following?
   A. Platelet transfusions
   B. Platelet transfusion with recombinant factor 7a
   C. Recombinant factor 7a alone
   D. Flow cytometry to confirm lack of GP2b/3a

2. A 20-year-old man with a lifelong history of excessive bleeding has recently obtained health insurance and presents to you for evaluation. Complete blood count (CBC) is notable for mild thrombocytopenia, and peripheral smear shows large platelets. Prothrombin time (PT)/partial thromboplastin time (PTT) and fibrinogen are within normal limits. He undergoes a platelet aggregation test, which shows normal response to platelet agonists (epinephrine, adenosine diphosphate [ADP], and collagen), but no response to ristocetin. Addition to plasma does not correct his response to ristocetin. How would you confirm his diagnosis?
   A. Send vWF:Ag, vWF:ristocetin and ristocetin-induced platelet aggregation (RIPA)
   B. Send serum protein electrophoresis (SPEP) to screen for plasma cell dyscrasia due to possible GPIbIX/V complex inhibitor
   C. Flow cytometry to assess for presence of GPIbIX/V complex on platelet surface membrane
   D. Review medications to rule out aspirin therapy

3. You are consulted for evaluation of thrombocytopenia in a 55-year-old man who is postoperative day 6 (POD6) after undergoing a three-vessel coronary bypass. He has been on a heparin drip since surgery. His platelets have dropped from 250,000 preoperatively to 75,000 on POD6. He has no evidence of thrombosis and he is overall recovering from his surgery well with the exception of an acute kidney injury (AKI) with creatinine up from baseline of 1 to 2.5 mg/dL. What is your management recommendation?
   A. Stop heparin and start Coumadin
   B. Stop heparin and start argatroban
   C. Stop heparin and start bivalirudin
   D. Stop heparin and start fondaparinux

4. A 65-year-old man with no known past medical history presents to your clinic for evaluation for macrothrombocytopenia. Peripheral blood smear reveals thrombocytopenia with large, pale-appearing platelets, in addition to nucleated red blood cells (RBCs), polychromasia, and teardrop cells. Bone marrow biopsy revealed significant reticulin fibrosis, and physical exam is notable for splenomegaly. His family history is remarkable for an older brother who died of myelofibrosis at the age of 55 years. What is the most likely diagnosis?
   A. Primary myelofibrosis
   B. Gray platelet syndrome associated with myelofibrosis
   C. Myelophthisis
   D. White platelet syndrome

5. A 45-year-old woman is admitted to the hospital for fever and confusion. Her hemoglobin was noted to be 8 with no known baseline. Platelets were 75,000 and white blood cells were 15,000. Prothrombin time (PT)/partial thromboplastin time (PTT) and fibrinogen were normal. Peripheral smear was remarkable for toxic granulation of the polymorphonuclear leukocytes (PMNs) and the presence of schistocytes. She was also noted to have a creatinine of 2.5 mg/dL, although her baseline remains unknown. What is your next step in management?
   A. Pulse high-dose steroids to suppress anti-ADAMTS13 antibodies
   B. Plasma exchange due to concern for thrombocytopenic purpura (TTP)
   C. Supportive care, with plan to keep platelets >10,000 and fibrinogen >100
   D. Send an ADAMTS14 level STAT

6. A 35-year-old woman with immune thrombocytopenia (ITP) previously responsive to steroids reported increasing petechiae with complete blood count (CBC) revealing platelet count of 20,000/mm^3. You recommend restarting high-dose prednisone. One week later, her platelet count is 15,000/mm^3. You administer intravenous immunoglobulin (IVIG; with transient response) and refer her to a surgeon for splenectomy. She presents today 4 weeks after her splenectomy with a platelet count of 25,000/mm^3. You recommend a thrombopoietin (TPO) agonist for refractory disease, and she is started on eltrombopag. All of the following are associated with eltrombopag except?

A. Eltrombopag's efficacy continues even after the drug is stopped
B. Patients receiving eltrombopag should have routine evaluation of liver function tests (LFTs)
C. Eltrombopag can increase risk of thrombosis
D. A lower dose of eltrombopag is indicated in patients of Asian decent

7. **A 67-year-old man presents with a history of myocardial infarction, for which he is on clopidogrel. What results would you expect from a platelet aggregation test?**
A. No primary or secondary wave response
B. Primary wave response only
C. No secondary wave only
D. No response to adenosine diphosphate (ADP) agonists, but response with ristocetin, epinephrine, and collagen

8. **A 21-year-old girl is sent to your clinic for evaluation of menorrhagia. She states that her maternal aunt also has menorrhagia, but no other known family history of bleeding. Blood work reveals microcytic anemia with hemoglobin (Hgb) of 10 and mean corpuscular volume (MCV) 65, but otherwise normal white blood cells (WBCs), platelets, fibrinogen, and prothrombin time (PT)/partial thromboplastin time (PTT). Bleeding time is prolonged, but platelet aggregation studies are normal. Which additional tests would help with her diagnosis?**
A. Ristocetin cofactor activity
B. von Willebrand antigen
C. Factor 8 activity
D. All of the above

9. **You are consulted for refractory severe thrombocytopenia (platelets ~5,000) in a 65-year-old man admitted with decompensated liver cirrhosis and gastrointestinal (GI) bleed. He was last hospitalized about 10 days ago for GI bleeding and received a red blood cell (RBC) transfusion. During that admission, his platelet count was ~80,000 (at his baseline). He had two prior admissions for GI bleed in the past 12 months, where he also received RBC and platelet transfusions. He has been evaluated by gastroenterologists, and no further procedures are recommended to help control his bleeding. Which of the following may help raise his platelet counts?**
A. Intravenous immunoglobulin (IVIG)
B. Correction of underlying coagulopathy related to liver disease
C. Splenectomy
D. Steroids

ANSWERS

1. **A. Platelet transfusions.** This patient has Glanzmann's thrombasthenia, which is an autosomal recessive mutation that results in defective or absent GP2b/3a, thereby inhibiting platelet aggregation and activation. Similar clinical scenarios can be seen with a GP2b/3a inhibitor or afibrinogenemia, except with the latter, PT/PTT is prolonged as well. In this young girl with no known autoimmune disease, an antibody inhibitor is less likely. Recombinant factor 7a may be considered in bleeding patients who have developed platelet refractoriness. Flow cytometry may be used to confirm disease diagnosis, but this can be completed concurrently or after administration of platelets for this bleeding patient with relatively substantial PRBC requirements. Of note, Glanzmann's thrombasthenia patients generally will have normal platelet counts and morphology, but defective platelet function as already noted.

2. **C. Flow cytometry to assess for presence of GPIbIX/V complex on platelet surface membrane.** This patient has Bernard-Soulier syndrome (BSS), which is an autosomal recessive condition with mutations in *GPIBA*, *GPIBB*, and *GP9* genes, resulting in a qualitative or quantitative defect in GPIbIX/V complex. Defects in this complex compromise *von Willebrand* (vWF) binding and contribute to shortening platelet survival and altering cellular structure, resulting in the macrothrombocytopenia characteristic of this disease. von Willebrand disease is ruled by the lack of platelet aggregation with ristocetin, which did not correct with the addition of plasma. An inhibitor is unlikely as patient is without a history suggestive of rheumatologic disease and unlikely to have plasma cell dyscrasia.

3. **B. Stop heparin and start argatroban.** This patient has a clinical scenario suspicious for heparin-induced thrombocytopenia (HIT) due to the drop in his platelets within 5 to 10 days of heparin exposure. His 4Ts score is 6 (>50% fall in platelet count [2 points], time of platelet drop within 5 to 10 days of heparin exposure (2 points), no thrombosis (0 points), and no other likely cause of thrombocytopenia (2 points), indicating a high pretest probability of HIT at 6. Therefore, all heparin products should be stopped and argatroban initiated. Bivalirudin is renally cleared, while argatroban is cleared by the liver, therefore an AKI does not prevent use of argatroban. Fondaparinux is not a Food and Drug Administration (FDA)-approved treatment for HIT, but has been shown to be effective and should be used as an alternative therapy in patients with contraindications or inability to receive parenteral argatroban. Once platelets have normalized, thereby indicating that the patient is no longer tipped into a procoagulant state, Coumadin can be started with an argatroban bridge until therapeutic *international normalized ratio* (INR).

4. **B. Gray platelet syndrome with associated myelofibrosis.** Gray platelet syndrome is an autosomal recessive disease with defective/absent alpha granules due to inability of the megakaryocyte to package the proteins into vesicles. Complications can be mild-to-moderate mucocutaneous bleeding. Platelet aggregation studies may have variable results, but

patients may over time develop myelofibrosis due to deposition of alpha granule proteins within the marrow. Primary myelofibrosis is less likely given the patient's family history and lack of evident concurrent myelodysplastic syndrome (MDS) that may be responsible for gray platelet appearance. White platelet syndrome is an autosomal dominant platelet secretory disease that is not associated with myelofibrosis.

5. **B. Plasma exchange due to concern for thrombocytopenic purpura (TTP).** Start plasma exchange due to concern for TTP. The normal PT/PTT and fibrinogen indicate lack of consumption and rules out disseminated intravascular coagulation (DIC) as a cause of the thrombotic microangiopathy (TMA). Since this is a potentially life-threatening condition, plasma exchange should be started while awaiting confirmation of diagnosis with ADAMTS13 levels, and corticosteroids for immune suppression of anti-ADAMTS13 antibody should not delay the initiation plasmapheresis for immediate removal of the immune complexes to prevent propagation of the end-organ damage created by TMA.

6. **A. Eltrombopag's efficacy continues even after the drug is stopped.** Efficacy of eltrombopag, a TPO agonist, is only present while the drug is being administered. It is associated with thrombosis, cataracts, and LFT abnormalities, and people of Asian descent do require a lower dose.

7. **D. No response to adenosine diphosphate (ADP) agonists, but response with ristocetin, epinephrine, and collagen.** Clopidogrel is an ADP inhibitor and therefore will interfere with ADP-mediated platelet activation through the secondary wave noted in platelet aggregation. Since it does not interfere with the function of epinephrine, GP1b, and collagen, there should be no impact on the activation of their subsequent pathways with their respective agonists.

8. **D. All of the above.** von Willebrand disease can be due to a qualitative or quantitative defect in von Willebrand factor. PT/PTT only measure coagulation factors and do not indicate von Willebrand factor (vWF) defect unless there is a corresponding drop in factor 8 to very low levels. The bleeding time can be prolonged in patients with vWF defects, but it is not a standard screening test due to extreme variability in performing the test. vWD screening tests are vWF antigen, a functional test like ristocetin cofactor activity to assess vWF ability to bind platelets, and factor 8 activity since vWF binds Factor 8 and increases its half-life.

9. **A. Intravenous immunoglobulin (IVIG).** IVIG is the first line of therapy for posttransfusion purpura, a condition characterized by alloimmunization most commonly to the HPA-1a antigen on donor platelets in HPA-1a–negative recipients. This is characterized by antibody-mediated consumption of donor and recipient platelets usually about 1 to 2 weeks after transfusion. First line of therapy is IVIG to help saturate Fc gamma receptors within the reticuloendothelial system, followed by plasmapheresis to remove the antibody if there is no response. The patient should avoid antigen-positive blood products in the future.

Hemostasis

8

Jordan K. Schaefer and Paula L. Bockenstedt

MOLECULAR BASIS OF COAGULATION

1. **What are the main sequences of events in the process of primary hemostasis?**

   A. **Primary hemostasis may be broken down into three phases:**

   Platelet adhesion, activation/secretion, and aggregation

   Platelet adhesion:

   i. Vessel injury leads to exposure of subendothelial matrix proteins, including collagen.
   ii. Platelets adhere to exposed subendothelial matrix, facilitated by interactions of the platelet GPIb complex (GP1b-GPV-GPIX) and von Willebrand factor (vWF).

   Platelet activation:

   i. Platelet GpVI and GP1a/IIa binding to collagen leads to platelet activation and calcium mobilization.
   ii. Platelet receptors interact with adenosine diphosphate (ADP), serotonin, platelet-activating factor, thromboxane A2, thrombin, and epinephrine originating from platelets or the surrounding cells at the site of vessel injury.
   iii. Platelet activation results in a cytoskeletal mediated shape change that facilitates subsequent platelet granule secretion.

   Platelet aggregation:

   i. The beta integrin αIIbβ3 (platelet GpIIb/IIIa receptor) is activated and binds soluble fibrinogen causing platelet aggregation and release of granules.

2. **Describe the contents of alpha granules and dense granules.**

   - Alpha granules contain fibrinogen, (vWF, PF4, p-selectin, clotting factors, adhesion molecules, and growth factors.
   - Delta or dense granules provide adenosine diphosphate (ADP), adenosine triphosphate (ATP), calcium, and serotonin.

3. **What are integrins?**

   - Integrins are transmembrane receptors on cells that facilitate cell–extracellular matrix adhesion and activate cellular signal transduction.
   - Examples of integrins in platelet-related hemostasis are the beta 1 integrins (α2β1, α5β1) and the β3 integrin, α2β3.

4. **What hereditary clotting disorders affect primary hemostasis?**
   - Hereditary disorders of platelet function or number (Chapter 7)
   - vWD

5. **What process is defective in Bernard-Soulier syndrome and why?**
   - BSS is an autosomal recessive disorder characterized by thrombocytopenia, large platelets, and decrease in the number of GpIb receptors or a functionally defective Gp1b complex.
   - Platelet adhesion is decreased.

6. **What process is defective in Glanzmann's thrombasthenia and why?**
   - Glanzmann's thrombasthenia is an autosomal recessive bleeding disorder with normal number and size of platelets.
   - The GpIIbIIIa complex is required for binding fibrinogen.
   - Platelet aggregation is decreased or absent due to a deficiency or absence of the GpIIb/IIIa heterodimer complex caused by mutations in either IIb or IIIa.
   - Clot retraction may also be impaired by defects in the interaction of GpIIbIIIa with the platelet cytoskeleton.

7. **How is congenital afibrinogenemia distinguished from Glanzmann's thrombasthenia?**
   - Both disorders result in decreased platelet aggregation to all agonists except ristocetin. Afibrinogenemia is associated with a prolonged prothrombin time (PT), activated partial thromboplastin time (aPTT), and thrombin time, whereas those laboratory tests are normal in Glanzmann's thrombasthenia.

8. **What is the role of vitamin K in clotting factor synthesis? What are the vitamin K–dependent clotting factors/cofactors?**
   - The cofactor vitamin K is necessary for terminal gamma-carboxylation in the synthesis of select clotting factor proteins to produce fully functional factors.
   - Vitamin K–dependent procoagulant factors are prothrombin (factor II) and factors VII, IX, and X.
   - Natural anticoagulant protein C and its cofactor, protein S, are also vitamin K dependent.

9. **What is secondary hemostasis?**
   - Secondary hemostasis occurs simultaneously with platelet adhesion and formation of the platelet plug. This is a series of enzymatic reactions mediated by coagulation factors to ultimately form fibrin to stabilize the platelet plug. This process occurs on the phospholipid membranes of cells through complexes.

10. **What is the sequence of procoagulant activation in secondary hemostasis?**
    - Exposed tissue factor (TF) in the damaged subendothelium binds to small amounts of circulating factor VII/VIIa resulting in a complex (extrinsic Xase), which binds and activates factor X to Xa. The TF/factor VIIa/factor Xa complex converts a small amount of prothrombin to thrombin causing an initial small burst of thrombin.

- An amplification loop is generated by thrombin activation of factors VIII, IX, and XI and this activates platelets leading to surface expression of platelet factor V. The TF/factor VIIa activation of factor IX is critical since the tissue factor pathway inhibitor, TFPI, inhibits the initial components of the extrinsic pathway.
- Activated factors IXa and VIIIa form the intrinsic Xase complex resulting in conversion of large amounts of factor X to Xa.
- Factor Xa complexed with platelet surface factor Va results in a burst of activation of prothrombin to thrombin and cleavage of factor I (fibrinogen) to fibrin monomers.
- Fibrin monomers assemble into fibrils forming a clot, which is stabilized by covalent cross-linking of fibrin monomers by thrombin-activated factor XIIIa and incorporation of thrombin-activatable fibrinolysis inhibitor (TAFI). The cellular location of these reactions, in proximity to platelets at the damaged endothelium, helps mediate the formation of a fibrin clot to the required location.

11. **What are the clotting factor activation steps that comprise the intrinsic pathway?**
    - In sequential order, factor XII (contact factor) is activated by kallikrein, formed from the cleavage of prekallikrein with high-molecular-weight kininogen (HMWK) as a cofactor to generate factor XIIa.
    - Factor XIIa promotes coagulation by then activating factor XI to XIa and also activates fibrinolysis by converting plasminogen to plasmin.
    - Factor XIa converts factor IX to IXa with factor VIIIa and calcium as cofactors.
    - Factor IXa, with factor VIIIa as cofactor, converts factor X to Xa.
    - At factor X, the intrinsic pathway joints the final common pathway.

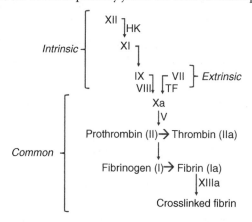

Simplified schematic of the classical model of the coagulation cascade. Cofactors (factor V, factor VIII, TF, HK) are shown in small font. For simplicity, the active and inactive factors of the extrinsic/intrinsic pathway have been condensed into one numeral representing both the active and inactive component; PK, inactive factor X and XIII are not shown.

HK, high-molecular-weight kininogen; PK, prekallikrein; TF, tissue factor.

12. **What are the clotting factor activation steps that comprise the extrinsic pathway?**
    - TF interacts with factor VIIa to activate factor X to Xa, joining the final common pathway.
    - Factor VIIa and TF also convert factor IX to IXa that then merges to the common pathway by converting factor X to Xa in the presence of factor VIIIa.

13. **What factors make up the final common pathway?**
    - Factor Xa binds to activated Va and forms the prothrombinase complex that converts prothrombin to thrombin (IIa). Thrombin cleaves fibrinogen into fibrin monomers. Fibrin monomers undergo polymerization. Factor XIIIa then cross-links the fibrin strands and stabilizes the thrombus.

14. **Where are the procoagulant factors synthesized?**
    - All procoagulant factors are made primarily in the liver hepatocytes, with the exception of factor VIII, which is synthesized in endothelial cells. Factor VIII circulates with vWF. vWF is synthesized extrahepatically by megakaryocytes and endothelial cells.

15. **By what endogenous mechanisms is coagulation regulated or inhibited?**
    a. Antithrombin (AT) inhibits thrombin (IIa), along with TF-VIIa, factor IXa, Xa, XIa, XIIa, and kallikrein. AT activity is enhanced 1,000 fold by endogenous or exogenous heparins.
    b. Thrombin is also inhibited by heparin cofactor II.
    c. Tissue factor pathway inhibitor (TFPI) inhibits factor Xa and the TF-VIIa-Xa complex, thus inhibiting the extrinsic pathway.
    d. Natural anticoagulant protein C is activated by binding to the thrombin-activated thrombomodulin receptor on the endothelial cell surface. Protein Ca complexes with its cofactor protein S and inactivates factors Va and VIIIa.

16. **What factor deficiencies are not associated with bleeding?**
    a. Factor XII, high-molecular-weight kininogen (HMWK), and prekallikrein deficiencies are not generally associated with bleeding.

17. **What events occur during fibrinolysis?**
    a. Tissue plasminogen activator (tPA) is released from the vessel wall at the site of injury. TPA activates plasminogen bound to fibrin to form plasmin. (Factor XIIa, XIa, and kallikrein are also able to convert plasminogen to plasmin, but at a slower rate.)
    b. Plasmin then breaks down fibrin to soluble fibrin degradation products, most notably the D-dimer.
    c. Urokinase is a second enzyme released from select tissue beds, which also activates plasminogen to plasmin and is important in tissue repair and remodeling.

18. **What factors regulate the activity of plasmin?**
    a. Plasminogen activator inhibitor (PAI) and a2-antiplasmin regulate plasmin to terminate plasmin-mediated fibrinolysis.

b. Thrombin-activatable fibrinolysis inhibitor incorporated in fibrin clot limits binding sites for plasminogen on fibrin, delaying fibrinolysis.

LABORATORY EVALUATION

1. **What should be considered when evaluating a new or unexpected reading of thrombocytopenia on a CBC from an otherwise asymptomatic patient?**

   - Pseudothrombocytopenia should be excluded. A CBC is performed using ethylenediaminetetraacetic acid (EDTA) anticoagulated blood. EDTA can cause platelet clumping that may result in a spuriously low platelet count. Clumping is often evident on review of a peripheral blood smear. Redrawing the blood in an alternate anticoagulant, like sodium citrate, yields the correct platelet count.

   - Exceptionally large platelets as seen in MYH9-related disorders or other macrothrombocytopenic conditions may not be counted due to the larger than normal size. This is recognized by a review of the blood smear.

2. **What causes a prolongation of the prothrombin time (PT)?**

   - A prolonged PT reflects abnormalities of the extrinsic pathway or common pathway and is caused by reduced levels of factor VII, factor X, factor V, prothrombin, fibrinogen, or an inhibitor.

   - Etiologies of an isolated prolonged PT include warfarin therapy (the assay is most sensitive to reductions in the vitamin K–dependent factors VII or X), mild vitamin K deficiency, liver disease, and hypofibrinogenemia.

3. **What causes a prolongation of the partial thromboplastin time (PTT)?**

   - A prolonged PTT reflects abnormalities of the intrinsic pathway or common pathway.

   - It can be caused by reduced levels of factor XII, prekallikrein, high-molecular-weight kininogen, factor XI, factor IX, factor VIII, factor X, factor V, prothrombin, or fibrinogen.

   - Etiologies of an isolated prolonged PTT include heparin, bivalirudin, the presence of a lupus anticoagulant, all procoagulant factor deficiencies except factor XIII and factor VII, interference from a paraprotein, or an inhibitor.

4. **What causes a prolongation of the thrombin time?**

   - The thrombin time is performed by adding thrombin and calcium to patient plasma and thus reflects the time to convert fibrinogen to fibrin. It can be prolonged by heparin, direct thrombin inhibitors, a quantitative deficiency, or a qualitative defect in fibrinogen.

   - Prolongation of the thrombin time may also be due to interference in fibrin polymerization by high quantities of fibrin degradation products or paraproteins and some inhibitors.

   - Some tumors produce heparin-like anticoagulants, which interact with antithrombin and prolong the thrombin time.

5. **What is the reptilase time and how does the reptilase time differ from the thrombin time?**

   - The reptilase time is similar to the thrombin clotting time in that the time to fibrin polymerization and clot formation after addition of reptilase to plasma is measured. Reptilase specifically cleaves only fibrinopeptide (a) from fibrinogen.
   - The reptilase time is not prolonged by heparin or direct thrombin inhibitors or tumor-related heparin-like substances, while the thrombin time is. Therefore, it can be used to detect heparin, argatroban, or dabigatran contamination. It is similarly prolonged with low fibrinogen levels, qualitative fibrinogen defects, or interference by fibrin degradation products.

6. **How is an abnormal PT or PTT further investigated?**

   - A mixing study is based on the principle that the PT or PTT test only begins to prolong when there is a 50% reduction in any given clotting factor. Hence, the plasma mixing study combines dilutions of patient plasma with normal plasma, and the PT and/or PTT is repeated immediately and up to 2 hours after incubating the mixture at 37°C.

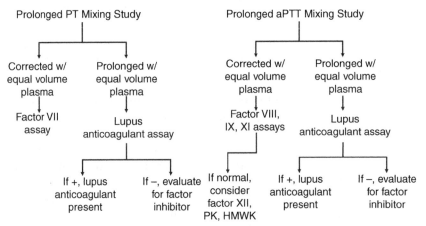

Evaluation of an isolated prolonged PT or activated aPTT. Note that if a prolonged clotting time fails to correct in the absence of a lupus anticoagulant, factor levels should be obtained to evaluate for a specific factor inhibitor.

aPTT, partial thromboplastin time; HK, high-molecular-weight kininogen; PK, prekallikrein; PT, prothrombin time; TF, tissue factor.

   - An abnormal PT or PTT test that corrects in the mixing study suggests a factor deficiency, and specific factor levels are then checked for deficiency.
   - A test that fails to correct with addition of normal plasma suggests an inhibitor (either lupus anticoagulant or specific factor inhibitor).
   - Effects of some coagulation factor inhibitors are most evident after incubation of the test samples. A mixing study performed on plasma containing a specific factor inhibitor may initially show correction but subsequently fail to correct the abnormal clotting time in the presence of 50% normal plasma when measured after incubation for up to 2 hours later.

7. How are specific procoagulant factor levels determined?

- Coagulation factors are assayed based on their activity levels. Coagulation factor assays can be performed either using chromogenic assays or more commonly using plasma clot–based methods.

- Factors of the extrinsic and common pathway can be assessed using a PT-based assay in which the patient's plasma is mixed with plasma that is deficient in the specific factor being tested, and the PT is determined. Similarly, the intrinsic pathway factors can be assayed with an aPTT-based assay using a similar method.

- Chromogenic clotting assays can be used to assay some clotting factors. These methods are less likely to have interference by a lupus anticoagulant, heparin, or a direct thrombin inhibitor.

- Screening for factor XIII deficiency relies on the fact that clots from factor FXIII–deficient patients are more soluble due to the lack of fibrin cross-linking. The urea clot solubility test is based on the time to dissolution of a patient's clot formed under controlled conditions compared to a control.

8. How is fibrinogen measured?

- Fibrinogen is measured by a modification of the thrombin time such that fibrinogen, rather than thrombin, is rate limiting in the reaction. Time to clot formation is calibrated against standard dilutions of fibrinogen.

- Fibrinogen is also measured antigenically by immunologic methods.

- Discrepancy between the fibrinogen activity level and fibrinogen antigen may indicate a dysfibrinogenemia.

9. What tests are used to screen for the presence of a lupus anticoagulant?

- Common screening tests are the dilute Russell viper venom time, hexagonal phase antiphospholipid assay, and the aaPTT. In the presence of a lupus anticoagulant, the prolonged clotting time should not correct to normal range with the addition of normal plasma. If a phospholipid-dependent lupus anticoagulant is present, adding excess phospholipid or hexagonal-phase phospholipid should correct the prolonged clotting time to normal range.

- These clot-based tests can be affected by anticoagulants, causing spurious results.

- Anticardiolipin antibodies and anti-β_2-glycoprotein I antibodies are enzyme-linked immunosorbent assay (ELISA)-based serological tests used to detect specific antibody phospholipid reactivities in the diagnosis of antiphospholipid antibody syndrome.

10. How are coagulation factor inhibitors measured?

- Coagulation factor inhibitors are most commonly assessed using assays modeled on the Bethesda inhibitor assay for factor VIII that assesses the remaining factor VIII activity in dilutions of the patient's plasma mixed with normal plasma compared to that of a control. Bethesda units are calculated as the amount of inhibitor that can neutralize 50% of 1 unit of factor VIII in normal plasma. It is multiplied by the dilution to determine the inhibitor titre.

11. What disorders can cause an abnormal fibrinogen level?

- Decreased fibrinogen can occur with consumption (as in disseminated intravascular coagulation [DIC]) or the breakdown of a clot (as seen after therapeutic tissue plasminogen activator [tPA]-mediated fibrinolytic therapy), snake venom, decreased production (as in liver disease or severe malnutrition), or a hereditary deficiency.
- Fibrinogen is an acute phase reactant and may be elevated in the setting of inflammation, tumors, vascular disease, or pregnancy.

12. How is platelet aggregometry used to detect platelet disorders?

- Platelet aggregometry is one method to determine platelet function. It is performed using platelet-rich plasma from a citrated blood sample. Agonists are added to the blood sample and the change in light transmittance is measured using a photometric device. Patients must be off interfering medications prior to the test.
- Typical agonists include collagen, ADP, epinephrine, ristocetin, and arachidonic acid. (See following table; Chapter 7.)

Condition	Aggregometry findings
Aspirin/Cox pathway defect	Aggregation reduced or absent for arachidonic acid and collagen. Primary wave only with epinephrine. Normal with thromboxane
Clopidogrel	Absent aggregation with ADP
Glanzmann thrombasthenia	Aggregation only with ristocetin (otherwise absent). Not corrected with the addition of plasma
von Willebrand disease	Aggregation normal with agonists except for ristocetin. RIPA generally corresponds with the level of ristocetin cofactor assay. Results normalize with the addition of plasma. Type 2B vWD shows aggregation with low-dose ristocetin
Bernard-Soulier syndrome	Aggregation normal with agonists except ristocetin, which is reduced. Results do not normalize with the addition of plasma

ADP, adenosine diphosphate; RIPA, ristocetin-induced platelet aggregation; vWD, von Willebrand disease.

13. **What additional reference lab tests are used to help establish a diagnosis of Bernard-Soulier syndrome (BSS) or Glanzmann thrombasthenia?**

    - Flow cytometry for decreased glycoprotein 1b-alpha (CD42b) or GpIX (CD42a) in the case of BSS or decreased GpIIb/IIIa (CD41, CD61) for Glanzmann thrombasthenia can be useful.
    - Genetic sequencing analysis of the GpIb-IX-V complex is available for confirmation of Bernard Soulier mutations.

14. **How is thromboelastography (TEG) used in the evaluation of bleeding disorders and assessment of hemostasis?**

    - TEG provides a global assessment of clot formation. A whole blood sample is added to a cup that rotates around a torsion wire (conventional TEG), or the pin rotates in the stationary cup of blood (ROTEM) measuring the force on the wire. This generates a real-time graphical display reflecting coagulation. Various additives to the blood can evaluate clotting through the extrinsic pathway, intrinsic pathway, the fibrinolytic system, and more. It can be used to guide blood product administration, assess anticoagulant drugs, and evaluate for disorders of hemostasis.

15. **What laboratory tests are used in the diagnosis of vWD?**

    - Diagnosis of vWD is based on abnormalities in vWF activity, antigen, factor VIII activity, and multimer analysis.
    - vWF platelet binding activity is measured by the use of a ristocetin cofactor assay. Ristocetin induces glycoprotein 1b–mediated platelet agglutination to vWF detected by aggregometry. Impaired ristocetin-induced platelet agglutination (RIPA) can be seen with a deficiency of vWF or with an impaired Gp1b or GpIX receptor, as in BSS. To eliminate the possibility of BSS, vWF activity is measured using patient plasma with ristocetin and normal control platelets. The slope of agglutination is compared to a reference standard of dilutions of vWF to estimate the relative vWF activity.
    - vWF antigen levels can be quantitated immunologically.
    - Factor VIII levels are typically checked when assessing for vWD due to the carrier function of vWF and to detect the abnormal vWF subtype type IIN or Normandy.
    - vWF multimeric analysis of plasma samples electrophoresed on agarose gel is helpful in subtyping vWD. Radiolabeled antibodies to vWF are used to determine the distribution of vWF multimer sizes on the gel. The patient sample is compared to a control.

Multmer analysis in vWD

Type 1	Normal pattern, reduced concentration
Type 1 Vincenza	Ultralarge multimers

(continued)

Multimer analysis in vWD	
Type 2A	**Absent/reduced intermediate–large multimers**
Type 2B	Absent/reduced of large multimers
Type 2M	Normal pattern
Type 2N	Normal pattern
Type 3	Absent
Platelet vWD	Reduced large multimers

- vWF collagen binding tests are enzyme-linked immunosorbent assay (ELISA) based and can help differentiate vWD type 2A or 2B that have abnormal collagen binding from vWD type 2N, which has normal collagen binding.
- Specific genetic sequencing is commercially available for confirmation of selected vWF subtypes such as type 2N, 2B, and 2M.

16. **What pathologic states can alter vWF activity and antigen assay results?**
    - vWF is an acute phase reactant and levels are affected by inflammation, stress, trauma, hormones, pregnancy, blood type, thyroid disease, exercise, and infection. A single normal test does not exclude the diagnosis, and abnormal results must be assessed according to context in which the result was drawn.

17. **Describe the implications of an abnormal euglobulin clot lysis time.**
    - The euglobulin protein fraction isolated from test plasma contains factor VIII, fibrinogen, factor XIII, plasminogen, and plasminogen activators. The euglobulin fraction is suspended, clotting is generated, and the time for clot dissolution is measured.
    - Increased times reflect reduced fibrinolysis. Shortened times can be a result of increased fibrinolysis as seen in disseminated intravascular coagulation (DIC), liver disease, with certain medications, or after thrombolysis.

HEREDITARY BLEEDING/VASCULAR DISORDERS

1. **What are the inheritance characteristics of hemophilia A and B?**
    - Hemophilia A and B are X-linked disorders resulting in decreased synthesis of factors VIII and IX, respectively.
    - Numerous points, frameshifts, deletions, and two inversion genetic mutations (hemophilia A) have been described leading to hemophilias A and B.
    - Thirty percent of factor VIII and IX mutations are de novo.
    - All daughters of hemophilic men are obligate carriers. No sons of hemophilic men and normal women will inherit hemophilia. Sons of obligate carrier mothers have a 50% chance of inheriting hemophilia. (See following diagram.)

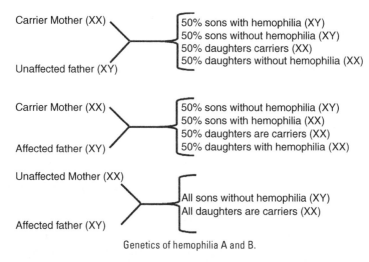

Genetics of hemophilia A and B.

2. **Are female carriers of hemophilia A or B symptomatic?**
   - Up to 20% of female carriers have levels less than 50% and are symptomatically affected due to situations of mosaicism, X chromosomal abnormalities, or imbalanced X chromosome inactivation (lyonization).

3. **What are the most frequent genetic mutations associated with severe hemophilia A?**
   - Nearly half of all severe hemophilia A cases result from two gross chromosomal inversions that involve introns 1 and 22 of the factor VIII gene, respectively. These inversions can be detected by specific polymerase chain reaction (PCR) testing and are useful for identifying carriers of severe hemophilia A.

4. **What are the clinical bleeding manifestations of hemophilia A and B?**
   - Delayed bleeding is the hallmark of a coagulation factor deficiency.
   - Spontaneous deep bruising, muscular hematomas, and intra-articular bleeding are characteristic of hemophilia. Spontaneous, nontraumatic intra-articular bleeding is not typically seen with factor VIII or IX levels of greater than 5% to 10%.

5. **How is the clinical severity of hemophilia A and B predicted?**
   - Severity of hemophilic bleeding is correlated with endogenous factor activity level.

Hemophilia severity	Percent factor level (factor VIII or IX)	Bleeding with...
Mild	5–40%	Major trauma or surgery, rarely spontaneous
Moderate	1–5%	Occasionally spontaneous, minor trauma or surgery
Severe	<1%	Spontaneous bleeding

6. **How are newborns born to known maternal carriers tested for hemo-philia A or B?**
   - Inherited hemophilia can be established at birth by measuring factor VIII or IX levels on cord blood.
   - Results may be affected by inflammation, level of deficiency, and the normal decreased neonatal synthesis of vitamin K–dependent factors.

7. **What are the inheritance characteristics and clinical features of factor XI deficiency?**
   - Factor XI deficiency is most common in patients who are of Ashkenazi Jewish descent where two specific mutations account for most of the deficiencies. However, the remaining reported cases are from all racial and ethnic groups.
   - Unlike hemophilia A or B, the factor XI activity level does not correlate with the degree of bleeding manifestations. Bleeding tendency is generally mild to moderate, with some patients not showing a bleeding phenotype despite a severe deficiency with levels less than 10%. When bleeding is present, it is often at sites of high fibrinolytic activity.
   - It is an autosomal recessive disease.

8. **What are the inheritance characteristics and clinical features of the rarer inherited factor deficiencies?**
   - Rare bleeding disorders due to other clotting factor deficiencies can be identified by clinical history and a laboratory workup guided by screening coagulation tests ([PT, PTT, and thrombin time). This includes deficiencies of fibrinogen, factor II, factor V, combined factor V/factor VIII, factor VII, factor X, and factor XIII. Factor VII and XI deficiencies will be most common, making up nearly two-thirds of this group (see following table).

Rare bleeding disorder	Frequency	Bleeding sites	Other features	Treatment
FVII deficiency	37.5%	Intracranial	Can have thrombosis	rFVIIa (R), factor VII concentrate* (PD)
FXI deficiency	26.5%	Surgery or trauma	—	FFP, FXI concentrate* (PD)
FV deficiency	9.0%	N/A	—	FFP, platelets
Fibrinogen deficiency	8.0%	N/A	Miscarriage, thrombosis, splenic rupture	Fibrinogen concentrate (PD), FFP, cryoprecipitate
FX deficiency	8.0%	Intracranial	—	Factor X concentrate (PD), PCC

(continued)

Rare bleeding disorder	Frequency	Bleeding sites	Other features	Treatment
FXIII deficiency	6.5%	Intracranial, umblilical stump, menorrhagia	Normal PT/PTT, poor wound healing	Factor XIII A-subunit (R), Factor XIII concentrate (PD), cryoprecipitate
FV + FVIII deficiency	3.0%	See FV and FVIII deficiency	—	FFP or platelets, Factor VIII
FII	1.5%	N/A	—	PCC

*Available outside of the United States.

FFP, fresh plasma; N/A, not applicable; PCC, prothrombin complex concentrate, often contain factors II, IX, X, and sometimes VII; PD, plasma derived; R, recombinant.

- Inheritance is typically autosomal recessive.
- Historical clues may include a history of parental consanguineous marriage or a socially or geographically restricted population.
- Combined factor V and VIII deficiency is distinct from factor V and VIII deficiencies individually. This disorder is typically related to a mutation in the gene encoding a component involved in intracellular transport of these factors, the *LMAN1* gene, or the *MCFD2* gene that codes a cofactor for *LMAN1*.
- Factor XIII deficiency bleeding manifestations include delayed bleeding from the umbilical stump, recurrent abortion, poor wound healing, menorrhagia, intra-articular bleeding, and severe delayed bleeding. Coagulation screening tests (PT/PTT/fibrinogen) are normal in factor XIII deficiency.

9. **Describe the clinical features of vWD.**

- vWD is the most common congenital bleeding disorder and is important for platelet adhesion.
- Patients have mucocutaneous bleeding, menorrhagia, as well as immediate and delayed postoperative or posttraumatic bleeding.

10. **What are the three major types of vWD and the testing profile for each?**

- Type 1 is the most common type, characterized by a reduced level of normally functioning vWF. It is generally autosomal dominant in inheritance with variable penetrance. Testing shows a reduced vWF antigen (<30), reduced ristocetin cofactor assay (<30), a ratio of ristocetin cofactor to antigen >0.5 to 0.7, and a normal or slightly decreased factor VIII. All vWF multimers are present but reduced in concentration. In the type I vWD Vincenza, patients have a rapid clearance of vWF.
- Type 2 vWD is characterized by a qualitative defect in vWF. There are four subtypes of type 2 vWD (see the following table). It is generally autosomal dominant (type 2A, 2B, 2M), but can be autosomal recessive (type 2N). Type 2N shows a normal vWF antigen, normal ristocetin cofactor activity, with a

significant decrease in factor VIII; this may be confused with a diagnosis of hemophilia A.

- Type 3 vWD shows a marked quantitative deficiency in vWF with markedly reduced levels of vWF antigen, ristocetin cofactor activity, and factor VIII. It is inherited in an autosomal recessive fashion.

		vWF:RCo (IU/dL)	vWF:Ag (IU/dL)	FVIII	vWF:RCo/ vWF:Ag ratio
Type 1	Partial reduction in vWF	<30	<30	Low or normal	>0.5–0.7
Type 2A	Decreased platelet adhesion	<30	<30–200	Low or normal	<0.5–0.7
Type 2B	Increased affinity for platelet GP1b	<30	30–200	Low or normal	<0.5–0.7
Type 2M	Decreased platelet adhesion	<30	30–200	Low or normal	<0.5–0.7
Type 2N	Decreased binding for FVIII	30–200	30–200	Very low	<0.5–0.7
Type 3	vWF deficiency	<3	<3	<10 IU/dL	–
Low vWF		30–50	30–50	Normal	>0.5–0.7
Normal		50–200	50–200	Normal	>0.5–0.7

vWF, von Willebrand factor.

11. **How are the four qualitative defects representing type 2 vWD distinguished?**

- Type 2A has an absence of high- and intermediate-molecular-weight multimers. Ristocetin-induced platelet agglutination (RIPA) is reduced.
- Type 2B results in vWF that binds platelets spontaneously, resulting in thrombocytopenia. High-molecular-weight multimers are decreased or absent. RIPA is increased and type 2B vWF can agglutinate platelets at lower ristocetin concentrations (0.5 mg/mL) than normal vWF.
- Type 2M, similar to type 2A, has reduced platelet adhesion. However, 2M has the full spectrum of multimers.
- Type 2N vWF has reduced binding of factor VIII, resulting in reduced factor VIII but normal vWF levels.

12. **What are inherited primary vascular disorders associated with bleeding manifestations?**

- Hereditary hemorrhagic telangiectasia (Osler-Weber-Rendu or HHT) is one of the most notable, autosomal dominant, hereditary vascular disorders, with several identified mutations resulting in recurrent epistaxis, mucocutaneous telangiectasias, arteriovenous malformations of the lungs, liver, and cerebral vasculature, and intestinal bleeding.

- Ehlers-Danlos syndrome (EDS) is a group of autosomal dominant connective tissue disorders that can affect joint mobility, tissue integrity, and wound healing. Skin and joint hypermobility with potential dislocations or subluxations are seen, along with poor wound healing and autonomic instability. In vascular EDS, vascular rupture or organ rupture is possible. Genetic testing is indicated.

- Marfan syndrome is also a genetic connective tissue disorder that is associated with aortic root dilation (potentially manifesting as aortic aneurysms, aortic regurgitation, and aortic dissection), joint hypermobility, characteristic facial features and skeletal changes, tall stature, lens dislocation, and dural ectasia. Treatment consists of cardiac and vascular monitoring, can include cardiovascular pharmacotherapy, and may involve surgery for related complications.

13. **What is the management for hereditary hemorrhagic telangiectasia (HHT)?**
    - Management involves assessing for sites of affected vasculature, local therapy for epistaxis, embolization of pulmonary or gastrointestinal (GI) tract, arteriovenous malformations (AVMs), and ligation or coiling of brain AVMs. Experimental systemic therapy with agents like the antivascular endothelial growth factor A, monoclonal antibody, bevacizumab, or thalidomide may be considered for severe cases.

14. **Other vascular disorders:**
    - Several other hereditary vascular conditions can result in abnormal hemangiomas, small arteries, cutaneous vascular anomalies, cavernous malformations, capillary malformations, lymphedema from lymphatic malformations, and more. Treatment for these depends on the underlying condition and is often supportive. Large vascular hemangiomas as in Kasabach-Merritt syndrome are associated with chronic DIC.

ACQUIRED BLEEDING DISORDERS

1. **What situations are associated with acquired factor deficiencies or inhibitors?**
   - An acquired coagulopathy can be seen with vitamin K deficiency (poor intake, malabsorption, altered gut flora, etc.), liver disease, medications, postpartum, with autoimmune conditions, amyloidosis, inflammatory bowel disease, consumptive coagulopathies (disseminated intravascular coagulation [DIC], fibrinolysis, etc.), antiphospholipid antibodies, malignancy, nephrotic syndrome, massive transfusion, and idiopathically.

2. **What factor deficiency is most commonly associated with amyloidosis?**
   - Factor X

3. **Describe the pathogenesis and clinical findings of disseminated intravascular coagulation.**

   - Disseminated intravascular coagulation describes a consumptive coagulopathy characterized by dysregulated endogenous anticoagulant pathways and fibrinolysis with imbalanced coagulation. It is partially mediated by tissue factor and cytokines. Clinically, this can manifest most commonly as bleeding but also with thrombosis.

4. **What conditions can lead to the development of DIC?**

   - Infection, obstetric conditions such as retained dead fetus, malignancy, trauma, transfusion reactions, liver disease, extremes of temperature, allergic reactions, snake bites, and vascular abnormalities (Kasabach-Merritt) are several entities that have been associated with DIC.

5. **What are characteristic laboratory features and management of DIC?**

   - DIC is associated with prolonged clotting times (PT/ PTT), reduced fibrinogen, elevated fibrin degradation products (d-dimer), and thrombocytopenia.
   - Therapy is directed at the underlying condition. Transfusion support is complex with judicious use of fresh frozen plasma (FFP), cryoprecipitate, and platelets. Heparin is considered only in very select cases in the setting of thrombosis.
   - Antifibrinolytics should not be used.

HEMOSTATIC DRUGS

1. **Name two drugs that work to inhibit fibrinolysis and describe how they work.**

   - Aminocaproic acid and tranexamic acid compete for lysine binding sites on plasminogen and plasmin, thus preventing them from binding fibrin. They can be given IV or orally. Caution is needed in genitourinary bleeding due to the possibility of precipitating urinary retention due to obstructing ureteral clot.

2. **What are the therapeutic agents used for the treatment of hemophilia A and B?**

   - For hemophilia A and B, both recombinant and plasma-derived factor preparations are available. Cryoprecipitate contains factor VIII but is not typically used for primary treatment due to the risk of blood-borne pathogens and large volume required. Cryoprecipitate is not used for factor IX deficiency.
   - Factor VIII is dosed as the ([desired factor VIII level – baseline level] multiplied by weight in kilograms), multiplied by 0.5; desired dosing level and frequency vary based on the bleed location/severity, the product being used, and patient-specific factors.
   - Desmopressin intravenously (IV) or intranasally can also be considered for minor bleeding episodes, as it causes the release of factor VIII and von Willebrand factor from endothelial stores. It acts through type 2 vasopressin receptors. Adverse effects include flushing, headaches, hypotension, and antidiuretic effects. Free water should be restricted to reduce the risk of hyponatremia.

- For hemophilia B, recombinant factor IX or plasma-derived product replacements are available. Adult dosage is calculated as ([desired factor IX level – baseline level] multiplied by weight in kilograms) multiplied by 1.2. Dosing is dependent on the clinical situation.
- Antifibrinolytic is a useful adjunctive therapy to improve clot integrity and reduce early degradation.

Hemophilia A Treatment Options

Type	Half-life
Recombinant	9–17 hours
Plasma derived, M-Ab purified	15–18 hours
Extended half-life	13–20 hours
DDAVP*	—
Hemophilia B Treatment Options	
Recombinant	16–26 hours
Plasma derived, solvent/detergent treated	18 hours
Plasma derived; M-Ab purified	23 hours
Extended half-life	54–104 hours

*DDAVP not appropriate for severe hemophilia.

DDAVP, desmopression; M-Ab, monoclonal antibody, half-lives depend on the specific factor replacement product and population. Treatment recommendations may differ between adults and children.

3. How are coagulation factor inhibitors treated in patients with congenital hemophilia A?

- Long-term management can include inducing immune tolerance in appropriately selected hemophilia A patients through high-dose factor infusions. Drugs like intravenous immunoglobulin (IVIG), cyclophosphamide, and rituximab have also been used.
- For active bleeding or necessary surgical procedures, bypassing agents such as activated factor VII or factor VIII inhibitor (an activated prothrombin complex concentrate) are often used. Plasmapheresis and high-dose factor VIII infusion is also a consideration depending on the clinical scenario and inhibitor titer.

4. How are rare factor deficiencies treated?

- Factor XII, high-molecular-weight kininogen, and prekallikrein do not lead to bleeding.
- Most rare factor deficiencies are managed with fresh frozen plasma (FFP) but this can be challenging due to excessive volume. For a 70-kg adult, four units of FFP raise a factor level by 10%.
- Plasma-derived concentrates of factors X, factor XI, and factor XIII are available.

- Cryoprecipitate and plasma-derived fibrinogen concentrates can be used for dysfibrinogenemias or fibrinogen deficiency.
- Recombinant concentrates of factor VIIa and factor XIII are available.

5. **How is vWD treated?**
- The subtype and bleeding event influences treatment options.
- Minor bleeding can often be managed with topical thrombin and local measures.
- Type 1 and some type 2 vWD patients who previously demonstrated a response to desmopressin can use IV DDAVP or intranasal DDAVP for minor procedures or bleeding.
- Desmopressin in type 2B vWD has the potential to lower platelet counts and potentially induce platelet aggregation. Therefore, its use in type 2B remains controversial and should probably be avoided. Patients with type 2M have a short duration of response.
- The mainstay of therapy for bleeding or bleeding prophylaxis in type 2 or type 3 vWD is vWF replacement therapy from plasma-derived or recombinant vWF products. Cryoprecipitate has been used in the past but is no longer the standard of care. Purified and recombinant factor VIII preparations do not contain sufficient vWF and are not used.
- Adjunctive measures may include oral contraceptives for menorrhagia and/or antifibrinolytic agents like tranexamic acid or aminocaproic acid.

QUESTIONS

1. A 34-year-old man with limited medical history presents with recurrent epistaxis and prolonged bleeding following a dental extraction. He notes a history of easy bruising. His nose bleeds last for up to an hour and he has required medical intervention on several occasions to control the bleeding. A complete blood count (CBC) shows mild thrombocytopenia (134×10^9/L) but is otherwise normal. Prothrombin time (PT) and partial thromboplastin time (PTT) are normal. Review of the peripheral blood smear shows giant platelets. Which of the following is most likely to support the diagnosis?
   A. Von Willebrand factor activity, von Willebrand factor antigen, factor 8, multimer analysis
   B. Platelet function testing showing no aggregation with ristocetin
   C. Platelet function testing showing no aggregation to all agonists except ristocetin
   D. Platelet electron microscopy

2. A 65-year-old female, G2P2, is referred after screening labs performed prior to an elective cholecystectomy revealed a prolonged activated partial thromboplastin time (aPTT) of 67 seconds. The patient denies a history of easy bruising or menorrhagia. She has tolerated numerous operations including a bowel resection and appendectomy without any bleeding complications. She has never required a blood transfusion and denies mucocutaneous bleeding. Review of her medical

records reveals her aPTT has been prolonged for many years, even before these operations. Physical exam is unremarkable. Complete blood count (CBC) and prothrombin time (PT) are normal. The aPTT corrects when mixed with an equal volume of normal plasma. Which is the most likely diagnosis?
A. Factor V deficiency
B. Factor VIII inhibitor
C. Factor XI deficiency
D. Factor XII deficiency

3. An 82-year-old man with moderate dementia is brought to the emergency department unresponsive with evidence of hematemesis after he was found down in his assisted living facility. His medications are unknown, but he has a reported history that includes hypertension, diabetes mellitus, transient ischemic attack (TIA), chronic back pain, coronary artery disease, and atrial fibrillation. The patient is afebrile, hypotensive, and has a rapid and irregular pulse. He is slow to respond. Physical exam is notable for small scattered ecchymoses and dried blood in the posterior oropharynx. Complete blood count (CBC) shows a hemoglobin of 6.8 g/dL and a normal platelet value. Prothrombin time (PT) is prolonged, corresponding to an international normalized ratio (INR) of 9.2. Activated partial thromboplastin time (aPTT) is prolonged at 52 seconds. The peripheral blood smear is normal. Aspartate aminotransferase (AST) is 76, alanine aminotransferase (ALT) is 64, and bilirubin and albumin are normal. CT head is negative. Laboratory testing is most likely to reveal which of the following?
A. Low fibrinogen related to hepatic synthetic dysfunction
B. Failure of the clotting times to correct by adding an equal volume of plasma
C. Low fibrinogen related to disseminated intravascular coagulation (DIC)
D. Reduced levels of factors II, VII, IX, and X

4. A 64-year-old male who is currently receiving adjuvant chemotherapy for colon cancer was recently hospitalized for neutropenic fever. In addition to thrombocytopenia, he was found to have an abnormal activated partial thromboplastin time (aPTT) of 52 seconds. Prothrombin time in the hospital was 12 seconds. He is referred for further evaluation. He denies any recent or historic bleeding, but has had a blood transfusion during the course of his colon surgery and chemotherapy. He has no personal or family history of thrombosis. Hemoglobin is 9.6 g/dL, platelets 136 × 10⁹/L, white blood cells (WBCs) 6.4 × 10⁹/L. His exam shows scattered small ecchymoses and no splenomegaly. What is the best next step for his evaluation?
A. Mixing study
B. Thrombin time and reptilase time
C. Factor XII assay
D. Repeat the lab from a peripheral blood draw

5. A 36-year-old woman with a longstanding history of menorrhagia, mucocutaneous bleeding, and easy bruising is referred for further evaluation. Hemoglobin is 9.8 g/dL, mean corpuscular volume (MCV) is 74 fL, platelets are 86,000 × 109/L, and white blood cell (WBC) count is normal. Prothrombin time (PT) and partial thromboplastin time (PTT) are normal. Further workup shows von Willebrand factor (vWF) activity (ristocetin cofactor assay) is 26%, vWF antigen is 58%, factor VIII is 96%. Multimer analysis reveals no high-molecular-weight multimers. Platelet aggregometry shows aggregation with 0.5 mg/mL of ristocetin. Which is the most likely diagnosis?
   A. Type 1 von Willebrand disease (vWD)
   B. Type 2A vWD
   C. Type 2B vWD
   D. Type 2M vWD

6. A 36-year-old female is admitted with a splenic laceration and intra-abdominal bleeding after being involved in a motor vehicle accident. She is unconscious on arrival and head CT shows a small subdural hematoma. Over the course of 6 hours, her hemoglobin dropped from 9.6 g/dL at presentation to 7.8 g/dL. Her platelet count is normal, as is the prothrombin time (PT) and activated partial thromboplastin time (aPTT). LDH, total bilirubin, and haptoglobin were normal. Reticulocytes are elevated and there are numerous polychromatophilic cells on peripheral smear. Her family reports and outside medical records confirm she has a history of factor XIII deficiency diagnosed after she had experienced menorrhagia. She has not required therapy since having a hysterectomy several years ago. She also had delayed umbilical cord bleeding and separation. The hospital has ordered recombinant factor XIII, but does not have any available. She has received 3 L of intravenous (IV) normal saline for low blood pressures and a blood transfusion has been initiated. What should be done for her factor deficiency?
   A. Supportive care until the arrival of the recombinant factor XIII
   B. Factor VIIa
   C. Cryoprecipitate
   D. Desmopressin

7. Which of the following facts about von Willebrand factor (vWF) is correct?
   A. von Willebrand disease (vWD) is the second most common congenital bleeding disorder.
   B. Thrombocytopenia is associated with type 2M vWD.
   C. Type 2N vWD presents with normal vWF antigen, normal vWF ristocetin cofactor activity, and reduced factor VIII level.
   D. vWF antigen and activity levels are higher in type 3 compared to type 1 vWD.

ANSWERS

1. **B. Platelet function testing showing no aggregation with ristocetin.**
   The bleeding history is suggestive of a platelet function disorder as it
   is out of proportion with the mild thrombocytopenia, and the smear
   reveals giant platelets. While family history is not discussed, an autosomal
   recessive pattern may be observed. Overall, this would be concerning for
   a diagnosis of Bernard-Soulier syndrome. Platelet function testing would
   be expected to show absence of aggregation in response to ristocetin.
   This is due to a defective glycoprotein Ib/IX/V receptor. Tests listed in
   choice A evaluate von Willebrand disease, which is not characterized
   by giant platelets. The platelet aggregation pattern in choice C is
   consistent with Glanzmann thrombasthenia. The platelet number,
   size, and morphology on light microscopy is normal in Glanzmann's
   thrombasthenia, which would be expected to have normal platelet values
   and morphology. Routine platelet electron microscopy, as in choice
   D, is generally performed to evaluate intracellular granules, which are
   decreased in a platelet storage pool deficiency.

2. **D. Factor XII deficiency.** This patient has a longstanding abnormal clotting time without any bleeding history. Of the choices, only D, factor XII
   deficiency, is not associated with bleeding and she can be cleared to
   proceed with surgery if the diagnosis is confirmed. Choice A, factor V,
   would affect both the aPTT and PT given that factor V is part of the final
   common pathway. Choice B, factor VIII inhibitor, would not be supported
   by the mixing study that suggests a factor deficiency. Factor XI deficiency,
   or hemophilia B, would be expected to be associated with bleeding,
   especially given the degree of prolongation of her aPTT.

3. **D. Reduced levels of factors II, VII, IX, and X.** The history is concerning
   for warfarin toxicity resulting in a gastrointestinal bleed. The patient has
   a history of atrial fibrillation and comorbidities that could indicate a need
   for warfarin. Warfarin results in a reduction in the vitamin K–dependent
   clotting factors. While the PT/INR is most sensitive to abnormalities in
   factor VII of the extrinsic pathway, reductions in the remaining vitamin
   K–dependent factors will impact the aPTT as well. For answer A, albumin
   and bilirubin are normal and there is no history to suggest liver disease.
   The PT and aPTT are higher than would be anticipated for isolated liver
   disease. Answer B describes a mixing study result that would implicate an
   inhibitor of a component of the common pathway or a lupus anticoagulant. Acquired spontaneous inhibitors of factors in the common pathway
   are rare. His known medical history does not include autoimmune disease, malignancy, or recent cardiac surgery in which bovine thrombin
   was used (associated with development of a factor V inhibitor). A mixing
   study could be obtained but would be more likely to indicate a factor
   deficiency. There are insufficient physical findings or laboratory evidence
   to suggest DIC. His normal platelet count and blood smear make a consumptive coagulopathy.

4. **D. Repeat the lab from a peripheral blood draw.** An abnormal lab is a common indication for referral. In this case, the patient has no bleeding or clotting history. It could be assumed that the lab may have been drawn through a chemotherapy port and thus may be prolonged by heparin contamination. Repeating the lab through a peripheral blood draw or, if that is not possible, through the port after adequate flushing of the line would obviate the need for more extensive or costly workup. If the prolonged aPTT was still felt to be heparin contamination (in this clinical setting, this is a valid concern), answer B could be a reasonable choice. Heparin contamination would be expected to prolong the thrombin time but not affect the reptilase time. If the patient had a significant bleeding history or heparin contamination was not suspected, a mixing study could be considered. Many mixing studies will include a thrombin time or use a heparinase to limit potential interference from heparin. Answer C, factor XII, could be an explanation for an isolated prolonged aPTT in this clinical setting but would not be the next best test.

5. **C. Type 2B vWD.** The patient has a clinical history consistent with vWD and likely a concurrent iron deficiency anemia. Patients with type 2B vWD have a gain-of-function mutation in the platelet GpIb binding domain on vWF that allows for vWF to bind spontaneously with platelets in vivo and in the presence of low concentrations of ristocetin in platelet aggregation assays. Spontaneous binding of vWF in vivo and clearance of vWF–platelet complexes by the spleen can result in thrombocytopenia. vWF multimer analysis shows absence of high molecular vWF multimers. The ratio of the vWF activity (ristocetin cofactor activity) to vWF antigen is less than 0.5, consistent with type 2 vWD. These labs are not consistent with the other choices.

6. **C. Cryoprecipitate.** A factor XIII level should be obtained, but the results would not be immediately available to guide management. A recombinant factor XIII A-subunit product is available in the United States, that when administered, combines with free factor XIII B-subunit to then function similar to endogenous factor XIII. However, given that it is not available, cryoprecipitate, based on weight, is the best option of the listed choices. Fresh frozen plasma could be considered but there would be concerns about the volume required in the setting of a severe bleed. Supportive care would not be appropriate given the critical nature of the bleed. Factor VIIa and desmopressin would not be the best choice in this situation. Animal studies showed thrombotic complications when factor VIIa and XIII A-subunit were given together at high doses. Desmopressin monotherapy would be insufficient for initial resuscitation.

7. **C. Type 2N vWD presents with normal vWF antigen, normal vWF ristocetin cofactor activity, and reduced factor VIII level.** vWD is the most common congenital bleeding disorder. Thrombocytopenia can be associated with type 2B vWD. vWF antigen and activity levels are lower in type 3 compared to type 1 vWD.

Thrombosis

9

Jordan K. Schaefer and Suman L. Sood

HEREDITARY THROMBOPHILIAS

1. **What are the five most common inherited thrombophilias and the mechanism by which they promote thrombosis?**
   - The five major inherited thrombophilias include factor V Leiden gene mutation, prothrombin gene mutation, and deficiency of the natural anticoagulants, protein C, protein S, and antithrombin. Combinations of these thrombophilias are possible.

   The Prevalence and Outcomes of Inherited Thrombophilias

	Population prevalence	Prevalence with VTE	RR for initial VTE	RR for recurrent VTE
1) Factor V Leiden	3%–7%	20%	3–5	1.4
2) Prothrombin 20210A mutation	0.7%–4%	5%	2–3	1.4
3) Protein C deficiency	0.2%	3%	4–6.5	1.4–1.8
4) Protein S deficency	0.03%–0.13%	2%	1–10	1.0–1.4
5) Antithrombin deficiency	0.02%	1%	5–10	1.9–2.6

   RR, relative risk; VTE, venous thromboembolism.

   - Factor V Leiden polymorphism confers resistance to activated protein C–mediated inactivation of activated factor V, therefore relatively increasing the amount of activated factor V available to convert prothrombin to thrombin. It is the most common inherited thrombophilia in Caucasians, but is less often seen in African American or Asian populations. It is most often seen in the heterozygous state (with 5–10 fold increase in thrombotic risk); homozygous individuals are at a significantly higher risk of venous thromboembolism. There is conflicting data on the effect of the mutation on arterial thrombosis; the vast majority of thrombosis will be venous.
   - Prothrombin G20210A mutation is a gain-of-function mutation that leads to increased levels of prothrombin (factor II). As a result, there is more thrombin available to convert fibrinogen to fibrin and interact with other elements of the coagulation cascade. Similar to factor V Leiden, a heterozygous status confers a modestly increased risk of venous thrombosis (2–3 fold) and this risk is higher when homozygous.

- Protein C deficiency is usually an autosomal dominant condition, and most adults are diagnosed in the heterozygous state. Protein C levels for these patients are typically about half of normal. The reduction in the amount of this "natural anticoagulant" leads to increased thrombotic rates. Recall that protein C is activated by thrombin complexed with thrombomodulin, and it exerts an anticoagulant effect by inactivating coagulation factors Va and VIIIa through the activated protein C complex (see factor V Leiden in the preceding text). A quantitative defect (type I) or a qualitative/functional defect of protein C (type II) may exist. Adults most often experience recurrent venous thromboembolism but neonatal purpura fulminans has been described in homozygous children with a severe deficiency. Given that warfarin decreases protein C faster than other coagulation factors, warfarin can precipitate skin necrosis by disturbing the balance between pro- and anticoagulant factors. Venous thromboembolic events are more common with protein C deficiency, but rarely arterial events may occur.

- Protein S deficiency is an autosomal dominant condition. Protein S circulates bound to C4b binding protein and as a free form. Deficiency can be a result of a quantitative disorder with proportionately reduced total protein S, free form, and activity (type I); a reduction in the activity, but with a normal total protein S and free form (type II); or a reduction in both the free protein S and the activity, but with a normal total protein S (type III). Clinically, it is similar to protein C deficiency. Neonatal purpura fulminans can occur in the homozygous state, and warfarin-induced skin necrosis can also occur.

- Antithrombin deficiency is an autosomal dominant condition with variable penetrance and can be either a quantitative defect (type 1) or a qualitative defect (type II) that is associated with recurrent venous thrombosis, both unprovoked and in association with other risk factors. The loss or impaired activity of antithrombin represents the loss of a "natural anticoagulant" and therefore disrupts the hemostatic balance. Recall that antithrombin inactivates several of the coagulation cascade enzymes, especially thrombin (factor IIa), factor IXa, and factor Xa, and that the activity of antithrombin is markedly increased by the activity of endogenous or exogenous heparins. Patients with antithrombin deficiency can demonstrate heparin resistance; this can be overcome by administering antithrombin. Pregnant patients with antithrombin deficiency are at an especially increased risk of thrombosis and can have adverse pregnancy outcomes. During pregnancy, antithrombin concentrates, along with low-molecular-weight heparin, are often considered. When evaluating patients for antithrombin deficiency, as with protein C and S deficiency, the timing of laboratory testing (discussed in the following text) is important, given that a variety of conditions can result in an acquired, rather than inherited, low antithrombin level.

2. **What are the general principles of evaluation and management for inherited thrombophilias?**

   - Family history is important in determining whom to screen for a thrombophilia, as penetrance and clinical expression of inherited thrombophilias is quite variable.

   - Management relies mostly on the clinical history of the particular patient and knowledge of a thrombophilia may not always change management. Asymptomatic individuals with a strong inherited thrombophilia (homozygous factor V Leiden, homozygous prothrombin gene mutation, heterozygous pro-thrombin gene mutation plus heterozygous factor V Leiden, or deficiency of antithrombin, protein C, or protein S) and no history of thrombosis should be considered for thrombosis prophylaxis during high-risk situations like pro-longed periods of travel, pregnancy, or postoperatively. Females considering estrogen-containing oral contraceptives should consider alternative contracep-tive options, given their increased risk of thrombosis.

- The presence of a strong thrombophilia (defined earlier) may influence deci-sions on length of anticoagulation in the setting of thrombosis (favoring long-term extended venous thromboembolism [VTE] prophylaxis). However, this is mostly based on expert opinion. See "Laboratory Testing and Imaging" section for indications of thrombophilia testing.

- As with any genetic condition, there are possible implications for children and family members when a diagnosis is made.

3. **What disorders of fibrinolysis can lead to increased rates of thrombosis?**
   - Deficient or defective plasminogen, tissue plasminogen activator, and increased levels of plasminogen activator inhibitor-1 can theoretically be associated with increased venous or arterial thrombosis. These are not widely tested clinically.
   - Dysfibrinogenemias are a group of generally autosomal dominant disorders in which an abnormal structure or function of fibrin impairs normal fibrinolysis and thus can be associated with thrombosis and/or bleeding.

ACQUIRED THROMBOTIC DISORDERS

1. **What situations are associated with an increased risk of venous throm-bosis?**
   - Situational factors include recent surgery or trauma, hospitalization, long peri-ods (generally greater than 4 hours) of travel, the presence of foreign material (like an intravascular device), pregnancy or exposure to estrogen, and immo-bility (e.g., using a cast).

2. **What diseases are associated with an increased risk of venous throm-bosis?**
   - Generally, any systemic inflammatory process like malignancy, infection, trauma, and many autoimmune disorders can increase the rate of thrombosis. Different malignancy subtypes are associated with a spectrum of thrombotic risk. Diseases associated with protein loss (nephrotic syndrome) may cause an acquired thrombophilia. Specific hematological disorders, including antiphos-pholipid antibody syndrome, myeloproliferative neoplasms, paroxysmal nocturnal hemoglobinuria, plasma cell dyscrasias, heparin-induced thrombo-cytopenia, and hemoglobinopathies are associated, to various degrees, with an increased risk of thrombosis through various mechanisms. There is conflicting evidence, but metabolic syndrome, chronic kidney disease, and vascular disease are also mildly associated with venous thromboembolism.

3. **What medications are associated with an increased risk of venous thrombosis?**
   - Hormonal contraceptives, hormone replacement, erythropoiesis-stimulating agents, testosterone, tamoxifen, bevacizumab, thalidomide or lenalidomide,

L-asparaginase, various other chemotherapeutic agents, and corticosteroids are all associated with venous thrombosis.

4. **What anatomic variations are associated with venous thrombosis and how are they managed?**

- Iliac vein compression syndrome (May-Thurner syndrome) generally results in a predisposition to left-sided venous thrombosis as a result of the right common iliac artery compressing the left common iliac vein against the lumbar spine. It most commonly occurs in young females and may require computed tomography venous (CTV) or magnetic resonance venous (MRV) imaging to diagnose due to the anatomic location of the defect. Management of symptomatic disease often involves endovascular therapy with possible stenting.

- "Effort-induced" upper extremity deep vein thrombosis (Paget-Schroetter syndrome) generally is the result of compression of the subclavian vein as it courses between the clavicle and first rib in the setting of repeated, often over-head activity of the ipsilateral upper extremity (e.g., a tennis player). Cervical ribs, anomalous tendon insertions, anterior scalene, or subclavius hypertrophy may contribute to the compression. The inflammatory response to the compression ultimately leads to upper extremity thrombosis that tends to propagate distally to the axillary veins. The mechanical obstruction may limit the risk of large central embolic events. Ultrasound is often used in the diagnosis, but CT or MR venography may be needed due to technical limitations with ultrasound. Therapy may include thrombolysis, systemic anticoagulation, and surgical thoracic outlet decompression.

- Congenital abnormalities of the inferior vena cava can also be associated with deep vein thrombosis. Anticoagulation is the mainstay of therapy for most abnormalities.

5. **What are other venous thrombosis risk factors?**

- Modifiable factors include obesity and smoking
- Nonmodifiable risk factors include age and male sex

6. **What are causes of arterial thrombosis? What evaluation can be done?**

- Arterial thrombosis can commonly result from a cardioembolic source as seen in atrial fibrillation or atrial flutter, endocarditis, cardiac tumors, and with a ventricular aneurysm, such as after myocardial infarction. A paradoxical embolism occurs when a venous thrombosis travels to the arterial side of circulation through a cardiac defect such as a patent foramen ovale. Arterial thromboemboli can also occur related to atherosclerotic plaque, typically at large-vessel bifurcations, or in association with vascular aneurysms. Other mechanical sources of arterial thrombosis include arterial dissection, fibromuscular dysplasia, vasculitis, arterial wall infection/arteritis, and from dislodgement of a thrombus after a procedure. Generally, any systemic inflammatory process like malignancy or inflammatory autoimmune disorders may also predispose to arterial thrombosis. Some specific considerations include cocaine use, cold agglutinins, cryoglobulinemia, dysfibrinogenemia, hyperviscosity, antiphospholipid antibody syndrome, paroxysmal nocturnal hemoglobinuria, heparin-induced thrombocytopenia, myeloproliferative neoplasms, and significant hyperhomocysteinemia, among others.

- Testing for these conditions can be considered, depending on the clinical situation. Inherited thrombophilias are rarely associated with arterial thrombosis and testing is generally of low yield.

7. What is the difference between atheroembolism and thromboembolism? What are the risk factors for atherosclerosis?

- Atherosclerosis can be a source of emboli, either from thromboembolism of a thrombus associated with an atherosclerotic plaque, or less commonly, atheroembolism from dislodgement of the material that makes up the plaque (cholesterol embolization syndrome). The latter (atheroembolism) is more commonly triggered by vascular intervention such as a cardiac catheterization, but can rarely occur spontaneously. Aortic thromboembolism needs to be distinguished from atheroembolism (cholesterol embolization) as the treatment is different. Thromboembolism often presents as sudden occlusion of a medium-to-large vessel and is often treated with anticoagulation or antiplatelet therapy. Atheroembolism often affects multiple locations and small arterioles ("blue toe syndrome"). It may be associated with eosinophilia and livedo reticularis.
- Risk factors for atherosclerosis include smoking, hypertension, hyperlipidemia, diabetes mellitus (metabolic syndrome), and age.

8. What is heparin-induced thrombocytopenia (HIT) and when should HIT be suspected?

- HIT is an adverse reaction to heparin that paradoxically leads to thrombosis rather than bleeding. The mechanism is complex but results from platelet factor 4, released from the alpha granules of platelets, binding to heparin, which triggers an immune response, resulting in an immunoglobulin G (IgG) class antibody targeted against the heparin–platelet factor 4 complex. This culminates in platelet activation through cross-linking FcγIIA receptors that promotes thrombosis; thrombocytopenia results from splenic clearance of the IgG complex.
- There is a greater risk of HIT in patients receiving unfractionated heparin relative to low-molecular-weight heparin, in those therapeutically anticoagulated relative to prophylactically, and in surgical patients over medical. Characteristically, it develops 5 to 14 days from exposure to heparin therapy. The platelets decrease in a characteristic pattern (typically an abrupt drop of 50%) and typically nadir at values above 20,000.
- Patients with a history of heparin exposure within the past 3 months can have a rapid onset (within 48 hours) of HIT upon reexposure to the drug due to previously formed antibodies.
- While overall the incidence is rare, given the severe consequences of the condition, it should be suspected with a declining platelet count for any patient receiving, or having received, heparin-based therapy. A 50% drop in platelet count should prompt consideration of HIT, even if it has not reached the level of absolute thrombocytopenia. Additionally, it should be in the differential with any clinical manifestations consistent with HIT (see the following text).

9. **What are some of the clinical manifestations of HIT?**

   - New or worsening venous thrombosis is one of the most common, severe complications of HIT. Arterial thromboses can also occur, manifesting as limb ischemia or organ infarction. Heparin-induced skin necrosis, typically at the injection site can occur. Some patients also will experience a systemic reaction (fevers, chills, vital sign changes, shortness of breath) after starting intravenous heparin. Despite the presence of thrombocytopenia and anticoagulation, bleeding is not common. Adrenal thrombosis and secondary hemorrhage has also been described.

10. **What is the "4Ts score" and how is it applied to the evaluation of suspected HIT?**

    - The 4Ts score is a risk prediction score for the diagnosis of HIT, which is composed of four elements, awarding 0 to 2 points based on clinical or laboratory parameters. The elements are thrombocytopenia, timing, thrombosis, and other causes of thrombocytopenia. Patients with ≤3 points are considered low risk, 4 to 5 points are intermediate risk, and ≥6 points are high risk (Chapter 7).

    - Other scoring systems are available but have not shown superior performance.

    - While clinical judgement is important, some providers use the 4Ts score to guide initial management, with a low-risk score not requiring additional testing. Those with intermediate- or high-risk scores typically are tested with an antiplatelet factor 4 enzyme-linked immunosorbent assay (ELISA) and possibly a serotonin release assay. During this time, there is strong consideration of stopping heparin anticoagulation and starting an alternative anticoagulant (direct thrombin inhibitor) while awaiting the result. Given the high risk of thrombosis in unrecognized HIT and the risk of bleeding with alternative anticoagulants in other causes of thrombocytopenia, initial management can be challenging, especially with intermediate-risk patients.

    - It is important to recognize that the diagnosis is based on clinical features in conjunction with laboratory findings. At times, the diagnosis can be made with an antiplatelet factor 4 ELISA in the right clinical setting, but the functional serotonin release assay is often required.

11. **How is HIT managed?**

    - Alternative, non-heparin anticoagulants (discussed in the following text) are used with diagnosed HIT or suspected HIT in patients at intermediate or higher risk. Ultrasounds of the upper and lower extremities should be considered to rule out the presence of a clot, as it would affect the duration of anticoagulation. Heparin should be strictly avoided (heparin flushes, prophylaxis, etc.) in diagnosed HIT and in those with suspicion of HIT. Warfarin should be avoided until the platelet count has normalized (>150,000), given the risk of venous limb gangrene. Once started, it should be overlapped for at least 5 days with another anticoagulant. Anticoagulation should continue for at least 3 months in the presence of thrombosis, and, while data is limited, at least 4 weeks in the absence of thrombosis.

- Patients with a remote history of HIT (>3 months in the past) and negative laboratory testing for HIT who require heparin, as with cardiopulmonary bypass, often can be briefly exposed to heparin for cardiac surgery and then use an alternative, non-heparin anticoagulant if needed postoperatively. For those who have positive HIT serologies or a more recent HIT diagnosis, when surgery cannot be delayed, performing the surgery using a direct thrombin inhibitor should be considered. Additionally, plasmapheresis can be considered.

12. When should antiphospholipid antibody syndrome (APLAS) be suspected?

- Antiphospholipid syndrome can be a primary autoimmune disorder or secondary to another condition like systemic lupus erythematosus.

- Clinical manifestations can range from asymptomatic to catastrophic antiphospholipid syndrome, which is characterized by diffuse thrombosis, affecting at least three organ systems simultaneously or within the course of a week. Catastrophic antiphospholipid syndrome can manifest similarly to thrombotic microangiopathies, heparin-induced thrombocytopenia, and disseminated intravascular coagulation.

- APLAS should be considered when a patient has venous, arterial, or small-vessel thrombosis, premature births related to preeclampsia or placental insufficiency, late miscarriages after 10 weeks, or recurrent embryonic losses (less than 10 weeks) without another explanation. Thromboses are most commonly venous. Some patients have associated neurologic symptoms like migraines, seizures, or strokes. Nonbacterial endocarditis has been reported and should be considered in the case of stroke. There is also an increased risk of myocardial infarction. Adrenal, cutaneous, ocular, osseous, and renal manifestations are also rarely associated.

- Generally, laboratory clues can include a mild-to-moderate thrombocytopenia, a false-positive test for syphilis, or an unexplained prolongation of the activated partial thromboplastin time.

13. What are the Revised Sapporo Antiphospholipid Syndrome Classification Criteria?

- The Sapporo Classification Criteria require at least one clinical criterion and one laboratory criterion. The laboratory criterion must be present on two occasions at least 12 weeks apart.

- Clinical criteria can be a vascular thrombosis or pregnancy morbidity. Vascular thromboses can be venous, arterial, or small vessel, in any tissue or organ. They should be confirmed on imaging, Doppler studies, or histopathology. Pregnancy morbidity can be one or more unexplained fetal deaths after 10 weeks gestation with a morphologically normal fetus; one or more premature births of a morphologically normal neonate (before 34 weeks gestation) due to eclampsia; severe preeclampsia or placental insufficiency; or finally, three or more unexplained consecutive spontaneous abortions before the 10th week of gestation.

- Laboratory criteria (reviewed in the "Laboratory Testing and Imaging" section) require medium- or high-titer immunoglobulin G (IgG) or IgM β_2Gp1 and/or anticardiolipin antibodies, or the presence of a lupus anticoagulant.

14. **What is the management of antiphospholipid syndrome? What can be added for catastrophic antiphospholipid syndrome?**

    • Treatment may vary depending on the clinical presentation and ongoing investigation. Initial management of thrombotic events is similar to that of other patients with thrombosis. Indefinite anticoagulation is recommended due to the high risk of recurrent thrombosis. Patients are often treated with long-term warfarin (target international normalized ratio [INR] 2–3) or low-molecular-weight heparin (LMWH), as studies are still pending with newer agents. A higher INR target has not shown superior outcomes in patients with an initial thrombotic event.

    • LMWH at therapeutic doses, as well as baby aspirin, is used in pregnancy for definite antiphospholipid syndrome and past thrombosis. Similar management is used for obstetric antiphospholipid syndrome during pregnancy (with the exception that prophylactic anticoagulation is often used in the absence of history of thrombosis). Some recent data suggest that women with obstetric APLAS remain at increased long-term risk to develop thrombosis even outside of pregnancy.

    • There is conflicting data on the additional benefit of adding aspirin to warfarin in antiphospholipid syndrome following an arterial thrombosis, but it is used in pregnancy as already mentioned.

    • Antibody-positive patients who do not have a history of clinical events (thus not meeting criteria for APLAS) are generally not anticoagulated. Treatment with hydroxychloroquine, often for a concurrent autoimmune condition, may lower thrombotic risk.

    • Laboratory monitoring of anticoagulation in antiphospholipid syndrome may be complicated by antibody interference with prothrombin times and activated prothrombin time. Chromogenic factor X assays or correlating factor II levels to the INR can be considered, among other strategies.

    • Catastrophic antiphospholipid syndrome has a high mortality rate. Therapy may include anticoagulation, steroids, plasma exchange, intravenous immunoglobulin (IVIG), and treating any potential provoking cause like infection. Some clinicians have added rituximab or eculizumab.

15. **What diagnoses should be considered in splanchnic vein thrombosis?**

    • Malignancy or other provoking factors (cirrhosis, pancreatitis, etc.) are the most common etiologies. These vascular territories can be associated with paroxysmal nocturnal hemoglobinuria and myeloproliferative neoplasms. Many clinicians consider testing for the JAK2 V617F mutation and consider exon 12, or further evaluation for a myeloproliferative disorder like polycythemia vera. Antiphospholipid antibodies are also considered.

16. **What diagnoses should be considered with cerebral vein thrombosis?**

    • Pregnancy or other hormonal therapy is the most common provoking factor. Paroxysmal nocturnal hemoglobinuria can also be associated with cerebral venous sinus. Additionally, myeloproliferative disorders and antiphospholipid antibody syndrome may be considered. There is some data to suggest that prothrombin gene mutation is seen with a higher incidence in cerebral vein thrombosis.

THROMBOSIS MANAGEMENT

1. **How long should a first, provoked, proximal deep vein thrombosis or pulmonary embolism be anticoagulated?**
   - At least 3 months. Thrombophilia workup is not indicated.

2. **How long should a first, unprovoked, proximal deep vein thrombosis or pulmonary embolism be anticoagulated?**
   - Indefinite anticoagulation should be considered in patients with acceptable bleeding risk. However, this may vary based on patient-specific recurrence risk, preferences, and comorbidities. Please note that after an initial period of 6 to 12 months, extended venous thromboembolism (VTE) prophylaxis may consist of either therapeutic or prophylactic dosing regimens, depending on the clinical situation.

3. **How long should a second, unprovoked, proximal deep vein thrombosis or pulmonary embolism be anticoagulated?**
   - Indefinite anticoagulation should, again, be considered depending on the particular circumstances.

4. **With what agent and for how long should a proximal deep vein thrombosis or pulmonary embolism be managed in the setting of active cancer?**
   - Low molecular weight heparin has shown a lower risk of recurrent venous thrombosis compared to warfarin, in patients with cancer. In the absence of renal impairment, low-molecular-weight heparin is therefore often utilized. Some evidence has supported the use of the direct oral anticoagulants edoxaban and rivaroxaban for cancer associated venous thrombosis. However, these anticoagulants may have a higher rate of bleeding. At least 3 to 6 months of therapy is indicated, but many providers continue anticoagulation as long as patients have ongoing risk factors (active cancer, immobility, etc.).

5. **What are the treatment options for distal/calf deep vein thromboses?**
   - Deep vein thromboses of the anterior/posterior tibial, peroneal, or muscular veins of the calf (gastrocnemius or soleal veins), in the absence of popliteal or more proximal involvement, may be anticoagulated similar to a proximal deep vein thrombosis. This is often done if patients have significant symptoms or risk factors for propagation (immobility, active cancer, history of thrombosis, etc.). Alternatively, reliable patients can be monitored with serial ultrasounds and anticoagulated if thrombus extension is observed. The ultrasound is often repeated at 7 to 14 days.

6. **What are the treatment options for superficial deep vein thrombosis?**
   - Management depends on the clinical scenario and veins affected. For a superficial vein thrombosis under 5 cm in length, distant from the confluence with the deep veins (the sapheno–femoral junction), supportive care is indicated. Surgical intervention or antibiotic therapy may be indicated in select situations.
   - For patients with superficial venous thrombosis that is close to the sapheno–femoral junction, or longer than 5 cm, anticoagulation is indicated, typically

for 45 days duration. Fondaparinux or rivaroxaban are commonly considered agents at prophylactic doses, but other direct oral anticoagulants, unfractionated heparin, and low-molecular-weight heparin are also likely effective.

7. **What considerations are needed for managing acute splanchnic vein thrombosis (hepatic vein, portal vein, mesenteric vein, splenic vein)?**
   - Given the potential for esophageal varices from underlying portal hypertension, management of or screening for varices may be indicated before starting anticoagulation. Optimal management is unclear, given limited data, but some providers do not anticoagulate asymptomatic, incidentally detected thromboses. Many of these patients are at high risk for bleeding, given underlying cirrhosis, malignancy, and/or thrombocytopenia from splenomegaly. Data for management of chronic thrombosis is controversial.

8. **What are absolute or relative contraindications to anticoagulation?**
   - Anticoagulation is often avoided or dose adjusted in the setting of thrombocytopenia (platelets less than $30{,}000\text{–}50{,}000 \times 10^9/\text{L}$), around the time of surgery, in the setting of intracranial hemorrhage, or with recent or active bleeding.
   - The risks and benefits of anticoagulation must be carefully considered with esophageal varices, altered drug metabolism as a result of liver or renal impairment, trauma, active labor, peptic ulcer disease, poor follow-up or social support, substance abuse, CNS lesions, and those at risk for falls or trauma.

9. **What should be considered in a patient with a venous thrombosis that cannot be anticoagulated?**
   - A temporary inferior vena cava (IVC) filter can be considered. This should be removed as soon as feasible to avoid long-term complications of IVC filters (perforation, increased lower extremity deep vein thrombosis [DVT], etc.).

10. **When should thrombolytic therapy be considered?**
    - The decision to pursue thrombolysis is very complex, patient specific, and generally beyond the scope of this review. It can be considered in the care of patients who are hemodynamically unstable as a result of massive pulmonary embolism, in carefully selected patients without contraindications who experience an ischemic stroke, in select cases of myocardial infarction, and in select episodes of arterial thrombosis. Thrombolytic therapy can be administered systemically or catheter directed.
    - Management decisions depend on the severity and clinical manifestations of the thrombotic event within the clinical context of the specific patient, especially bleeding risk, given the potential for catastrophic bleeding complications. Mechanical thrombectomy alone may be used in some situations. Care is often multidisciplinary, influenced by institutional resources and expertise.

THROMBOSIS COMPLICATIONS

1. **What diagnosis should be considered if a patient is found to have pulmonary hypertension or unexplained exertional dyspnea? What imaging should be considered? What is the treatment?**

- Chronic thromboembolic pulmonary hypertension (CTEPH) can be a complication of longstanding obstruction of the pulmonary arteries, eventually leading to pulmonary hypertension and right-sided heart failure. Ventilation perfusion scans and CT angiography are usually the initial diagnostic imaging tests. Echocardiography and right heart catheterization are often part of the evaluation. There are several other differential diagnoses that should be excluded in the workup. Treatment includes anticoagulation, consideration of surgical intervention, and pulmonary hypertension therapies.

2. **How is post-thrombotic syndrome diagnosed? What treatments are available?**

- Post-thrombotic syndrome (PTS) is a complication of deep venous thrombosis that results from damage to the valves within the vein that normally help in returning blood back to the heart, culminating in aberrant venous flow, resulting in symptoms including extremity pain, skin color change, swelling, and when severe, ulceration.
- The diagnosis is largely clinical and may utilize a clinical score like the Villalta score. Treatment can include compression garments, leg elevation, skin care, and when severe, endovascular or surgical intervention.

LABORATORY TESTING AND IMAGING

1. **What initial labs could be assessed with a patient experiencing venous or arterial thrombosis?**

- For most patients, a laboratory evaluation will include a comprehensive blood count, and a creatinine and liver function tests. Baseline coagulation tests (prothrombin time [PT], activated partial thromboplastin time [aPTT]) are also considerations. This is used less often to determine the cause of the thrombosis than to guide management.
- Renal and hepatic function may have implications for anticoagulant choice. They also may suggest a primary or secondary renal or hepatic disease. Erythrocytosis or anemia, thrombocytosis or thrombocytopenia, or abnormal white blood cell values may require further investigation. As examples, thrombocytopenia may suggest portal hypertension or a marrow replacing process and may influence bleeding risk when determining anticoagulation. Thrombocytosis may be indicative of iron deficiency, inflammation, or a myeloproliferative neoplasm. Erythrocytosis can be seen with polycythemia vera or a variety of secondary causes like testosterone use. Anemia also has a broad differential but could suggest a hematologic malignancy, a marrow infiltrative disorder, blood loss, or a variety of other conditions; as with thrombocytopenia, severe anemia may be a consideration when considering anticoagulation risk.
- An elevated baseline PT/international normalized ratio (INR) can be indicative of liver disease, vitamin K deficiency, and more. A prolonged aPTT, at baseline, can be associated with the presence of lupus anticoagulant. These tests can influence subsequent anticoagulation monitoring and diagnostic testing. Fibrinogen can be tested if there is a concern for disseminated intravascular coagulation or as part of an evaluation for dysfibrinogenemia.
- A peripheral blood smear can be considered to investigate abnormalities on the CBC and may be informative of hemolysis (as in disseminated intravascular

coagulation, paroxysmal nocturnal hemoglobinuria, thrombotic thrombocy-topenic purpura [TTP]/hemolytic uremic syndrome [HUS], etc.), evidence of myelophthisis or marrow involvement, pseudothrombocytopenia, and more.

- Patients with recent heparin exposure may be tested for heparin-induced thrombocytopenia, using an antiplatelet factor 4 assay and/or a serotonin release assay.

- A d-dimer is often considered for diagnostic purposes. Patients with a low pretest probability of DVT, as determined by a clinical decision rule like the Wells score, generally do not need further workup if the d-dimer is negative. Similarly, a negative high-sensitivity d-dimer can negate the need for further workup in a patient with a moderate pretest probability of DVT.

- Inflammation markers like an erythrocyte sedimentation rate and C-reactive protein can be useful when considering malignancy or inflammatory conditions like inflammatory bowel disease.

- A urinalysis can screen for proteinuria as is seen in nephrotic syndrome and can assess for hematuria, hemoglobinuria (as seen in paroxysmal nocturnal hemoglobinuria), or urine sediment.

- Depending on the clinical situation, serum or urine protein electrophoresis, tumor markers, tests for rheumatic conditions, and imaging may be entertained.

- In an otherwise asymptomatic individual, extensive screening for malignancy beyond what is indicated by age has been shown to be low yield and is therefore discouraged.

2. **What imaging is used in the diagnosis of venous thromboembolism?**

- Compression venous ultrasonography is the primary test for extremity venous thrombosis. Negative whole-leg compression ultrasonography does not require further investigation if a more proximal venous thrombosis is not suspected. If only a proximal ultrasound is performed, a repeat ultrasound at 1 week may be indicated based on patient risk and biomarker testing.

- Deep vein extremity thrombosis can also be assessed with CT venography or MR venography, and conventional contrast venography. The contrast agent or use of a magnet may be contraindicated in some patients. Conventional venography is invasive and can cause complications, including provoking thrombosis.

- MR venography or CT venography are the tests of choice for cerebral venous thrombosis.

- Splanchnic venous thrombosis can be diagnosed with CT, MR, or ultrasound with Doppler depending on the clinical situation and vascular bed of concern.

- Ventilation perfusion scans are considered to diagnose suspected pulmonary embolism when CT angiography is contraindicated, as with severe renal insufficiency. This is limited when patients have preexisting lung disease. MR pulmonary angiography, echocardiography, and conventional catheter-directed angiography are other imaging modalities considered for the diagnosis of pulmonary embolism.

3. **When is thrombophilia testing indicated?**

- Generally, thrombophilia testing should only be considered when it would change management. Testing for inherited thrombophilias is discouraged by several organizations, including the Choosing Wisely Initiative, for venous thromboembolism that occurs around a transient risk factor like surgery. Testing is low yield when an alternative explanation is present like an active malignancy, for women with pregnancy complications (pregnancy loss, abruption, preeclampsia, and intrauterine growth restriction) in the absence of a history of thrombosis (testing for antiphospholipid syndrome that is not inherited may be indicated), and in general for arterial thrombosis, especially at an older age.

- Testing for an inherited thrombophilia is often considered with a strong family history of venous thromboembolism. Some clinicians consider testing for thrombophilia in young patients, those with recurrent events, or when it is a non-extremity venous thrombosis (splanchnic vein or cerebral vein).
- Protein C or S deficiency is commonly considered with warfarin-induced skin necrosis.

4. What are the tests for the most common hereditary thrombophilias?

- Factor V Leiden and prothrombin G20210A mutation can be tested directly with genetic testing and the tests are therefore not affected by anticoagulant therapy. Alternatively, to screen for factor V Leiden mutation, some clot-based tests for activated protein C resistance are used. A positive test shows a reduced anticoagulant effect in patient plasma from the addition of a standard amount of activated protein C, most often due to factor V Leiden mutation. Functional tests can be affected by the presence of a lupus anticoagulant or direct factor inhibitors. While most commonly due to factor V Leiden mutation, activated protein C resistance can result from protein S deficiency, high levels of factor VIII, in the setting of malignancy, and more.
- Recall that protein C deficiency can be a quantitative defect (type 1) or a functional defect of protein C (type II). Deficiency is most often evaluated using functional assays that can detect both types of disease but immunoassays are also available. Furthermore, anticoagulation, vitamin K deficiency, liver disease, and consumption from acute thrombosis or acute illness can affect levels, making the diagnosis more challenging.
- Protein S deficiency is challenging to diagnose. Recall that protein S circulates bound to C4b-binding protein and as a free form. Given that C4b-binding protein is an acute phase reactant, and the potential for interference with functional assays due to activated protein C resistance and elevated factor VIII activity, the diagnosis often cannot be made around an acute thrombosis. Immunoassays are often used, given that they can detect both free protein S and total protein S. As with protein C deficiency, caution is needed evaluating for this condition because vitamin K deficiency, pregnancy or estrogen hormones, liver disease, times of increased utilization, and anticoagulants can influence results.
- Antithrombin deficiency is commonly assessed using functional assays, as they can detect both types of disease (quantitative—type 1 and qualitative—type 2), but immunoassays are also available. Caution is necessary, given that anticoagulants can influence the results and a variety of conditions (nephrotic syndrome, extracorporeal membrane oxygenation [ECMO], asparaginase, liver disease, acute thrombosis, etc.) can cause an acquired antithrombin deficiency. While ideally tested away outside from acute thrombosis, a rapid evaluation may be needed, especially if considering heparin therapy, given the potential for heparin resistance.

5. **What is the cause and significance of an elevated serum homocysteine value? Is therapy indicated to reduce the risk of venous thrombosis?**
   - An elevated homocysteine level can be hereditary or acquired. Hereditary causes are most commonly due to mutations in the methylene tetrahydrofolate reductase (*MTHFR*) gene that result in reduced enzymatic activity. Acquired causes of hyperhomocysteinemia include folic acid, B6, or B12 deficiencies.
   - Significantly elevated homocysteine levels have been suggested as a risk factor for cardiovascular, cerebrovascular, peripheral arterial, and venous thromboembolic disease; however, this is controversial. Screening for elevated homocysteine is not routinely suggested for primary or secondary prevention of venous thromboembolism based on trials not showing evidence of benefit for treating these patients with vitamin supplementation. *MTHFR* mutations are not associated with increased risk of thrombosis and should not be tested for in patients with thrombosis. Treatment of thromboses is the same as that in the general population.

6. **What laboratory tests are used for the diagnosis of heparin-induced thrombocytopenia?**
   - When testing is indicated, antiplatelet factor 4 antibody testing by ELISA is often used to screen for heparin-induced thrombocytopenia due to the high sensitivity. However, it has a low specificity. A platelet ^{14}C-serotonin release assay is considered the "gold standard" laboratory test for heparin-induced thrombocytopenia due to the high sensitivity and specificity.

7. **What tests are used for the diagnosis of antiphospholipid antibody syndrome?**
   - While clinical correlation is necessary for a diagnosis of antiphospholipid antibody syndrome, laboratory abnormalities must be present on two occasions, at least 12 weeks apart
   - The presence of a lupus anticoagulant is indicated by the prolongation of a phospholipid-dependent coagulation test (like the activated partial thromboplastin time, dilute prothrombin time, dilute Russell viper venom time, or kaolin clotting time) plus failure of that prolonged clotting time to correct with normal plasma but correction with excess phospholipids. Exclusion of other coagulation defects is also required
   - A high-titer (>99th percentile) immunoglobulin G (IgG) or IgM isotype anticardiolipin antibodies by ELISA
   - A positive high-titer (>99th percentile) test of IgG or IgM isotype β_2Gp1 antibodies by ELISA
   - Positivity for all three tests and higher titers of antibodies predict a higher thrombotic risk

8. **What tests can indicate the presence of a dysfibrinogenemia?**
   - Elevated thrombin and reptilase times can be suggestive of a dysfibrinogenemia. Testing fibrinogen by an immunologic method often gives a higher value than a functional method; therefore, an elevated ratio of a fibrinogen antigen to activity can be suggestive. Genetic testing can be performed.

9. **What tests could suggest a diagnosis of paroxysmal nocturnal hemoglobinuria (PNH)? What test confirms the diagnosis?**

- Labs in PNH will typically show findings consistent with a hemolytic anemia and thrombocytopenia. The urine is notable for hemosiderinuria and potentially hemoglobinuria. Urine dipstick will often be positive for blood, but microscopy will be negative for hematuria.

- The diagnosis is established with flow cytometry showing an absence or reduction in glycosylphosphatidylinositol (GPI)-linked proteins like CD 59 or CD 55. The presence of the GPI anchor is assessed using fluorescent aerolysin (FLAER).

ANTIPLATELET AND ANTICOAGULANT DRUGS

1. **What is the mechanism of action and half-life of aspirin? How can the effect of aspirin be reversed?**

   - Aspirin acetylates and irreversibly inhibits cyclooxygenase, ultimately resulting in a reduction of thromboxane A_2, interfering with platelet aggregation. It has a half-life of about 20 minutes at low doses.

   - After about 7 to 10 days, new platelets will replace those acetylated by aspirin, giving the option of holding aspirin for 5 to 10 days before a nonemergent procedure. If it has been a short time since aspirin ingestion, platelet transfusion can be considered for urgent bleeding.

2. **What is the mechanism of action of clopidogrel, prasugrel, and ticagrelor? Can the effect be reversed?**

   - These drugs act primarily on the adenosine diphosphate (ADP) receptor and thus reduce platelet activation and aggregation. They have a half-life of about 7 to 10 hours and the drugs can be held in nonurgent scenarios. In critical bleeding, platelet transfusion can be considered, but the antiplatelet drugs or their metabolites could inhibit the transfused platelets.

3. **What is the mechanism of action of abciximab, eptifibatide, or tirofiban?**

   - These intravenous drugs act on the Gp IIb/IIIa receptor and can work to prevent platelet aggregation. Recall that this is the receptor that is defective in Glanzmann thrombasthenia.

4. **What is the mechanism of action of heparin or low-molecular-weight heparin (LMWH)? Can the effect be reversed? How are these drugs monitored?**

   - Unfractionated heparin exerts an anticoagulant effect by binding antithrombin and potentiating its effects. This results in the inactivation of several clotting factors, in particular thrombin (factor IIa) and factor Xa. Heparin is processed in the reticuloendothelial system and ultimately degraded in the liver. It is a highly charged molecule and binds nonspecifically to plasma proteins and cells. It can be monitored by anti-Xa heparin levels or by following regular activated partial thromboplastin times and adjusting the infusion by a standard nomogram. Reversal can be achieved by protamine sulfate; there is a small risk of anaphylaxis. Heparin resistance can be seen with antithrombin deficiency or by nonspecific binding of heparin to off-target cells or proteins (especially in an inflammatory state), with an inadequate amount left for therapy.

   - LMWHs also bind antithrombin but their smaller size results in less inactivation of thrombin (factor IIa) relative to unfractionated heparin, thus resulting in greater activity against factor Xa relative to thrombin (factor IIa). Due to limited thrombin inhibition, the activated partial thromboplastin time cannot be used to monitor therapy. However, anti-Xa levels can be used for this purpose and may be considered in obese patients. LMWHs have a more predictable pharmacokinetic profile and clearance. Therefore, they can be given once or twice daily as a subcutaneous formulation. LMWH should be dose adjusted or avoided in the setting of renal insufficiency. It can be partially reversed with protamine sulfate.

5. **What is the mechanism of fondaparinux? Can the effect be reversed? How can it be monitored?**

   ● Fondaparinux similarly binds to antithrombin and primarily acts to facilitate the inactivation of factor Xa. It is administered subcutaneously once daily based on weight. It should be avoided in the setting of renal insufficiency. It can be monitored using anti-Xa levels and does not have a standardized reversal strategy at this time.

6. **What is the mechanism of action of argatroban and bivalirudin? How can these drugs be monitored?**

   ● These drugs are intravenous direct thrombin inhibitors, most commonly used for suspected or confirmed heparin-induced thrombocytopenia. They have short half-lives and currently do not have a formal reversal agent. Argatroban is hepatically cleared, while bivalirudin is renally cleared. They can be monitored by the activated partial thromboplastin time, but they also notably affect the prothrombin time, which must be considered when transitioning to warfarin. Some chromogenic antifactor IIa assays can be used to monitor these drugs as well.

7. **What is the mechanism of action of warfarin? What patient counseling is needed? How is warfarin monitored?**

   ● Warfarin inhibits the enzymes necessary to reduce vitamin K, which is required for the γ-carboxylation of coagulation factors II, VII, IX, and X and the anticoagulant proteins C and S. It has numerous drug interactions and dietary interactions with a relatively narrow therapeutic window. Monitoring of warfarin is done with the prothrombin time, which is standardized using the international normalized ratio (INR). An INR of 2 to 3 is targeted for most indications, but a higher target is used in some situations, like mechanical heart valves. When starting warfarin for an acute VTE, it is advised to have about 5 days of overlap with a parenteral anticoagulant, given the potential for a transient period of hypercoagulability, as the natural anticoagulant proteins C and S decrease prior to achieving therapeutic levels of the remaining vitamin K–dependent clotting factors. Warfarin can be effectively used in patients with renal disease; PT-/INR-based monitoring may be challenging in advanced hepatic disease.

   ● Warfarin is teratogenic and appropriate measures should be taken to prevent pregnancy for patients with childbearing potential. Patients should be educated on maintaining a consistent amount of dietary vitamin K and caution for interacting drugs. Given the long half-life, low-molecular-weight-heparin or intravenous (IV) heparin is considered for "bridging" anticoagulation in patients with high thrombotic risk when warfarin must be interrupted (surgery or procedures).

- Warfarin that needs to be reversed due to bleeding, supratherapeutic levels, or surgery can be managed by holding the drug, oral or intravenous vitamin K, fresh frozen plasma, or prothrombin complex concentrates. The intensity and method of reversal depends on the clinical situation, balancing bleeding and thrombotic risk.

8. **What are the direct oral anticoagulants (DOACs) and their mechanisms of action? What are their dosing schedules, toxicities, and general management?**

- The DOACs include apixaban, edoxaban, rivaroxaban, and dabigatran. Dabigatran is a direct thrombin inhibitor, while the first three inhibit factor Xa. They all have a rapid time (hours) to peak onset of action and a half-life around 10 to 14 hours. Dabigatran and apixaban are dosed twice daily while the others are daily. Notable differences include dabigatran being associated with dyspepsia, rivaroxaban needs to be taken with food, and apixaban has the least renal clearance. Both dabigatran and edoxaban were studied with 5 days of bridging parenteral anticoagulation for acute venous thromboembolism, while apixaban and rivaroxaban were given at higher initial doses in the beginning without parental anticoagulation bridging.

- Patients are generally not bridged on the DOACs for procedures or surgeries.

- Dabigatran is the most renally cleared. Reversal depends on the clinical situation but it could include idarucizumab (direct reversal agent), oral charcoal if recent ingestion, dialysis, or simply holding the medication. Reversal of the remaining DOACs can be managed by holding the drugs or giving prothrombin complex concentrates (limited data). A direct reversal agent for the anti-Xa medication is in clinical trial.

Anticoagulant	Target	Dosing	Half-life*	Uses	Features
Apixaban	Xa	Oral BID	~12 hours	AF, VTE	Least renal clearance of DOACs
Edoxaban	Xa	Oral daily	~12 hours	AF, VTE	—
Rivaroxaban	Xa	Oral daily	~12 hours	AF, VTE	Need to take with food
Dabigatran	IIa	Oral BID	~15 hours	AF, VTE	Associated with dyspepsia
Argatroban	IIa	IV	~1 hour	HIT	Hepatic clearance
Bivalirudin	IIa	IV	~<1 hour	PCI (w/ HIT)	—
Heparin	IIa, Xa	IV	~1.5 hours	ACS, AF, VTE	Monitor aPTT or anti-Xa to dose

(continued)

Antiplatelet	Target	Dosing	Half-life*	Uses	Features
LMWH	Xa>IIa	SubQ daily— BID	~6 hours	ACS, VTE	Renal clearance, weight-based dosing
Fondaparinux	Xa	SubQ daily	~19 hours	VTE	Weight-based dosing, renally cleared
Warfarin	II, VII, IX, X, Protein C + S	Oral daily	~40 hours, variable	AF, VTE	Drug/dietary interactions, monitor with INR
Aspirin (low dose)	COX	Oral Daily	~20 min	AF, CAD, VTE, PAD, PP	Affects platelets for 7–10 days
Clopidogrel, prasugrel, ticagrelolr	ADP	Oral daily to oral BID	~7–10 hours	ACS	—
Abciximab, eptifibatide, tirofiban	Gp IIb/ IIIa	IV	Min–hours	PCI	—

*plasma half life.

ACS, acute coronary syndrome; ADP, adenosine diphosphate; AF, atrial fibrillation; aPTT, activated partial thromboplastin time; BID, twice daily; CAD, coronary artery disease; COX, cyclooxygenase; DOAC, direct oral anticoagulant; Gp, glycoprotein; HIT, heparin-induced thrombocytopenia; INR, international normalized ratio; PCI, percutaneous coronary intervention; PP, primary prevention; SubQ, subcutaneously; VTE, venous thromboembolism.

QUESTIONS

1. A 27-year-old male with a history of an unprovoked right lower extremity proximal deep vein thrombosis 3 years ago is admitted with a severely symptomatic left lower extremity deep vein thrombosis. He is started on intravenous (IV) heparin with a bolus. He has consistently subtherapeutic activated partial thromboplastin times but is ultimately discharged on warfarin. He does well until he experiences a recurrent event when bridging back to warfarin after an urgent appendectomy. He is referred for further evaluation. Which of the following is the most likely etiology of his thrombosis?
   A. May-Thurner syndrome (iliac vein compression syndrome)
   B. Antithrombin deficiency
   C. Factor V Leiden gene mutation
   D. Paroxysmal nocturnal hemoglobinuria

2. A 54-year-old male is admitted after a motor vehicle accident. He has a splenic laceration, a nondisplaced humerus fracture, and several

fractured ribs. His admission labs show a hemoglobin of 13.6 g/dL, white blood cell count of 6.5 × 10⁹/L, and platelets are 285 × 10⁹/L. He receives supportive care with analgesics and immobilization of his arm. He is discharged to inpatient rehabilitation after one week of inpatient care. At that point, he complains of left lower extremity pain, and a lower extremity ultrasound confirms an acute deep vein thrombosis of the left lower extremity. Repeat complete blood count (CBC) shows a hemoglobin of 11.4 g/dL, white blood count of 8.2 × 10⁹/L, and platelets are 141 × 10⁹/L. Renal function, hepatic function, and a baseline set of coagulation tests are normal. He denies any bleeding and has had an otherwise uncomplicated hospital course. The patient is started on intravenous heparin. What would you suggest for the next step in management?

A. Bridge to warfarin for 3 months for provoked deep vein thrombosis (DVT)
B. Send a hypercoagulable workup
C. Change to a non-heparin anticoagulant and test for heparin-induced thrombocytopenia (HIT)
D. Discharge on twice-daily rivaroxaban

3. A 65-year-old male with a history of obesity, nicotine dependence, obstructive sleep apnea, and coronary artery disease presents with a 3-day history of worsening abdominal pain. A CT abdomen shows an acute, occluding portal vein thrombosis but an otherwise normal-appearing liver. Labs show a hemoglobin of 17.6 g/dL, hematocrit of 50%, white blood cell count of 9.2 × 10⁹/L, and platelets are 395 × 10⁹/L. Renal and liver function tests are normal. Lactate dehydrogenase (LDH), haptoglobin, and a peripheral blood smear are normal. Urine dipstick and microscopy are also normal. Which of the following is the most likely to explain the cause of this patient's thrombosis?

A. Liver biopsy
B. Anticardiolipin antibodies, lupus anticoagulant, and anti-beta-2 glycoprotein antibodies
C. Flow cytometry for paroxysmal nocturnal hemoglobinuria (PNH)
D. *JAK2 V617F* mutation

4. A 62-year-old female was found to have bilateral segmental pulmonary emboli on a routine follow-up scan for stage IV, metastatic adenocarcinoma of the lung. Her chronic shortness of breath has been unchanged and she has recently been receiving palliative chemotherapy. A complete blood count (CBC) shows a hemoglobin of 9.2 g/dL, white blood cell count of 4.2 × 10⁹/L, and platelets are 90 × 10⁹/L. These values are consistent with her labs after past cycles of chemotherapy. Renal function and hepatic function are normal. Which of the following would you suggest?

A. Warfarin with a goal international normalized ratio (INR) of 2 to 3
B. Dabigatran
C. Low-molecular-weight heparin
D. No therapy given that it is asymptomatic

5. A 71-year-old male with a past medical history of hypertension, transient ischemic attack, coronary artery disease, type 2 diabetes mellitus, and gastroesophageal reflux disease presents for routine follow-up. He has been on warfarin for several years for his atrial fibrillation but would like to transition to a direct oral anticoagulant (DOAC). He travels frequently and does not eat regular or large meals. He has no liver disease or renal disease. He is on several medications that he takes twice daily but none has drug interactions with the DOACs. His international normalized ratios (INRs) have been stable in the range of 2 to 3. His body mass index (BMI) is 28 kg/m². Which anticoagulant would you suggest?
   A. Apixaban
   B. Dabigatran
   C. Rivaroxaban
   D. Continue warfarin

6. A 37-year-old female is admitted for a right segmental pulmonary embolism from which she had pleuritic chest pain and shortness of breath. She had delivered her second child about 9 months ago and recently drove 3 hours for her job in pharmaceutical sales. She has no significant medical history but does note that she had preeclampsia with both of her previous pregnancies. Additionally, she had one miscarriage at 11 weeks gestation. Physical exam is normal. Labs show a normal complete blood count and comprehensive metabolic panel. Pregnancy test is negative. She is started on intravenous (IV) heparin and is planned to transition to warfarin. Homocysteine is elevated at 22 mcmol/L, protein S antigen is 67%, anti-cardiolipin antibodies and beta-2 glycoprotein 1 antibodies are strongly positive. Protein C and antithrombin activity are within the reference range, and no mutation of factor V Leiden or the prothrombin gene is seen. The patient has no history of thrombosis. What is the best next step in management?
   A. Suggest long-term warfarin for antiphospholipid syndrome
   B. Suggest warfarin for protein S deficiency for 3 months. Recheck protein S after holding anticoagulation at 3 months
   C. Test for the methylene tetrahydrofolate reductase (*MTHFR*) gene mutation for hyperhomocysteinemia
   D. Suggest warfarin therapy with repeat testing for anti-cardiolipin, beta-2 glycoprotein 1 antibodies, and a lupus anticoagulant in 3 months

7. A 32 year old, G1P0 woman with a history of obesity is at approximately 28 weeks gestation with an uncomplicated pregnancy to date. She presents to the emergency room with a primary concern of shortness of breath and pleuritic chest discomfort. She endorses a one week history of left calf pain and swelling. She has no personal or family history of venous thromboembolism. Her heart rate is 105 with a normal blood pressure. Physical exam shows her chest to be clear but confirms left lower extremity pain and tenderness. Which is the best next step in management?

A. Computed tomography pulmonary angiography
B. Ventilation perfusion scan
C. D-dimer
D. Venous compression ultrasonography of the lower extremities

8. A 56 year old male presents for a routine follow-up appointment eight weeks after having a right knee arthroscopy. He notes an area of warmth, pain, and swelling on the inner aspect of his right calf. He has no history of venous thromboembolism. Exam shows swelling and warmth over the right calf but no varicose veins or evidence of infection. Labs include a normal complete blood count, liver function tests, and a normal creatinine. Lower extremity venous ultrasonography shows no evidence of deep vein thrombosis but does confirm a superficial vein thrombosis that is reported to be nearly 6 cm in length. It is not in close proximity to the saphenofemoral junction. You are asked for management recommendations. Which of the following would be the best next step in management?
A. Repeat ultrasound in 7-10 days
B. Enoxaparin bridge to warfarin, continue anticoagulation for at least three months
C. Enoxaparin bridge to warfarin, continue anticoagulation for at least 45 days
D. Fondaparinux, prophylactic dose for at least 45 days

ANSWERS

1. **B. Antithrombin deficiency.** The patient had a clot at a young age with no clear provoking factors. His labs suggested resistance to IV heparin. Of the choices listed, this would be most consistent with antithrombin deficiency. A heparin resistance phenomenon can also be observed with elevated heparin binding proteins (i.e., inflammation), increased heparin clearance, and when other coagulation factors are elevated. May-Thurner syndrome would be expected to cause left lower extremity clots. While factor V Leiden mutation is a common thrombophilia, it does not explain this patient's heparin response. Paroxysmal nocturnal hemoglobinuria is similarly not suggested in this scenario.

2. **C. Change to a non-heparin anticoagulant and test for heparin-induced thrombocytopenia (HIT).** The patient in this vignette has a presentation concerning for HIT. Over a course of 5 to 10 days, he experienced a 50% drop in his platelets, and developed a new thrombosis. There are other possible explanations for the thrombocytopenia. The 4Ts score is there-fore 7. Further evaluation and empiric management for HIT is indicated. Transitioning to warfarin in the setting of potential HIT would not be appropriate and risks complications of warfarin-like warfarin-induced skin necrosis. A hypercoagulable workup is not indicated as this DVT may be provoked by a hospitalization or potentially HIT. The direct oral anticoag-ulants (DOACs), including rivaroxaban, have insufficient evidence for use in HIT or suspected HIT at this time.

3. **D. *JAK2 V617F* mutation.** The patient presents with a portal vein throm-bosis in the setting of an elevated hemoglobin and hematocrit. While the patient has risk factors for secondary erythrocytosis, this is concerning for a myeloproliferative disorder like polycythemia vera. Testing for the *JAK2* mutation would be appropriate to evaluate for this. PNH and antiphos-pholipid antibody syndrome could also be associated with a portal vein thrombosis. However, there is no evidence of hemolysis or suggestion of hemoglobinuria as could be seen with PNH. Antiphospholipid syndrome would not explain the elevated hemoglobin.

4. **C. Low-molecular-weight heparin.** The patient is diagnosed incidentally with a cancer-associated thrombosis (CAT). Low-molecular-weight hepa-rin has been shown to be superior to warfarin for the treatment of CAT. Studies have shown that select direct oral anticoagulants are non-inferior to low-molecular-weight heparin. However, there is currently no data to support the use of dabigatran. Therapy is indicated for this segmental pulmonary embolism, even in the absence of symptoms.

5. **A. Apixaban.** Of the listed DOACs, apixaban would be the most appro-priate. Given the history of gastroesophageal reflux disease, dabigatran could be avoided as it is more likely to exacerbate this condition. Dabigatran is coated in tartaric acid to help adsorption, and gastrointesti-nal symptoms were a common reason for discontinuation in clinical trials. Rivaroxaban has to be taken with meals and should be dosed daily. Given

that the patient does not eat regular meals, it may be best to use something that can be taken on a regular schedule. Apixaban is twice daily, but the patient is already taking twice-daily medications. The patient has expressed a preference to transition to a DOAC. As long as the patient understands the risks and benefits of the DOACs, transitioning from warfarin would be reasonable. However, with certain drug interactions, liver disease, renal impairment, compliance concerns, a history of a mechanical heart valve, if a reversal agent was needed, or the patient had an extreme in body weight, continuing warfarin may be best.

6. **D. Suggest warfarin therapy with repeat testing for anti-cardiolipin, beta-2 glycoprotein 1 antibodies, and a lupus anticoagulant in 3 months.** This patient could have antiphospholipid syndrome based on the strongly positive antibodies and the history of miscarriage. Furthermore, she had a pulmonary embolism without a strong provoking factor. However, the diagnosis requires the laboratory testing to be positive on two occasions, at least 12 weeks apart. Therefore, repeating the testing is indicated. Long-term warfarin would likely be suggested in the setting of antiphospholipid syndrome. In the setting of acute thrombosis, testing for protein S deficiency can be misleading, and taking the patient off anticoagulation could be risky. This patient has another potential explanation for her pulmonary embolism and further evaluation of the low protein S level may not change management. If this patient was being considered for discontinuing anticoagulation, retesting could be considered either off of warfarin for 4 weeks (which lowers protein S) or on heparin/low-molecular-weight heparin therapy. If the protein S level was very low, warfarin may not be the best choice of anticoagulant, given some potential risk for warfarin-induced skin necrosis. This is unlikely, given the mild reduction in protein S here. *MTHFR* is the enzyme-involved folate metabolism that is commonly mutated and can result in hyperhomocysteinemia. However, MTHFR mutations are not associated with an increased risk of thrombosis.

7. **D. Venous compression ultrasonography of the lower extremities.** The patient is pregnant and has clinical symptoms suggestive of a lower extremity deep vein thrombosis and pulmonary embolism. To avoid the radiation associated with a computed tomography scan or ventilation perfusion scan, many clinicians favor lower extremity ultrasound. If the diagnosis of venous thromboembolism is confirmed, anticoagulation can be initiated without additional diagnostic testing that may have risk. Given the higher pre-test probability of venous thromboembolism in pregnancy, d-dimer is avoided in pregnant patients and this patient would be considered high risk based on presentation.

8. **D. Fondaparinux, prophylactic dose for at least 45 days.** Given the length of the superficial vein thrombosis, anticoagulation is generally pursued for symptomatic patients with an acceptable bleeding risk. Most often, prophylactic dosed anticoagulation can be given for approximately 45 days with repeat clinical assessment. Repeat ultrasound can be considered in the case of patients with shorter segment superficial

vein thromboses that remain away from the saphenofemoral junction, and that do not have extensive risk factors for deep vein thrombosis, like active malignancy. While warfarin would likely be effective, studies have supported the use of prophylactic doses of anticoagulation for a short duration. Therefore, prophylactic fondaparinux would be the most appropriate choice of the listed options.

Myeloproliferative Neoplasms 10

Brittany Siontis and Rami N. Khoriaty

Chronic Myelogenous Leukemia (CML)

EPIDEMIOLOGY

1. **What is the median age at diagnosis of CML?**
   - Sixty-seven; incidence increases with age.

ETIOLOGY AND RISK FACTORS

1. **What is the one known causative factor?**
   - Ionizing radiation

2. **What two genes are involved in the hallmark Philadelphia (Ph) chromosomal translocation of CML and what chromosomes are they on?**
   - *Breakpoint cluster region* (*BCR*) on chromosome 22 and *ABL1* proto-oncogene on chromosome 9

3. **What is the protein product of balanced translocation between the long arms of chromosomes 9 and 22?**
   - The BCR-ABL1 oncoprotein

DIAGNOSTIC CRITERIA

1. **What is required to make a diagnosis of CML?**
   - Identification of
     - t(9;22) in cytogenetic analysis of bone marrow (BM), or
     - The BCR-ABL1 fusion gene by fluorescence in situ hybridization (FISH), or
     - The BCR-ABL1 transcript by quantitative reverse transcriptase polymerase chain reaction (RT-PCR)
   - ~2% to 5% of CML patients have transcript variants that are not detected by PCR, but would be detected by FISH or cytogenetics
   - Less than 5% of patients present with clinical and morphologic features of CML, but with no detectable BCR-ABL1 fusion on any of the above tests. It is debatable how to treat these patients, but some reports suggest the latter patients might benefit from tyrosine kinase inhibitors, as do patients with Ph+ CML. This chapter focuses on Ph+ CML.

2. **Name two other hematologic malignancies that can harbor t(9;22).**
   - Ph+ acute lymphoblastic leukemia
   - Ph+ acute myeloid leukemia

STAGING

1. **What are the three phases of CML, and what characterizes each phase by the World Health Organization (WHO) criteria?**

Chronic Phase (CP)	Accelerated Phase (AP)	Blast Phase (BP)
No features of accelerated or blast phase	Peripheral or marrow blasts 10%–19%, peripheral blood basophils ≥20%, platelets <100,000 unrelated to therapy, platelets >1,000,000 unresponsive to therapy, increasing spleen size and white blood cell (WBC) count unresponsive to therapy, additional chromosomal abnormalities in Ph+ cells at diagnosis (second Ph, trisomy 8, isochromosome 17q, trisomy 19, complex karyotype, or abnormality of 3q26.2), any new chromosomal abnormality in Ph+ cells occurring during therapy	Peripheral or marrow blasts ≥20%, extramedullary blasts, large clusters or foci of blasts in bone marrow (BM)

SIGNS AND SYMPTOMS

1. **What are the symptoms and physical exam findings at presentation?**
   - Asymptomatic neutrophilia (± left shift) on routine complete blood count
   - Weight loss and/or night sweats
   - Splenomegaly and its symptoms: early satiety, left upper quadrant fullness/pain
   - Gradual onset of fatigue
   - Rare manifestations:
     - Gout
     - Bleeding (due to thrombocytopenia)
     - Thrombosis (due to thrombocytosis and/or leukocytosis)

2. **Are infections rare or common at presentation?**
   - Rare, because neutrophil function is preserved

3. **What are the characteristic findings on a complete blood count (CBC) at diagnosis?**
   - Leukocytosis (20,000 to as high as 700,000) with left shift and circulating myeloblasts, myelocytes, metamyelocytes, and band forms
   - Basophilia (± eosinophilia): a hallmark feature of CML
   - Mild normochromic, normocytic anemia
   - Normal or elevated platelet count

PROGNOSTIC FACTORS

1. **What is the most important prognostic factor?**
   - Disease status at diagnosis: Patients with accelerated phase chronic myeloid leukemia (AP-CML) and blast phase chronic myeloid leukemia (BP-CML) have worse outcomes than patients with chronic phase chronic myeloid leukemia (CP-CML) do, and are treated differently.

2. **What prognostic factors are associated with worse outcomes in CP-CML?**
   - Age, spleen size, platelet count, and blast percentage on the peripheral blood (all included in the Sokal risk assessment score)
   - In addition to these prognostic factors, peripheral blood basophil and eosinophil percentages have prognostic values in the Hasford scoring system

TREATMENT

1. **How are patients with newly diagnosed CP-CML treated?**
   - Tyrosine kinase inhibitor (TKI) therapy: Nilotinib (300 mg BID), dasatinib (100 mg daily), and imatinib (400 mg daily) are the three Food and Drug Administration (FDA)-approved TKIs for first-line treatment of CP-CML
   - Consider hydroxyurea for patients with white blood cell (WBC) count greater than 100,000 (only temporarily until WBC count goes down)
   - Addition of allopurinol 300 mg daily until blood counts normalize

2. **What should be taken into consideration when selecting one of the three tyrosine kinase inhibitors (TKIs; dasatinib, nilotinib, imatinib) in the first-line treatment of CP-CML?**
   - Side effects of the different TKIs (see Questions 3–6)
   - Patient comorbidities
   - Sokal and Hasford prognostic scores: Consider nilotinib or dasatinib, rather than imatinib, in patients with intermediate- or high-risk disease
   - Patient preference and cost/insurance coverage

3. **What are some characteristic toxicities associated with nilotinib?**
   - QT prolongation, gastrointestinal (GI) upset, pancreatitis, hyperglycemia, hypercholesterolemia, liver toxicity
   - Increased risk of arterial thrombotic events
   - Nilotinib is the only TKI that needs to be taken twice a day
   - Patients cannot have PO intake for 2 hours before or 1 hour after each dose of nilotinib

4. **What are some characteristic toxicities associated with dasatinib?**
   - QT prolongation, thrombocytopenia, gastroesophageal reflux disease (GERD), pleural effusion, bleeding from platelet dysfunction, pulmonary hypertension

5. **What are some characteristic toxicities associated with imatinib?**
   - Skin rash, muscle cramps, diarrhea, periorbital swelling, edema, liver function test abnormalities, hypophosphatemia, QT prolongation.

6. **Which of the three TKIs approved in first-line CP-CML (imatinib, dasatinib, nilotinib) should be avoided in the following conditions?**
   - History of pancreatitis: Avoid nilotinib
   - History of pericardial/pleural disease: Avoid dasatinib
   - History of (or significant risk factors for) arterial thrombotic events: Avoid nilotinib
   - Patients on anticoagulants: Avoid dasatinib
   - Patient with pulmonary hypertension: Avoid dasatinib
   - Patients who are not able to fast for 3 hours twice a day (2 hours before and 1 hour after each dose of medication): Avoid nilotinib

7. **What are the treatment response criteria for CP-CML patients treated with first-line TKIs?**

Response	Definition	Recommended Monitoring
Hematologic response	**Complete hematologic response (CHR):** Platelet count <450,000, WBC <10,000, no peripheral blood immature granulocytes, basophils <5%, no palpable splenomegaly	CBC: every 1 week for first 6 weeks, then every 2 weeks until CHR, then every 3 months (M)
Cytogenetic response (CyR)	**Minor (mCyR):** Ph+ cells 36%–65% **Partial (PCyR):** Ph+ cells 1%–35% **Complete (CCyR):** Ph+ cells 0%	BM cytogenetics: at diagnosis; if failure to achieve milestones; at any sign of loss of response
Molecular response (MR)	**Early (EMR):** BCR-ABL1:Control gene ratio <10% at 3 and 6 M **Major (MMR):** BCR-ABL1:Control gene ratio <0.1% **Complete (CMR):** BCR-ABL1 transcripts undetectable in a lab where polymerase chain reaction (PCR) sensitivity of at least 4.5 logs below standardized baseline	qPCR: at diagnosis; every 3 M for 2 years after BCR-ABL 0.1%–1% (or 2 years after CCyR), then every 3–6 M; if there is 1-log increase in BCR-ABL with MMR, repeat in 1–3 M
BCR-ABL kinase domain mutation analysis		If failure to achieve response milestones; at any sign of loss of response; if there is 1-log increase in BCR-ABL with loss of MMR; at disease progression to AP or BP

AP, accelerated phase; BM, bone marrow; BP, blast phase; CBC, complete blood count; qPCR, quantitative polymerase chain reaction; WBC, white blood cell.

8. **What are the treatment response goals for CP-CML patients treated with first-line TKIs?**

Time	Optimal Response	Treatment Failure
3 M	CHR	No CHR
	Ph+ <35% (BM cytogenetics)	Ph+ >95% (BM cytogenetics)
	BCR-ABL <10%	
6 M	Ph+ 0% (BM cytogenetics)	Ph+ >35% (BM cytogenetics)
	BCR-ABL <1%	BCR-ABL >10%
12 M	BCR-ABL <0.1%	Ph+ >0% (BM cytogenetics)
		BCR-ABL >1%
Anytime	BCR-ABL <0.1%	Loss of CHR
		Loss of CCyR
		Confirmed loss of MMR
		Clonal chromosomal abnormalities

BM, bone marrow; CCyR, complete cytogenetic response; CHR, complete cytogenetic response; M, month; MMR, major molecular response.

9. **What is a practical approach to monitor CP-CML after first-line TKI therapy?**
   - Complete blood count (CBC) every 1 to 2 weeks until complete cytogenetic response (CHR), then every 3 months. After 3 months of the start of therapy, if no CHR, then this is treatment failure (see Question 11 for treatment). For patients in CHR by 3 months, proceed with monitoring as follows.
   - At 3 months: Perform peripheral blood quantitative polymerase chain reaction (qPCR; or bone marrow [BM] cytogenetics if qPCR is not available):
     - If BCR-ABL transcripts ≤10% (or if partial cytogenetic response [PCyR] is achieved): This is optimal response. Continue the same treatment and monitor qPCR every 3 months.
     - If BCR-ABL transcripts >10% (or if no PCyR): This is suboptimal response. Evaluate for compliance, drug interactions, and check for ABL kinase mutation.
       - If patient was on imatinib, consider switching to nilotinib or dasatinib (recommended) or increasing the imatinib dose to a maximum of 800 mg a day if not a candidate for the second-generation TKIs. Evaluate for allogeneic stem cell transplant (ASCT).
       - If patient was on dasatinib or nilotinib, consider switching to the other second-generation TKI or keeping the same course. Do not switch from second-generation TKI to imatinib. Evaluate for ASCT.
       - Caveat: If the BCR-ABL transcript is only slightly >10% with a steap decline from baseline, patients might achieve BCR-ABL<10% at 6 months and might therefore have a favorable outcome.

- At 6 months: Perform peripheral blood qPCR (or bone marrow [BM] cytogenetics if qPCR is not available):
  - If BCR-ABL transcripts ≤10% (or if PCyR is achieved): Continue the same treatment and monitor qPCR in 3 months. BCR-ABL transcripts <1% constitute optimal response.
  - If BCR-ABL transcripts >10% (or if no PCyR): This is treatment failure.
- At 12 months: Perform peripheral blood qPCR (or BM cytogenetics if qPCR is not available):
  - If BCR-ABL transcripts ≤1% (or if complete cytogenetic response [CCyR] is achieved): Continue same treatment. Monitor qPCR every 3 months for 2 years after achieving transcript ≤1% (or after CCyR), then every 3 to 6 months afterward.
  - If BCR-ABL transcripts >1%: This is treatment failure. Switch to an alternate TKI (see the following text) and evaluate for ASCT.
- Despite the ease of PCR monitoring, BM biopsy is typically still recommended at diagnosis and if there is suspicion of loss of response. A BM biopsy should be considered to document CCyR.

10. What are the management options for patients with TKI intolerance?

- Patients with intolerance to one TKI can be switched to one of the other three TKIs approved in first-line treatment. An additional option is bosutinib, a second-generation TKI, Food and Drug Administration (FDA) approved for patients with intolerance or resistance to imatinib, dasatinib, or nilotinib.

11. What are the management options for patients in CP-CML who fail first-line TKI therapy?

- Evaluate for compliance and drug interactions.
- Test for *ABL* kinase mutations to help guide the choice of the second-line TKI (see Question 13): ~50% of patients with treatment failure have mutations in the *ABL* kinase.
- For most patients, switching to a/another second-generation TKI is appropriate. Patients treated with first-line dasatinib or nilotinib should not be switched to imatinib.
- In other words, patients who fail first-line imatinib can be treated with dasatinib, nilotinib, or bosutinib. Patients who fail first-line dasatinib can be treated with nilotinib or bosutinib, while patients who fail first-line nilotinib can be treated with dasatinib or bosutinib.
- The specific choice of the second-line TKI should be guided by the *ABL* kinase mutation status (see following Questions 12 and 13).
- Ponatinib is only used as a second-line TKI if the patient has the T315I *ABL* mutation.
- Third-line treatment options include any of the remaining second-generation TKIs, ponatinib, and allogeneic stem cell transplant (ASCT). Further options for patients not eligible for ASCT include clinical trials, omacetaxine, and interferon alpha.

- All patients who fail first-line TKI should be evaluated for ASCT (indications for ASCT are included in Question 16).

12. **What ABL kinase mutation confers resistance to all first- and second-generation TKIs imatinib, nilotinib, dasatinib, and bosutinib?**

- *T315I* mutation
- Patients with treatment failure due to T315I mutation should be considered for early allogeneic stem cell transplant (ASCT) and could be treated with the third-generation TKI ponatinib (or with omacetaxine as a less favorable alternative) while a donor is identified or if ASCT is not an option

13. **What ABL kinase mutations help with the choice of second-line TKI?**

- Patients without the *T315I* can be switched to a second-generation TKI (dasatinib, nilotinib, or bosutinib).
- The *V299L* mutation predicts a better response to nilotinib than dasatinib or bosutinib do.
- The *T315A, F317L/V/I/C* mutations are more sensitive to nilotinib or bosutinib than to dasatinib.
- The *Y253H, E255K/V,* and *F359V/C/I* mutations predict a better response to dasatinib or bosutinib than nilotinib does.

14. **What are some characteristic toxicities associated with ponatinib?**

- Arterial thrombotic events (significantly high risk, and the reason it is only used in very rare/specific situations), heart failure, hepatotoxicity, QT prolongation, pancreatitis, fluid retention

15. **What are some characteristic toxicities associated with bosutinib?**

- Diarrhea, nausea/vomiting, hepatotoxicity, rash, low incidence of pleural effusion, vascular events, and cardiac toxicity. In contrast to other TKIs, bosutinib has minimal QT prolongation

16. **What is the role of allogeneic stem cell transplant (ASCT) in CML?**

- Reserved as third- or fourth-line treatment after TKI failure in chronic phase CP-CML patients
- ASCT should be prioritized in patients with low probability of response to second-generation TKIs (patients with no cytogenetic response to imatinib or second-generation TKIs or patients with mutations predicting low sensitivity to second-generation TKIs)
- Indicated for AP-CML or BP-CML after best response to TKI is achieved (regardless of the depth of response)
- Should be considered and discussed with patients younger than 30 years of age, given that it is the only curative option for CML

17. **How successful is ASCT for CML?**

- Cure rate of ~65% for patients transplanted in chronic phase chronic myeloid leukemia (CP-CML)
- Transplant-related mortality and relapse are higher in patients transplanted in (AP-CML or BP-CML

18. **Can TKI be stopped in CP-CML?**

   - In general, TKI discontinuation should not be done, except if within a clinical trial.
   - If TKI discontinuation is considered, consultation with a CML expert center should be done.
   - TKI discontinuation could be considered (after expert consultation) in patients who fulfil ALL the following criteria:
     ○ More than 18 years of age
     ○ Patients in CP-CML, with no prior AP-CML or BP-CML
     ○ No history of resistance of any TKI
     ○ Prior evidence of quantifiable BCR-ABL
     ○ Patients who have been on an approved TKI for at least 3 years
     ○ Evidence of complete molecular response (CMR; on at least 4 tests) over the past 2 years
     ○ Access to BCR-ABL polymerase chain reaction (PCR) testing with a sensitivity of detection of at least 4.5 logs (with results reported within 2 weeks of blood draw)
   - Patients who fit all these criteria and decide to discontinue TKI should be monitored with monthly PCR for the first 6 months, followed by PCR every 2 months during months 7 to 24, and PCR every 3 months afterward indefinitely.
   - Patients in whom the TKI is stopped, must remain in major molecular response (MMR) while off the TKI. If MMR is lost, patients should resume the TKI immediately with monthly PCR monitoring for 6 months followed by PCR monitoring every 3 months indefinitely.
     ○ If MMR is not achieved within 3 months of restarting the TKI or if the disease progresses to AP-CML or BP-CML, the expert CML center that initially consulted on the patient should be immediately informed/consulted again.

19. **How should AP-CML be treated?**

   - Patients presenting with AP-CML should be treated with dasatinib 140 mg daily, nilotinib 400 mg BID, or bosutinib 500 mg daily (and less favorably imatinib 600 mg PO daily), followed byASCT (if eligible) as soon as the best response is achieved with the TKI.
   - Patients who progress from CP-CML to AP-CML should have their new TKI chosen based on the ABL mutation analysis.
   - Patients with AP-CML who achieve an optimal response (see Question 8) to the TKI (particularly if within 6 months of starting therapy) might choose to be monitored very carefully with deferring ASCT until the first sign of disease progression. This relapse requires another TKI followed by ASCT.

20. **How are patients with BP-CML treated?**

   - Patients in BP-CML should undergo ABL kinase mutation analysis to help select the best TK. All patients should be evaluated for ASCT.

- Patients with lymphoid blast crisis are generally treated with combination chemotherapy (acute lymphoblastic leukemia [ALL]-type induction regimen) with second-generation TKI, followed by ASCT. Alternatively, patients could be treated with a second-generation TKI + steroids, followed by ASCT. CNS prophylaxis should be done in patients with lymphoid blast crisis.
- Myeloid blast crisis does not typically respond well to AML induction regimens. Patients in de novo myeloid blast crisis CML are generally treated with a second-generation TKI (with or without AML-type chemotherapy) until best response, followed by ASCT. Patients with blast crisis CML that develops on TKI therapy are treated with combination chemotherapy + more potent TKI, followed by ASCT.

Myeloproliferative Neoplasms (General)

1. What characterizes a myeloproliferative neoplasm (MPN)?

- Clonal hematopoietic stem cell disease with overproduction of one or more blood cell lines
- Normal maturation with effective hematopoiesis and extramedullary hematopoiesis
- Risk for leukemic transformation

2. What are the eight MPNs recognized by the 2016 WHO?

- BCR-ABL1–positive cCML
- Polycythemia vera (PV)
- Essential thrombocythemia (ET)
- Primary myelofibrosis (PMF)
- Chronic neutrophilic leukemia
- Chronic eosinophilic leukemia, not otherwise specified
- MPNs, unclassifiable

3. What is the most common gene mutated in PV, ET, and PMF?

- *JAK2*

4. What is *JAK2*'s normal function?

- Tyrosine kinase critical in intracellular signaling for the erythropoietin, thrombopoietin, interleukin-3, granulocyte colony-stimulating factor (G-CSF), and granulocyte macrophage colony-stimulating factor (GM-CSF) receptors

5. What *JAK2* mutations are tested for in MPN?

- *JAK2* V617F (most common mutation) and *JAK2 exon 12* mutations
- *JAK2* V617F mutation causes constitutive activation of downstream messengers through the JAK-STAT, PI3K, and AKT pathways

6. **In which MPN is *JAK2* mutation most prevalent?**
   - Polycythemia vera (98%–99%), essential thrombocythemia (ET; ~60%), primary myelofibrosis (PMF; ~55%)

7. **Name two additional frequently mutated genes in ET and PMF.**
   - *MPL* (mutation in the transmembrane domain of the thrombopoietin receptor)
   - *CALR*
   - *JAK2*, *CALR*, and *MPL* mutations are generally mutually exclusive

8. **What thrombophilic condition should raise the suspicion of a *JAK2* mutation?**
   - Budd-Chiari syndrome (as well as other abdominal vein thromboses)

9. **Which gene is characteristically mutated in chronic neutrophilic leukemia?**
   - *CSF3R*

Polycythemia Vera

EPIDEMIOLOGY

1. **What is the median age at diagnosis of PV?**
   - Approximately 60 years, but occurs in all age groups

2. **What is the median survival of PV patients?**
   - Median survival is ~14 years (and ~24 years in patients <60 years)

3. **What are prognostic factors for worse survival in PV?**
   - Risk factors predicting worsening survival in PV are age >57 years (with age >67 being even higher risk), leukocytosis (white blood cell [WBC] count >15,000), venous thrombosis, and abnormal karyotype.

4. **What are the risks of transformation to myelofibrosis and risk of leukemic transformation in PV?**
   - Transformation to myelofibrosis occurs in 12% to 21% of PV patients
   - Risk of transformation to AML: ~8% at 20 years

5. **What characterizes PV pathophysiologically?**
   - Growth factor (erythropoietin [EPO])-independent proliferation of erythroid cells, producing an elevated red cell mass

DIAGNOSTIC CRITERIA

1. **What are the WHO diagnostic criteria for PV?**

2016 WHO criteria*	
Major	A1. Hemoglobin (Hb) >16.5 g/dL (men) or Hb >16 g/dL (women), hematocrit (Hct) >49% (men) or Hct >48% (women), or red blood cell mass >25% above mean normal predicted value
	A2†. Hypercellular (age-adjusted) bone marrow (BM) with panmyelosis and pleomorphic mature megakaryocytes
	A3. Presence of *JAK2* mutation
Minor	B. Subnormal EPO level

*PV diagnosis requires meeting criteria A1 to A3, or meeting criteria A1 to A2 and B.

†BM biopsy might not be necessary if Hb is >18.5 (or Hct >55.5) in men or if Hb >16.5 (or Hct >49.5) in women, if all the other criteria (A1, A3, and B) are met.

WHO, World Health Organization.

2. What features help distinguish PV from secondary polycythemia?
- Splenomegaly
- Leukocytosis
- Thrombocytosis
- Low EPO level
- Bone marrow (BM) panhyperplasia
- Normal arterial oxygen saturation
- Increased vitamin B_{12} level

SIGNS AND SYMPTOMS

1. What are the common presenting signs/symptoms in PV?
- Incidental polycythemia (± thrombocytosis ± leukocytosis) on CBC, pruritus aggravated by hot shower, erythromelalgia, gout, kidney stones, palpable sple-nomegaly (50%–70%), early satiety, joint pain, thrombosis symptoms (arterial or venous), and neurologic symptoms such as headache and confusion

TREATMENT

1. What subset of PV patients should be treated with aspirin?
- All PV patients who do not have a contraindication should be treated with aspirin 81 mg daily.
- Similarly, all patients should have their cardiovascular risk factors strictly controlled.

2. In addition to aspirin, what are the treatment options for patients with PV in the first-line setting and what is the target hematocrit?
- Phlebotomy and cytoreduction with hydroxyurea
- The target hematocrit, whether the patient is getting phlebotomies or hydrox-yurea, is <45%

3. **How do we choose between phlebotomy and hydroxyurea to achieve the hematocrit goal of <45%?**
   - Patients with low-risk disease—<60 years of age and with no prior history of thrombosis—are treated with phlebotomy.
   - Patients with high-risk disease—≥60 years of age or with a prior history of thrombosis—are treated with hydroxyurea.
   - Additional potential indications for cytoreductive therapy include frequent need for phlebotomy with poor tolerance of phlebotomy, symptomatic or progressive splenomegaly, symptomatic thrombocytosis, progressive leukocytosis, progressive disease-related symptoms (e.g., pruritus, night sweats, fatigue), disease-related major bleeding.
   - Patients with acquired von Willebrand disease (vWD) should also be considered for cytoreduction. Always check vWF activity if platelets are >1 million before administering aspirin (see "Essential Thrombocythemia (ET)" section).

4. **In addition to aspirin, which therapy in polycythemia vera (PV) has demonstrated the greatest reduction in thrombotic events?**
   - Hydroxyurea

5. **What is an alternative agent to hydroxyurea for cytoreduction in the first-line setting?**
   - Interferon alpha or peginterferon alpha could be considered for younger patients, pregnant patients who require cytoreductive therapy, or patients who defer hydroxyurea.

6. **What are the indications to change the cytoreductive agent to a second-line agent?**
   - Intolerance or resistance for first-line cytoreductive agent
   - New thrombosis or disease-related major bleeding
   - Frequent need for phlebotomy with poor tolerance of phlebotomy
   - Symptomatic or progressive splenomegaly
   - Symptomatic thrombocytosis
   - Progressive leukocytosis
   - Progressive disease-related symptoms (e.g., pruritus, night sweats, fatigue)

7. **What are second-line treatment options for PV?**
   - Ruxolitinib (particularly if significant splenomegaly or constitutional symptoms)
   - Interferon alpha or peginterferon alpha (if not previously used)
   - Hydroxyurea (if not previously used)
   - Clinical trial

8. **Is allogeneic stem cell transplantation indicated for PV?**
   - Allogeneic stem cell transplantation is the only curative option, but is almost never indicated in PV, unless the disease progresses to myelofibrosis or acute leukemia (for treatment of post-PV myelofibrosis, please refer to the "Primary Myelofibrosis" section)

Essential Thrombocythemia

EPIDEMIOLOGY

1. **What is the typical age at presentation of patients with ET?**
   - The age at presentation has a bimodal distribution: one peak around age 30 years with a second (larger) peak at age 50 to 60 years.
   - Women:men ratio is 1.5 to 2:1 in the early peak.

2. **What is the median survival of ET patients?**
   - Median survival is ~20 years (and ~33 years in patients <60 years of age); in some reports, survival comparable to that of age-matched population

3. **What percentage of ET patients have mutations in *JAK2, MPL,* or *CALR*?**
   - *JAK2* mutation (~60% of patients)
   - *CALR* mutation (~22% of patients)
   - *MPL* mutation (~3% of patients)

4. **What are prognostic factors for worse survival in ET?**
   - Risk factors predicting worse survival in ET are age >60 years, leukocytosis (white blood cell [WBC] count >11,000), and history of thrombosis.

5. **What percentage of ET patients transform to myelofibrosis or AML?**
   - Risk of transformation to myelofibrosis: ~5% to 10 % at 15 years
   - Risk of transformation to AML: <5% at 20 years

6. **Does *CALR* mutation result in a similar risk compared to *JAK2* mutations in ET?**
   - Patients with *CALR* mutations have a lower risk of thrombosis compared to patients with *JAK2*-mutated ET.
   - Patients with *CALR* mutations appear to have a comparable risk of transformation to myelofibrosis (MF) or acute myeloid leukemia (AML) compared to patients with *JAK2*-mutated ET.

DIAGNOSTIC CRITERIA

1. **What are the WHOdiagnostic criteria for ET?**

	2016 WHO criteria*
Major criteria	A1. Platelet count >450,000
	A2. Megakaryocyte proliferation with large and mature morphology (with hyperlobulated nuclei), with no or little granulocyte or erythroid proliferation, and very rarely minor (grade 1) reticulin fibrosis

(continued)

2016 WHO criteria*	
	A3. Not meeting WHO criteria for CML, PV, PMF, myelodysplastic syndrome (MDS), or other myeloid neoplasm
	A4. Presence of *JAK2, CALR,* or *MPL* mutation
Minor criteria	B1. Presence of a clonal marker or absence of evidence of reactive thrombocytosis

*ET diagnosis requires meeting criteria A1 to A4, or meeting criteria A1 to A3 and the B criterion.

CML, chronic myeloid leukemia; PMF, primary myelofibrosis; PV, polycythemia vera; WHO, World Health Organization.

SIGNS AND SYMPTOMS

1. **What are the most common presenting signs/symptoms in ET?**
   - Asymptomatic (50%)
   - Vasomotor symptoms: visual changes, lightheadedness, headaches, palpitations, typical/atypical chest pain, erythromelalgia, livedo reticularis, acral paresthesias
   - Palpable splenomegaly and its symptoms: early satiety or left upper quadrant abdominal pain
   - Thrombosis (~15% at presentation)

2. **In addition to the thrombosis risk and the risk of transformation to myelofibrosis and acute myeloid leukemia (AML), what are other complications of ET?**
   - Major hemorrhage (5%–10%) from acquired von Willebrand disease
   - Recurrent first trimester abortions

TREATMENT

1. **How are patients in the different risk categories treated?**
   - Patients with very-low-risk disease (age ≤60 years, no *JAK2* mutation, and no prior history of thrombosis) and patients with low-risk disease (age ≤60 years with *JAK2* mutation and no prior history of thrombosis) are treated with aspirin 81 mg po daily or observation. Of note, in one report, aspirin use did not affect the risk of thrombosis in patients with *CALR*-mutated low-risk ET but was associated with higher bleeding risk. The latter has not been confirmed in a prospective clinical trial
   - Patients with intermediate-risk disease (age >60 years with no *JAK2* mutation and no prior history of thrombosis): aspirin 81 mg po daily
   - Patients with high-risk disease (age >60 years with *JAK2* mutation or history of thrombosis at any age): aspirin 81 mg po daily + cytoreduction
   - All patients should have their cardiovascular risk factors monitored and strictly managed
   - Potential indications for cytoreductive therapy regardless of the ET risk group include symptomatic or progressive splenomegaly, symptomatic

thrombocytosis, progressive leukocytosis, progressive disease-related symptoms (e.g., pruritus, night sweats, fatigue), disease-related major bleeding, vasomotor/microvascular disturbances not responsive to aspirin (e.g., headaches, chest pain, erythromelalgia)

2. **In what situation should aspirin be avoided in ET?**
   - In patients with acquired vWD)
   - In patients with platelets ≥ 1 million/microL, check *von Willebrand factor* *(vWF)* ristocetin cofactor activity before starting aspirin. Patients with vWF ristocetin activity $\leq 30\%$ have an increased bleeding risk with aspirin. The latter patients are treated with platelet cytoreduction to result in vWF ristocetin activity $\geq 30\%$ before starting aspirin

3. **What are the first-line cytoreduction options in ET?**
   - Hydroxyurea (the most commonly used first-line treatment in ET)
   - Interferon alpha (or peginterferon alpha) could be considered for younger patients, pregnant patients who require cytoreductive therapy, or patients who defer hydroxyurea
   - Anagrelide

4. **When is plateletpheresis indicated in ET?**
   - Plateletpheresis is indicated in patients with significantly elevated platelet counts in the setting of acute and serious thrombotic or hemorrhagic events (such as stroke, ischemic limb, significant hemorrhagic event due to acquired vWD).
   - The effect of plateletpheresis on reducing platelet count is transient, and patient should be started at the same time on a platelet cytoreductive agent.

5. **What are the indications to change the cytoreductive agent to a second-line agent?**
   - Intolerance or resistance to first-line cytoreductive agent
   - New thrombosis, acquired vWD, or disease-related major bleeding
   - Symptomatic or progressive splenomegaly
   - Symptomatic thrombocytosis
   - Progressive leukocytosis
   - Progressive disease-related symptoms (e.g., pruritus, night sweats, fatigue)
   - Vasomotor/microvascular disturbances not responsive to aspirin (e.g., headaches, chest pain, erythromelalgia)

6. **What are second-line cytoreductive agents in ET?**
   - Hydroxyurea (if not previously used)
   - Interferon alpha (if not previously used)
   - Anagrelide (if not previously used)
   - Clinical trial

7. **What is the mechanism of action of anagrelide?**
   - Interferes with terminal differentiation of megakaryocytes

8. **In what group of patients should anagrelide therapy be avoided and why?**
   - In those with cardiovascular comorbidities because it can cause fluid retention, palpitations, and pulmonary hypertension

9. **Is allogeneic stem cell transplantation indicated for ET?**
   - Allogeneic stem cell transplantation is almost never indicated in ET, unless the disease progresses to myelofibrosis or acute leukemia (for treatment of post-ET myelofibrosis, please refer to the "Primary Myelofibrosis" section)

Primary Myelofibrosis

EPIDEMIOLOGY

1. **In addition to PMF, which two hematologic disorders most commonly lead to secondary myelofibrosis?**
   - Myelofibrosis could be a primary disease (PMF) or secondary to ET or PV.
   - Fibrosis in the bone marrow (BM) could also result from other etiologies such as hairy cell leukemia, metastatic solid tumor to the bone marrow, autoimmune or other chronic inflammatory conditions, and so forth.

2. **What is the median survival of patients with PMF?**
   - Median survival: ~6 years (but highly variable, see prognostic factors in the following text).

DIAGNOSTIC CRITERIA

1. **What are the WHOdiagnostic criteria for PMF?**

	2016 WHO Criteria*
Major	A1. Megakaryocyte proliferation and atypia accompanied by reticulin and/or collagen fibrosis (grades 2–3 on 0–3 scale). **In prefibrotic/early PMF**, the megakaryocytic changes are not accompanied by fibrosis, and the BM shows increased cellularity with granulocytic proliferation and often decreased erythropoiesis
	A2. Not meeting WHO criteria for CML, PV, ET, MDS, or other myeloid neoplasm
	A3. Demonstration of *JAK2*, *CALR*, or *MPL* mutation or other clonal marker or no evidence of reactive marrow fibrosis. In rare situations, a next-generation sequencing panel that detects recurrently mutated genes in myeloid malignancies might help in establishing clonality, if the diagnosis remains in question after routine workup

(continued)

2016 WHO Criteria*	
Minor	B1. Leukoerythroblastosis (absent in prefibrotic PMF)
	B2. Increased serum LDH
	B3. Anemia
	B4. Palpable splenomegaly
	B5. Leukocytosis (WBC >11,000)

Note: *PMF diagnosis requires meeting criteria A1 to A3 and at least 1 B criterion.

BM, bone marrow; CML, chronic myeloid leukemia; ET, essential thrombocythemia; LDH, lactate dehydrogenase; MDS, myelodysplastic syndrome; PMF, primary myelofibrosis; PV, polycythemia vera; WBC, white blood cell; WHO, World Health Organization.

2. **What are the three most commonly mutated genes in PMF?**
   - *JAK2* (~55% of patients)
   - *CALR* (~27%): improved overall survival (OS) and lower thrombosis risk compared to patients with *JAK2* mutations
   - *MPL* W515L (~7% of patients)
   - ~10% of patients with PMF do not have any of these mutations. These patients have inferior leukemia-free survival compared to patients with *JAK2* or *CALR* mutations and inferior overall survival compared to patients with *CALR* mutations.

3. **What raises the suspicion of progression of PV or ET to myelofibrosis?**
   - Progressive cytopenias
   - New or progressive splenomegaly
   - Fevers, night sweats, unintentional weight loss
   - Leukoerythroblastosis on the peripheral blood smear
   - A BM biopsy should be performed to confirm post-PV or post-ET myelofibrosis, if suspected
   - Of note, post-PV or post-ET myelofibrosis is treated like PMF

SIGNS AND SYMPTOMS

1. **Name several common presenting symptoms of PMF.**
   - Fatigue, anemia, abdominal discomfort and early satiety (from splenomegaly), fever, night sweats, weight loss, bone pain, pruritus, complications of portal hypertension (such as variceal bleed, ascites)

2. **What are the two most common physical exam findings in patients with PMF?**
   - Palpable splenomegaly and hepatomegaly

3. **What does the classic peripheral blood smear of PMF show?**
   - Leukoerythroblastosis (immature cells of the granulocytic series and nucleated red blood cells) and teardrop-shaped red blood cells (seen in fibrotic PMF)

PROGNOSTIC FACTORS

1. **What are the factors associated with decreased survival in PMF based on the Dynamic International Prognostic Scoring System-plus (DIPSS-plus)?**
   - Age >65 years
   - Presence of constitutional symptoms
   - Anemia, hemoglobin (Hgb) ≤10 g/dL
   - Leukocytosis, WBC count greater than $25,000 \times 10^6/L$
   - Presence of ≥1% circulating peripheral blasts
   - Presence of unfavorable karyotype (complex karyotype, +8, −7/7q−, i(17q), inv(3), −5/5q, 12p−, or 11q23 rearrangement)
   - Platelet count <100,000/microL
   - Red blood cell transfusion need (patients with red cell transfusion need will automatically get 2 points because their Hgb would be <10 g/dL)

2. **How are patients with PMF risk stratified? What is the median survival of patients in each risk group?**
   - Risk factors (from the prior question) are added up
     - Low-risk group: zero risk factors; median survival is ~15.4 years
     - Intermediate-1-risk group: one risk factor; median survival is ~6.5 years
     - Intermediate-2-risk group: two or three risk factors; median survival is ~2.9 years
     - High-risk group: at least four risk factors; median survival is ~1.3 years

TREATMENT

1. **What is the goal of treatment in PMF?**
   - Palliation in most cases, except in patients who are candidates for bone marrow transplantation, where cure might be attained (see the following text).

2. **How do you treat patients with low-risk PMF?**
   - Asymptomatic patients should be observed or treated on a clinical trial.
   - Symptomatic patients are treated with ruxolitinib, interferon (or peginterferon) alpha, hydroxyurea (if cytoreduction would be symptomatically beneficial), or on a clinical trial.

3. **How do you treat patients with intermediate-1-risk PMF?**
   - Asymptomatic patients can be observed or treated on a clinical trial.
   - Symptomatic patients should be treated with ruxolitinib or on a clinical trial.
   - Allogeneic stem cell transplantation should be considered in patients with low platelet count, complex karyotype, or high-risk mutations (ex *ASXL1*, *EZH2*, *IDH1/2*, *SRSF2*, *TP53*). This is one reason why next-generation sequencing for a select panel of genes might be helpful in patients with myelofibrosis.

4. **How do you treat patients with intermediate-2- or high-risk PMF?**

   - Transplant candidates should undergo allogeneic stem cell transplantation.
   - Non-transplant candidates with platelets ≥50K can be treated with ruxolitinib (certainly if symptomatic) or on a clinical trial. Those with platelets <50K should be treated on a clinical trial.
   - Non-transplant candidates with symptomatic anemia only should be worked up for other etiologies of anemia. If no other cause is identified, erythropoietin levels should be obtained.
     - If EPO is <500 mU/mL, patients can be treated with an erythropoiesis-stimulating agent or on a clinical trial. Avoid erythropoiesis-stimulating agents in patients with significant splenomegaly, because they might worsen the splenomegaly.
     - If EPO is ≥500 mU/mL, the options include danazol, lenalidomide or thalidomide ± prednisone, or a clinical trial. Use lenalidomide particularly in the presence of del 5q. Splenectomy can be considered in refractory cases with significant splenomegaly; however, this decision should not be taken lightly because of the morbidity and mortality associated with the procedure (~10% perisurgical mortality) and because a subset of patients develop compensatory hepatomegaly, some of whom might die of liver failure.

5. **How is myelofibrosis-associated pulmonary hypertension diagnosed and treated?**

   - Diagnosis is confirmed by a technetium 99m sulfur colloid scintigraphy.
   - Single-fraction whole-lung radiation (100 cGy) has been shown to be effective.

QUESTIONS

1. A 70-year-old woman with a past medical history notable for hypertension, diabetes, and stroke is found to have leukocytosis (white blood cell [WBC] count of 25,000) on routine labs. Hemoglobin is mildly reduced at 11.5 g/dL and platelet count is mildly elevated at 500,000. She notes some mild fatigue but is otherwise asymptomatic. Examination is notable for a spleen tip palpable 3 cm below the left costal margin. Further testing reveals BCR-ABL by fluorescence in situ hybridization (FISH) to be positive. You calculate her Sokal score, and she is found to be high risk. What is the next best step in management?
   A. Initiation of hydrea
   B. Initiation of imatinib
   C. Initiation of nilotinib
   D. Initiation of dasatinib

2. A 63-year-old gentleman with a history of chronic myeloid leukemia (CML) on imatinib presents to clinic for routine follow-up. Labs are notable for a white blood cell (WBC) count of 50,000 (10,000 6 months ago) and platelet count of 650,000 (normal 6 months ago). Quantitative polymerase chain reaction (qPCR) for BCR-ABL returns

elevated at 5% (previously undetected), and this result was confirmed by repeat testing. The patient confirms that he is taking imatinib religiously and has not missed any dose. What is the next best step in management?

A. Continue imatinib and repeat PCR again in 1 month
B. Start nilotinib
C. Perform a molecular mutation analysis
D. Switch to ponatinib

3. A 67-year-old woman with a past medical history notable for hypertension, glaucoma, and diabetes presents to clinic for evaluation of 2 months of progressive fatigue, early satiety, and weight loss. Labs are obtained and complete blood count (CBC) shows a white blood cell (WBC) count of 95,000 with basophilia (22%). Hemoglobin (Hgb) is 9.5 and platelets are 650,000. WBC differential reveals 12% blasts. Fluorescence in situ hybridization (FISH) for BCR-ABL is positive. Bone marrow biopsy shows 15% blasts, with cytogenetics revealing the Philadelphia chromosome in 20 out of 20 cells examined. What is the next best step in management?

A. Admit to hospital for cytotoxic chemotherapy
B. Initiate second-generation tyrosine kinase inhibitor (TKI)
C. Refer for consideration of allogeneic stem cell transplantation
D. B and C

4. A 55-year-old woman is referred to hematology for evaluation of a hemoglobin of 16.8/hematocrit of 51% found on routine labs. White blood cell (WBC) and platelet counts are normal. Upon further questioning, she reports minimal pruritus following a hot bath but denies burning and erythema of her hands. Her past medical history is otherwise notable for mild hypertension and tobacco dependency. She denies any family history of hematologic disorders. There is no personal or family history of thrombosis. Physical examination is unremarkable. What is the next best step in management?

A. Initiate JAK2 inhibitor therapy and evaluate for etiology
B. Immediately phlebotomize and evaluate for etiology
C. Evaluate for etiology
D. Initiate hydrea and evaluate for etiology

5. A 46-year-old man presents with polycythemia (hemoglobin 18.7, hematocrit 56%). He does not have a history of prior thromboembolic events. Workup demonstrated negative *JAK2 V617F* mutation. Bone marrow biopsy demonstrated increased cellularity with panmyelosis and pleomorphic mature megakaryocytes. EPO level is low. How should this patient be managed?

A. Initiate JAK2 inhibitor therapy
B. Aspirin and phlebotomy
C. Aspirin only
D. Observation and optimizing risk factors for thrombosis

6. A 68-year-old woman is found to have a platelet count of 800,000 on routine labs. She is asymptomatic. She has no history of arterial or venous thrombotic events. Physical examination is notable for a palpable spleen tip 2 cm below the costal margin. Testing for *JAK2 V617F* is positive. Bone marrow biopsy demonstrates findings consistent with essential thrombocythemia (ET) and rules out other possible disorders. What is the next best step in management?
   A. Hydrea and aspirin
   B. Interferon alpha
   C. Anagrelide
   D. Aspirin monotherapy
   E. Check von Willebrand factor (vWF) activity. No therapy is needed because she is asymptomatic

7. A 78-year-old man with a past medical history of diabetes, coronary artery disease, heart failure (ejection fraction [EF] 35%), and hypertension presents for evaluation of fatigue, night sweats, unintentional weight loss, left upper quadrant abdominal pain, and early satiety. The patient developed these symptoms gradually over the past 6 months. Physical exam is notable for splenomegaly (spleen tip palpated about 15 cm below the left costal margin). Labs obtained were a white blood cell (WBC) count of 14,000 (2% circulating blasts), hemoglobin (Hb) 11 g/dL, and platelet count of 160,000. Peripheral smear is notable for teardrop cells. *JAK2 V617F* and *exon 12* mutations are negative, as is *MPL* mutation. The patient has a *CALR* mutation identified. Infections are ruled out. What is the best management option for this patient?
   A. Supportive care with transfusions as needed
   B. Hydroxyurea
   C. Ruxolitinib
   D. Bone marrow transplantation

8. A 65-year-old man presents with left abdominal fullness and early satiety. On physical exam, he is noted to have splenomegaly. His complete blood count (CBC) shows a white blood cell (WBC) count of 9, hemoglobin 18.2, hematocrit 54.6%, and a platelet count of 350,000. He reports that he was diagnosed with a deep vein thrombosis (DVT) the year prior and completed 6 months of anticoagulation. Workup reveals a *JAK2 V617F* mutation. Bone marrow biopsy reveals a hypercellular marrow for age with panmyelosis and pleomorphic mature megakaryocytes. What is the best management for this patient?
   A. Aspirin alone
   B. Aspirin and phlebotomy
   C. Aspirin and cytoreduction with hydroxyurea
   D. Interferon alpha

9. A 65-year-old woman with high-risk essential thrombocythemia (ET) has been receiving hydroxyurea and aspirin for the past few years. She presents to clinic for evaluation due to left upper abdominal discomfort over the past 2 to 3 months. She reports increased fatigue and new-onset night sweats for the past 3 months. Of note, for the past year, due to a drop in hemoglobin and platelet counts, she has been requiring hydrea dose reduction. Her hydrea dose about a year ago was 1,000 mg po BID but her hydrea dose was slowly decreased for the past year and then hydrea was completely stopped about a month ago. Her complete blood count (CBC) currently shows white blood cell (WBC) count 30,000, hemoglobin (Hb) 9, and platelets 140,000. CBC from 6 months ago demonstrated WBC 12,000, Hb 11, and platelets 350,000. Recent workup for anemia was negative for iron/vitamin deficiencies. She has no infection of signs/symptoms of infection or inflammation to explain the worsening leukocytosis. On physical exam, her spleen is palpable about 6 cm below the left costal margin (a new finding). Bone marrow biopsy demonstrates megakaryocyte proliferation and atypia accompanied by reticulin fibrosis (grade 2–3).

What is the best step in management?
A. Observation
B. Switch to anagrelide
C. Refer for allogeneic stem cell transplantation
D. Start interferon alpha

10. A 65-year-old woman presents to the emergency department and was found on a complete blood count (CBC; performed for another reason) to have a platelet count of 1,800,000 (with white blood cell [WBC] 10 and hemoglobin [Hb] 12.5). She has no medical problems and takes no medications or supplements. *JAK2 V617F* mutation is positive. Bone marrow biopsy is consistent with essential thrombocythemia (ET). What is the best step in the management of this patient?
A. Ruxolitinib
B. Referral for allogeneic stem cell transplantation
C. Assess for *von Willebrand factor* (vWF) ristocetin activity
D. Hydrea + aspirin
E. Aspirin alone

ANSWERS

1. **D. Initiation of dasatinib.** The patient is high risk based on her Sokal score; therefore, outcomes are improved with nilotinib or dasatinib compared to imatinib. She has a history of arterial events (as well as multiple risk factors for arterial thrombosis), making nilotinib a less desirable option. Therefore, the best option for this patient is dasatinib. Hydrea is typically considered briefly (in addition to tyrosine kinase inhibitor [TKI]) for patients with WBC >100K who need immediate leukoreduction.

2. **C. Perform a molecular mutation analysis.** Patients who show resistance to imatinib should be evaluated for mutations in the ABL kinase domain. Certain mutations may guide therapy and therefore this test should be done before transitioning to a second-generation TKI. Continuing current therapy would not be a good choice given the loss of response to the current therapy. Ponatinib should be limited to specific clinical situations, given its high risk of arterial thrombosis.

3. **D. B and C.** This patient has accelerated phase chronic myeloid leukemia (CML). Patients in accelerated phase CML should be treated with a second-generation TKI followed by ASCT after best response is obtained. Cytotoxic chemotherapy is not indicated.

4. **C. Evaluate for etiology.** Patients who present with elevated hematocrit should be evaluated for the etiology prior to initiation of therapy directed at the etiology. If the patient has polycythemia secondary to hypoxemia, for example, dropping the hemoglobin/hematocrit might result in respiratory compromise.

5. **B. Aspirin and phlebotomy.** Patients who present with polycythemia and exhibit typical bone marrow abnormalities for PV as well as low EPO level, have a diagnosis of polycythemia vera (PV). *JAK2 V617F* mutation is present in most patients with PV, but ~5% to 7% of patients with PV have the *JAK2 exon 12* mutation instead, while ~1% to 2% of patients with PV do not have either *JAK2 V617F* or *JAK2 exon 12* mutations. In these patients, the typical bone marrow findings coupled with a low EPO level clinch the diagnosis. This patient is <60 years of age and has no prior history of thromboembolic events; therefore, he should be treated with aspirin and PRN phlebotomy (goal hematocrit <45%).

6. **A. Hydrea and aspirin.** This is a patient with high-risk ET given her age >60 years with *JAK2* mutation. She needs to be treated with aspirin and hydrea. Hydrea is teratogenic but this not a problem in this patient (age 68 years). Patients of childbearing age who desire to become pregnant should be counseled about pregnancy while on hydrea and should employ safe contraception methods that do not increase risk of thrombosis, and hydrea should be stopped before pregnancy. Interferon could be used instead of hydrea in patients planning to become pregnant. Interferon and anagrelide monotherapy (without aspirin) is not adequate. vWF activity should be checked in patients with very high platelet count (>1 million) prior to aspirin administration.

7. **C. Ruxolitinib.** This patient meets criteria for higher risk (intermediate-2-/high-risk) primary myelofibrosis. He is not a candidate for allogeneic stem cell transplantation given his age and comorbidities. He has symptomatic splenomegaly and constitutional symptoms; therefore, he would benefit from ruxolitinib therapy as opposed to supportive care alone or hydrea.

8. **C. Aspirin and cytoreduction with hydroxyurea.** All patients with polycythemia vera should be on aspirin. In addition, this patient has high-risk polycythemia vera based on age and history of thrombotic events. Therefore, cytoreductive therapy is indicated. Aspirin alone or in combination with phlebotomy is not appropriate for patients with high-risk disease. Interferon alpha is an alternative agent for cytoreduction, though typically reserved for younger patients or during pregnancy, but certainly interferon alpha alone (without aspirin) is not an appropriate option.

9. **C. Refer for allogeneic stem cell transplantation.** This patient has post-ET myelofibrosis. According to Dynamic International Prognostic Scoring System-plus (DIPSS-Plus), the disease is in the intermediate-2-/high-risk category. Patients in this category have reduced life expectancy due to their disease and are best treated with allogeneic stem cell transplantation if they are candidates.

10. **C. Assess for von Willebrand factor (vWF) ristocetin activity.** This is a 65-year-old woman with newly diagnosed ET. She falls in the high-risk category (age >60 years and positive *JAK2 V617F* mutation). Patient with high-risk ET are generally treated with aspirin + cytoreduction. However, when the platelet count is >1,000,000, vWF ristocetin activity should be done (and confirmed to be >30%) before aspirin can be safely started. Patients with vWF ristocetin activity ≤30% have an increased bleeding risk with aspirin. The latter patients are treated with platelet cytoreduction to result in *von Willebrand disease* (vWD) ristocetin activity ≥30% before starting aspirin.

Acute Leukemia

11

Lyndsey Runaas, Rami N. Khoriaty, and Dale Bixby

Acute Myeloid Leukemia

EPIDEMIOLOGY

1. What is the median age at diagnosis?

- Sixty-seven

2. What is the incidence of acute myeloid leukemia (AML)?

- There were an estimated 21,380 new cases of AML in the United States in 2017.

ETIOLOGY AND RISK FACTORS

1. What are the common risk factors for acute myeloid leukemia (AML)?

- Increasing age
- Prior chemotherapy:
  - Topoisomerase II inhibitors: latency of 1 to 3 years, associated with rearrangement of the histone-lysine n-methyltransferase 2A (*KMT2A*) gene (previously known as the mixed lineage leukemia [*MLL*] gene; 11q23)
  - Alkylating agents: latency period of 3 to 7 years, associated with the del 5q/-5 and/or del 7q/-7 chromosomal abnormalities as well as complex cytogenetic changes
- Antecedent hematologic disorder: myelodysplastic syndrome, myeloproliferative neoplasms
- Toxins/chemicals: benzene, pesticides, petroleum products
- Radiation exposure: toxic or therapeutic
- Congenital disorders: Down syndrome, Bloom syndrome, Fanconi anemia, dyskeratosis congenita, GATA2 deficiency, Shwachman-Diamond syndrome, Diamond-Blackfan anemia, and others

PATHOLOGY—CLASSIFICATION

1. What are the subtypes of AML according to the WHO classification?

AML and related neoplasms

AML with recurrent genetic abnormalities

> AML with t(8;21)(q22;q22.1); *RUNX1-RUNX1T1*

> AML with inv(16)(p13.1q22) or t(16;16)(p13.1;q22); *CBFB-MYH11*

(continued)

AML and related neoplasms

APL with *PML-RARA*

AML with t(9;11)(p21.3;q23.3);*MLLT3-KMT2A*

AML with t(6;9)(p23;q34.1);*DEK-NUP214*

AML with inv(3)(q21.3q26.2) or t(3;3)(q21.3;q26.2); *GATA2, MECOM*

AML (megakaryoblastic) with t(1;22)(p13.3;q13.3);*RBM15-MKL1*

AML with mutated *NPM1*

AML with biallelic mutations of *CEBPA*

Provisional entity: AML with BCR-ABL1

Provisional entity: AML with mutated *RUNX1*

AML with myelodysplasia-related changes

Therapy-related myeloid neoplasms

AML, NOS

AML with minimal differentiation

AML without maturation

AML with maturation

Acute myelomonocytic leukemia

Acute monoblastic/monocytic leukemia

Pure erythroid leukemia

Acute megakaryoblastic leukemia

Acute basophilic leukemia

Acute panmyelosis with myelofibrosis

Myeloid sarcoma

Myeloid proliferations–related Down syndrome

Transient abnormal myelopoiesis (TAM)

Myeloid leukemia associated with Down syndrome

NOS, not otherwise specified

SIGNS AND SYMPTOMS

1. What are the common signs and symptoms of AML?

- Fever
- Infections
- Bleeding
- Fatigue and other symptoms of anemia
- Leukostasis: central nervous system (CNS) manifestations, cardiopulmonary symptoms, retinal hemorrhage, priapism
- Disseminated intravascular coagulation (DIC)

- Tumor lysis syndrome (TLS)
- Leukemia cutis (cutaneous involvement)

Please see Chapter 20 for management of the hematologic emergencies of leukostasis, DIC, and TLS

DIAGNOSTIC WORKUP

1. **Define the diagnostic criteria for AML.**
   - Marrow and/or peripheral blood containing ≥20% myeloid blasts
   OR
   - Presence of t(15;17), t(8;21), inv(16), or t(16;16) regardless of the blast percentage
   Myeloid lineage is established if *any* of the following is identified:
   - Auer rods
   - Blasts are myeloperoxidase positive (by flow cytometry, immunohistochemistry, or cytochemistry)
   - Monocytic differentiation (with at least two of the following: nonspecific esterase, CD11c, CD14, CD64, lysozyme)

PROGNOSTIC FACTORS

1. **How are patients with AML stratified into different risk groups?**
   - Age and cytogenetics are independent prognostic factors (older age is a poor prognostic factor).

Risk Status	Cytogenetics/Molecular Abnormalities
Favorable risk	t(8;21) without *c-KIT* mutation
	inv(16) or t(16;16) without *c-KIT* mutation
	t(15;17)
	Normal cytogenetics with *NPM1* mutation in the absence of *FLT3-ITD* or isolated double-mutated *CEBPA*
Intermediate risk	Normal cytogenetics (without favorable- or poor-risk gene mutation)
	+8
	t(9;11)
	Cytogenetic changes not associated with favorable or poor risk
	T(8;21) or inv(16)/t(16;16) with a *c-KIT* mutation
Poor risk*	Complex cytogenetics (at least 3 chromosomal abnormalities)
	Monosomy karyotype
	−5/5q-
	−7/7q-

(continued)

Risk Status	Cytogenetics/Molecular Abnormalities
	11q23(some evidence suggests that t(9;11) may be associated with an intermediate risk, though this is controversial)
	inv(3)/t(3;3)
	t(6;9)
	t(9;22)
	Normal cytogenetics with *FLT3-ITD* mutation
	TP53 mutation

*Poor-risk acute myeloid leukemia (AML): also includes patients with antecedent hematologic disease evolving into AML and treatment-related AML. Collectively, these are known as secondary AML (sAML).

2. How are the patients with APL risk stratified?

- Sanz criteria

Low-risk APL	WBC <10,000 and platelet >40,000
Intermediate-risk APL	WBC <10,000 and platelet <40,000
High-risk APL	WBC >10,000

APL, acute promyelocytic leukemia; WBC, white blood cell.

TREATMENT

AML

1. **What are the induction treatment options for younger patients (<60 years old) with non-acute promyelocytic leukemia (non-APL) AML?**
   - Standard-dose cytarabine (100–200 mg/m^2 infusion over 7 days) + idarubicin (12 mg/m^2) or daunorubicin (60–90 mg/m^2) × 3 days
   - Standard-dose cytarabine (200 mg/m^2 infusion over 7 days) + daunorubicin 60 mg/m^2 × 3 days and cladribine 5 mg/m^2 × 5 days
   - High-dose cytarabine 2 g/m^2 every 12 hours × 6 days or 3 g/m^2 every 12 hours × 4 days + idarubicin 12 mg/m^2 or daunorubicin 60 mg/m^2 × 3 days
   - Standard-dose cytarabine 200 mg/m^2 continuous infusion × 7 days with daunorubicin 60 mg/m^2 × 3 days and oral midostaurin 50 mg every 12 hours, days 8 to 21—for FLT3-mutated AML
   - Fludarabine 30 mg/m^2 intravenous (IV) days 2 to 6, cytarabine 2 g/m^2 over 4 hours starting 4 hours after fludarabine on days 2 to 6, idarubicin 8 mg/m^2 IV days 4 to 6, and granulocyte colony-stimulating factor (G-CSF) subcutaneous (SC) daily days 1 to 7
   - Dual-drug liposomal encapsulation of cytarabine 100 mg/m^2 and daunorubicin 44 mg/m^2 IV over 90 minutes on days 1, 3, and 5 (therapy-related AML or AML with myelodysplasia-related changes)

- Standard-dose cytarabine 200 mg/m² continuous infusion × 7 days with daunorubicin 60 mg/m² and gemtuzumab ozogamicin 3 mg/m² (up to one 4.5 mg vial) on days 1, 4, and 7 (CD33 positive)
- Clinical trial (especially for patients with antecedent hematologic disorder or therapy-related AML)

2. **How do we evaluate the efficacy of induction therapy?**
   - Obtain a bone marrow biopsy 14 to 21 days after start of induction therapy
     - Aplastic marrow (<5% cellular and <5% blasts): Await count recovery and consider growth factor support
     - Significant cytoreduction and low-percentage blasts:
       - Standard-dose cytarabine + idarubicin or daunorubicin
       - Standard-dose cytarabine with daunorubicin and midostaurin
       - Dual-drug liposomal encapsulation of cytarabine 100 mg/m² and daunorubicin 44 mg/m² IV over 90 minutes on days 1 and 3 (therapy-related acute myeloid leukemia [AML] or AML with myelodysplasia-related changes)
       - High-dose cytarabine-based regimen
     - Significant residual blasts:
       - Cytarabine 1.5 to 3 g/m² every 12 hours × 6 days
       - Standard-dose cytarabine with idarubicin or daunorubicin (3 days)
       - Standard-dose cytarabine with daunorubicin and midostaurin
       - Dual-drug liposomal encapsulation of cytarabine 100 mg/m² and daunorubicin 44 mg/m² IV over 90 minutes on days 1 and 3 for subsequent cycles (therapy-related AML or AML with myelodysplasia-related changes)
   - If the day 14 marrow is ambiguous, could repeat a bone marrow biopsy in 5 to 7 days before proceeding with further treatment
   - Obtain the next marrow at count recovery (absolute neutrophil count [ANC] ≥1.0 and platelet count ≥100,000)

3. **What are the induction treatment options for older patients (>60 years) with non-APLAML?**
   - Candidate for intensive remission induction therapy:
     - De novo AML without unfavorable cytogenetics/molecular markers and no antecedent hematologic disorder /therapy-related AML:
       - Standard-dose cytarabine (100–200 mg/m² continuous infusion × 7 days) with idarubicin 12 mg/m² or daunorubicin 60 to 90 mg/m² × 3 days or mitoxantrone × 3 days
       - Standard-dose cytarabine 200 mg/m² continuous infusion × 7 days with daunorubicin 60 mg/m² and gemtuzumab ozogamicin 3 mg/m² (up to one 4.5 mg vial) on days 1, 4, and 7(CD33 positive)
     - Unfavorable cytogenetic/molecular markers OR antecedent hematologic disorder OR therapy-related AML:

- ■ Lower intensity therapy (5-azacytidine, decitabine)
- ■ Standard-dose cytarabine (100–200 mg/m^2 continuous infusion × 7 days) with idarubicin 12 mg/m^2 or daunorubicin 60 to 90 mg/m^2 × 3 days or mitoxantrone 12 mg/m^2 × 3 days
- ■ Standard-dose cytarabine 200 mg/m^2 continuous infusion × 7 days with daunorubicin 60 mg/m^2 × 3 days and oral midostaurin 50 mg every 12 hours, days 8 to 21—for FLT3-mutated AML
- ■ Dual-drug liposomal encapsulation of cytarabine 100 mg/m^2 and daunorubicin 44 mg/m^2 intravenous (IV) over 90 minutes on days 1, 3, and 5 (therapy-related AML or AML with myelodysplasia-related changes)
- ■ Clofarabine ± standard-dose cytarabine
- Patients not candidates for intensive remission induction therapy:
  - ○ Lower intensity therapy ([5-azacytidine, decitabine] preferred, low-dose cytarabine)
  - ○ Gemtuzumab ozogamicin 6 mg/m^2 on day 1 and 3 mg/m^2 on day 8 (CD33 positive)
  - ○ Enasidenib (*IDH2*-mutated AML)
  - ○ Best supportive care (hydroxyurea, transfusion support)

4. **How does the bone marrow result 14 to 21 days after beginning induction therapy in patients *older than 60 years* guide therapy?**
   - Aplastic marrow (<5% cellular and <5% blasts): Await count recovery and consider growth factor supplementation
   - Significant cytoreduction with low-percentage blasts:
     - ○ Additional standard dose cytarabine + anthracycline
     - ○ Standard-dose cytarabine with daunorubicin and midostaurin
     - ○ Dual-drug liposomal encapsulation of cytarabine 100 mg/m^2 and daunorubicin 44 mg/m^2 intravenous (IV) over 90 minutes on days 1 and 3 for subsequent cycles (therapy-related AML or AML with myelodysplasia-related changes)
     - ○ Intermediate-dose cytarabine-based regimen (1 to <2 g/m^2)
     - ○ Reduced-intensity hematopoietic stem cell transplantation (HSCT)
     - ○ Await count recovery

5. **When is complete remission (CR) evaluated and how is it defined?**
   - Evaluation of CR requires that a bone marrow biopsy be performed after count recovery—ANC ≥1,000 and platelets ≥100,000 (independent of transfusions)

   Morphologic CR: marrow blasts less than 5%, no Auer rods, no persistence of extramedullary disease

   Cytogenetic CR: normal cytogenetics in patients who had abnormal cytogenetics at diagnosis

   Incomplete CR (CRi): CR with persistence of cytopenia (usually thrombocytopenia)

6. **What is the post-remission treatment of choice for younger patients (<60 years old) with non-APL AML in complete remission?**
   - Favorable-risk AML:
     - High-dose cytarabine (3 g/m^2) over 3 hours every 12 hours on days 1, 3, and 5 for three to four cycles
     - Cytarabine $1,000 \text{ mg/m}^2$ every 12 hours on days 1 to 4 + daunorubicin 60 mg/m^2 on day 1 (first cycle) or days 1 to 2 (second cycle) + gemtuzumab ozogamicin 3 mg/m^2 (up to one 4.5 mg vial) on day 1 × 2 cycles
   - Intermediate-risk AML:
     - Allogeneic stem cell transplantation—matched sibling or alternative donor
     - High-dose cytarabine ($2-3 \text{ g/m}^2$) over 3 hours every 12 hours on day 1, 3, and 5 for three to four cycles
     - High-dose cytarabine (3 mg/m^2) over 3 hours every 12 hours on days 1, 3, and 5 with oral midostaurin 50 mg every 12 hours on days 8 to 21—*FLT3*-mutant AML
     - Dual-drug liposomal encapsulation cytarabine 65 mg/m^2 and daunorubicin and 29 mg/m^2 intravenous (IV) over 90 minutes on days 1 and 3 (therapy-related AML or AML with myelodysplasia-related changes)
     - Cytarabine $1,000 \text{ mg/m}^2$ every 12 hours on days 1 to 4 + daunorubicin 60 mg/m^2 on day 1 (first cycle) or days 1 to 2 (second cycle) + gemtuzumab ozogamicin 3 mg/m^2 (up to one 4.5 mg vial) on day 1 × 2 cycles (CD33 positive)
   - Poor-risk AML:
     - Allogeneic HSCT—matched sibling or alternative donor
     - High-dose cytarabine (3 gm/m^2) over 3 hours every 12 hours on days 1, 3, and 5 with oral midostaurin 50 mg every 12 hours on days 8 to 21—*FLT3*-mutant AML
     - Dual-drug liposomal encapsulation cytarabine 65 mg/m^2 and daunorubicin and 29 mg/m^2 IV over 90 minutes on days 1 and 3 (therapy-related AML or AML with myelodysplasia-related changes)

7. **What is the post-remission treatment of choice for older patients (>60 years old) with non-APL AML in complete remission?**
   Previous intensive therapy:
   - Reduced-intensity allogeneic HSCT—matched sibling or alternative donor
   - Standard-dose cytarabine ($100-200 \text{ mg/m}^2/\text{day}$) × 5 to 7 days ± idarubicin/daunorubicin for one to two cycles
   - Intermediate-dose cytarabine ($1-1.5 \text{ g/m}^2$) over 3 hours × 4–6 doses for 1 to 2 cycles for patients with good PS, normal renal function, and better-risk or normal karyotype
   - Intermediate-dose cytarabine ($1-1.5 \text{ gm/m}^2$) over 3 hours every 12 hours on days 1, 3 and 5 with oral midostaurin 50 mg every 12 hours on days 8 to 21—*FLT3*-mutant AML

- o Dual-drug liposomal encapsulation cytarabine 65 mg/m^2 and daunorubicin and 29 mg/m^2 intravenous (IV) over 90 minutes on days 1 and 3 (therapy-related AML or AML with myelodysplasia-related changes)
- o Cytarabine 1,000 mg/m^2 every 12 hours on days 1 to 4 + daunorubicin 60 mg/m^2 on day 1 (first cycle) or days 1 to 2 (second cycle) + gemtuzumab ozogamicin 3 mg/m^2 (up to one 4.5 mg vial) on day 1 × 2 cycles (CD33 positive)
- Continue azacytidine or decitabine every 4 to 6 weeks until toxicity or disease progression
- Observation

Previous lower intensive therapy:

- Reduced-intensity HSCT
- Continue hypomethylating regimen until progression
- Gemtuzumab ozogamicin 2 mg/m^2 on day 1 every 4 weeks up to eight continuation courses

8. What is the surveillance strategy in AML?

- Complete blood count (CBC) every 1 to 3 months for 2 years, then every 3 to 6 months until 5 years
- Bone marrow aspirate and biopsy only if cytopenias or abnormalities on peripheral smear
- Donor search at relapse (if not already done)

9. What is the treatment strategy for relapsed (non-APL AML patients?

Aggressive therapy for appropriate patients:

- Cladribine + cytarabine + granulocyte colony-stimulating factor (G-CSF) ± mitoxantrone or idarubicin
- High-dose cytarabine (HIDAC; if not received previously in treatment) ± (idarubicin or daunorubicin or mitoxantrone)
- Fludarabine + cytarabine + G-CSF ± idarubicin
- Etoposide + cytarabine ± mitoxantrone
- Clofarabine ± cytarabine + G-CSF ± idarubicin
- Dual-drug liposomal encapsulation of daunorubicin and cytarabine

Less aggressive therapy:

- Hypomethylating agents (5-azacytidine or decitabine)
- Low-dose cytarabine

Therapy for AML with *FLT3-ITD* mutation

- Hypomethylating agents (5-azacytidine or decitabine) + sorafenib

Therapy for AML with *IDH-2* mutation

- Enasidenib

Therapy for CD33-positive AML

- Gemtuzumab ozogamicin

10. **What are the induction and consolidation treatment options for patients with *high-risk* APL?**

Able to Tolerate Anthracyclines

- *Induction*: All-trans retinoic acid (ATRA) 45 mg/m^2 in divided doses until clinical remission + daunorubicin 50 mg/m^2 × 4 days + cytarabine 200 mg/m^2 × 7 days
  - *Consolidation (after CR)*: arsenic 0.15 mg/kg/day × 5 days for 5 weeks × 2 cycles, then ATRA 45 mg/m^2 × 7 days + daunorubicin 50 mg/m^2 × 3 days for two cycles
- *Induction*: ATRA 45 mg/m^2 (days 1–36, divided) + age-adjusted idarubicin 6 to 12 mg/m^2 on days 2, 4, 6, and 8 + arsenic trioxide 0.15 mg/kg (days 9–36 as 2-hr intravenous [IV] infusion)
  - *Consolidation*: ATRA 45 mg/m^2 × 28 days + arsenic trioxide 0.15 mg/kg/day × 28 days × 1 cycle then ATRA 45 mg/m^2 × 7 days every 2 weeks × 3 + arsenic trioxide 0.15 mg/kg/day × 5 days for 5 weeks × 1 cycle
- *Induction*: ATRA 45 mg/m^2 in divided doses + daunorubicin 60 mg/m^2 × 3 days + cytarabine 200 mg/m^2 × 7 days
  - *Consolidation (after CR)*: daunorubicin 60 mg/m^2 × 3 days + cytarabine 200 mg/m^2 × 7 days for one cycle, then cytarabine 1.5 to 2 g/m^2 (2 g/m^2 for age <50 years or 1.5 g/m^2 for age 50–60 years) every 12 hours × 5 days + daunorubicin 45 mg/m^2 × 3 days for one cycle and 5 doses of intrathecal chemotherapy
- *Induction*: ATRA 45 mg/m^2 in divided doses + idarubicin 12 mg/m^2 on days 2, 4, 6, and 8
  - *Consolidation (after CR)*: ATRA 45 mg/m^2 × 15 days + idarubicin 5 mg/m^2 and cytarabine 1 g/m^2 × 4 days for one cycle, then ATRA × 15 days + mitoxantrone 10 mg/m^2/day × 5 days for one cycle, then ATRA × 15 days + idarubicin 12 mg/m^2 for 1 dose + cytarabine 150 mg/m^2/8 h × 4 days for one cycle
- *Induction*: ATRA 45 mg/m^2 in divided doses daily + arsenic trioxide 0.15 mg/kg/day IV + gemtuzumab ozogamicin 9 mg/m^2 on day 1
- Consolidation: Arsenic trioxide 0.15 mg/kg IV daily 5 days/week for 4 weeks every 8 weeks for a total of four cycles + ATRA 45 mg/m^2 for 2 weeks every 4 weeks for a total of seven cycles. If ATRA or arsenic trioxide discontinued due to toxicity, gemtuzumab ozogamicin 9 mg/m^2 once every 4 to 5 weeks until 28 weeks from CR

Not Able to Tolerate Anthracyclines

- Induction: ATRA 45 mg/m^2 in two divided doses daily + arsenic trioxide 0.15 mg/kg IV daily
  - Consolidation: Arsenic trioxide 0.15 mg/kg/day IV 5 days/week for 4 weeks every 8 weeks for a total of 4 cycles, and ATRA 45 mg/m^2/d PO for 2 weeks every 4 weeks for a total of seven cycles
- Induction: ATRA 45 mg/m^2 in divided doses daily + arsenic trioxide 0.3 mg/kg IV on days 1 to 5 of cycle 1 and 0.25 mg/kg twice weekly in weeks 2 to 8

○ Consolidation: ATRA 45 mg/m² in divided doses daily + arsenic trioxide 0.3 mg/kg IV on days 1 to 5 of cycles 1 to 7 and 0.25 mg/kg twice weekly in weeks 2 to 4 of four cycles

- Induction: ATRA 45 mg/m² in two divided doses daily + gemtuzumab ozogamicin 9 mg/m² day 1 (for patients not able to tolerate arsenic trioxide for reasons that may include prolonged QTc)

  ○ Consolidation: ATRA 45 mg/m² in divided doses daily during weeks 1 to 2, 5 to 6, 9 to 10, 13 to 14, 17 to 18, 21 to 22, and 25 to 26 Gemtuzumab ozogamicin 9 mg/m² monthly until 28 weeks from CR

    ■ Patients started on an induction regimen according to one treatment protocol should receive consolidation and maintenance following the same protocol. Switching from one protocol to another should not be done.

    ■ All patients with high-risk acute promyelocytic leukemia (APL) should be considered for CNS prophylaxis with four to six doses of IT chemotherapy. The first lumbar puncture (LP) is performed at count recovery after induction therapy.

11. **What is the treatment of choice for patients with *low-/intermediate-riskAPL*?**

- *Induction*: All-trans retinoic acid (ATRA) 45 mg/m² in divided doses + arsenic trioxide 0.15 mg/kg intravenous (IV) daily

  ○ *Consolidation:* Arsenic trioxide 0.15 mg/kg/day intravenous (IV) 5 days/week for 4 weeks every 8 weeks for a total of four cycles, and ATRA 45 mg/m²/day for 2 weeks every 4 weeks for a total of seven cycles

- *Induction*: ATRA 45 mg/m² in divided doses daily + idarubicin 12 mg/m² on days 2, 4, 6, and 8

  ○ *Consolidation*: ATRA 45 mg/m² × 15 days + idarubicin 5 mg/m² × 4 days × 1 cycle, then ATRA × 15 days + mitoxantrone 10 mg/m²/day × 3 days × 1 cycle, then ATRA × 15 days + idarubicin 12 mg/m² × 1 dose × 1 cycle

- *Induction*: ATRA 45 mg/m² in divided doses daily + arsenic trioxide 0.3 mg/kg IV on days 1 to 5 of cycle 1 and 0.25 mg/kg twice weekly in weeks 2 to 8

  ○ *Consolidation*: ATRA 45 mg/m² in divided doses daily + arsenic trioxide 0.3 mg/kg IV on days 1 to 5 of cycles 1 to 7 and 0.25 mg/kg twice weekly in weeks 2 to 4 of four cycles

    ■ Patients started on an induction regimen according to one treatment protocol should receive consolidation and maintenance following the same protocol. Switching from one protocol to another should not be done.

12. **How are patients with APL monitored after consolidation and what is the postconsolidation therapy if polymerase chain reaction (PCR) is negative?**

- Bone marrow biopsy should be performed to document cytogenetic/molecular remission after consolidation.

- If PCR is negative, patients should receive maintenance therapy per the initial treatment protocol.
- PCR monitoring should be performed every 3 months for a minimum of 2 years.

13. How should patients with PCR-positive disease (after consolidation or if PCR turns positive during postconsolidation therapy) be treated?

- PCR should be repeated in 2 to 4 weeks for confirmation. If it is confirmed positive, patients are considered in first relapse.
  - ○ No prior exposure to arsenic trioxide or early relapse (≤6 months) after arsenic trioxide–containing regimen:
    - Arsenic trioxide 0.15 mg/kg intravenous (IV) daily ± all-trans retinoic acid (ATRA) 45 mg/m² in two divided doses daily ± **gemtuzumab until count recovery with marrow** confirmation of remission
  - ○ Early relapse (<6 months) after ATRA and arsenic trioxide only (no anthracycline):
    - Anthracycline-based regimen as given in high-risk APL
  - ○ Late relapse (≥6 months) after arsenic trioxide–containing regimen:
    - Arsenic trioxide 0.15 mg/ kg IV daily ± ATRA 45 mg/m² in two divided doses daily ± anthracycline ± gemtuzumab until count recovery with marrow confirmation of remission
- Those who achieve second morphologic remission should be strongly considered for CNS prophylaxis.
- If the PCR turns negative, patients should be treated with autologous stem cell transplantation (or with arsenic consolidation for a total of six cycles if not candidates for transplantation).
- If the PCR stays positive, patients should be treated with allogeneic stem cell transplantation (or on a clinical trial if not transplant candidates).
- Patients who do not achieve second morphologic remission are treated on a clinical trial or with allogeneic stem cell transplantation.

14. What is a unique medical emergency that can occur in the treatment of APL?

- *Differentiation syndrome*: develops in APL (ATRA and arsenic are risk factors)
  - ○ The signs and symptoms are fever, weight gain, edema, dyspnea, hypoxia, worsening renal function, opacities on chest imaging, pleural/pericardial effusions, and hypotension.
    - Patients need to be treated with dexamethasone 10 mg twice daily.
    - If differentiation syndrome is severe, ATRA (and arsenic) needs to be held and resumed only after it resolves.
    - Consider differentiation syndrome prophylactic therapy with dexamethasone when starting ATRA in patients with white blood cell (WBC) count greater than 30,000.

Acute Lymphoblastic Leukemia (ALL)

EPIDEMIOLOGY

1. What is the median age at diagnosis?

- Fifteen years
- ALL has a bimodal age distribution with a peak occurring during early childhood and a second peak after age 45 years. Fifty-seven percent of patients are diagnosed at age less than 20 years, and 27% are diagnosed at age 45 years or older

2. What is the incidence of ALL?

- There were an estimated 5,970 new cases of ALL in the United States in 2017.

ETIOLOGY AND RISK FACTORS

1. What are the common risk factors for ALL?

- Hispanics > Whites > African Americans
- Men > women
- Environmental exposure: nuclear radiation
- Prior chemotherapy exposure
- Congenital disorders: Down syndrome, ataxia-telangiectasia, Bloom syndrome

PATHOLOGY—CLASSIFICATION

1. How is ALL classified?

B-lymphoblastic leukemia/lymphoma

B-lymphoblastic leukemia/lymphoma NOS

B-lymphoblastic leukemia/lymphoma with recurrent genetic abnormalities

- with t(9;22)(q34.1;q11.2); BCR-ABL1
- with t(v;11q23.3); KMT2A
- with t(12;21)(p13.2;q22.1); ETV6-RUNX1
- with hyperdiploidy
- with hypodiploidy
- with t(5;14)(q31.1;q32.3);IL3-IGH
- with t(1;19)(q23;p13.3);TCF3-PBX1
- *Provisional entity, BCR-ABL1-like*
- *Provisional entity, with iAMP21*

T-lymphoblastic leukemia, lymphoma

T-lymphoblastic leukemia/lymphoma, NOS

Provisional entity, early T-cell precursor lymphoblastic leukemia

NOS, not otherwise specified.

SIGNS AND SYMPTOMS

1. What are the common signs and symptoms of ALL?

- Lymphadenopathy and/or hepatosplenomegaly
- Fever and other constitutional symptoms
- Infections
- Bleeding
- Fatigue and other symptoms of anemia
- Leukostasis: CNS manifestations, cardiopulmonary symptoms, retinal hemorrhage, priapism
- DIC
- Tumor lysis syndrome (TLS)
- Painless testicular swelling
- Mediastinal mass
- Musculoskeletal pain

Please see Chapter 20 for management of the hematologic emergencies of leukostasis, DIC, and TLS.

DIAGNOSTIC WORKUP

1. What are the diagnostic criteria for ALL?

- Marrow and/or peripheral blood and/or lymph node involvement with lymphoid blasts
  - Typically, there will be 20% lymphoblasts in the marrow at the time of diagnosis
- Phenotypic and genetic determination of the lymphoblasts to allow for appropriate subclassification as outlined earlier

PROGNOSTIC FACTORS

1. How are patients with ALL stratified into different risk groups?

	Adverse Risk	Standard Risk
Age	<1 y or >35 y	>1 y but <35 y
Immunophenotype	ETP	T cell
	Pro-B (especially CD20+)	pre-B
WBC count	>100,000 for T cell	<100,000 for T cell
	>30,000 for B cell	<30,000 for B cell

(continued)

	Adverse Risk	Standard Risk
Genetic aberrations	Complex (≥5 changes)	Hyperdiploidy (>50 chromosomes)
	low hypodiploidy (30 to 39 chromosomes)/ near triploidy (60 to 78 chromosomes)	t(1;14)
		t(12;21)
	t(9;22) or BCR-ABL	
	MLL rearrangement especially t(4;11)	
	14q32/IGH translocation	
CNS involvement	Present	Absent
Response to therapy	Time to CR >4 weeks	
	Minimal residual disease present after induction	

CNS, central nervous system; CR, complete remission; ETP, early T precursor; MLL, mixed lineage leukemia; WBC, white blood cell.

TREATMENT

1. **How are adult patients with Philadelphia chromosome–positive (Ph+) ALL treated?**
   - Adolescent and young adult (AYA; age 15–39 years)
     - Induction chemotherapy + tyrosine kinase inhibitors (TKI). If CR is achieved, patients should undergo consideration for an allogeneic stem cell transplantation followed by consideration of maintenance TKI following the transplant. If no donor is available or the patients are ineligible for a transplant, they should be continued on consolidation multiagent chemotherapy + TKI followed by maintenance therapy + TKI.
     - Examples include COG AALL-0031, EsPhALL regimen, TKI + hyperCVAD, TKI, + multiagent chemotherapy, TKI + corticosteroids, TKI + dexamethasone + vincristine.
   - Patients ≤65 years without major comorbidities:
     - Induction chemotherapy + TKI. If CR is achieved, patients should undergo consideration for an allogeneic stem cell transplantation followed by consideration of maintenance TKI following the transplant. If no donor is available or the patients are ineligible for a transplant, they should be continued on consolidation multiagent chemotherapy + TKI followed by maintenance therapy + TKI.
     - Examples include TKI + hyperCVAD, TKI + multiagent chemotherapy, TKI + corticosteroids, TKI + dexamethasone + vincristine.
   - Patients >65 years old or with significant comorbidities:
     - Induction therapy with TKI + steroids or TKI + chemotherapy. If they achieve CR, they should be continued on TKI as consolidation.

2. **How are adult patients with (Ph− ALL treated?**
   - Adolescent and young adult (AYA; age 15–39 years)
     - Pediatric-inspired regimens
     - Multiagent chemotherapy
     - Examples include C10403, COG AALL-0232, COG AALL 0434, DFCI ALL 00-01regimen
     GRAALL 2005 regimen, PATHEMA ALL-96 regimen, hyperCVAD, and USC-CCG 1882 regimen
     - If CR is achieved, patients should continue multiagent chemotherapy as consolidation followed by maintenance therapy or undergo allogeneic stem cell transplantation if a donor is available (if high risk as outlined in table in the preceding text)
   - Patients <65 years old without major comorbidities:
     - Induction with multiagent chemotherapy
     - Examples include CALGB 8811, Linker 4-drug regimen, hyper-CVAD, MRC UKALLXII/ECOG2993
     - If CR is achieved, patients should continue multiagent chemotherapy as consolidation followed by maintenance therapy or undergo allogeneic stem cell transplantation if a donor is available (if high risk as outlined in table in the preceding text)
   - Patients who are ≥65 years old or older or with substantial comorbidities:
     - Induction with multiagent chemotherapy or steroids. If they achieve CR, they should receive consolidation with chemotherapy followed by maintenance therapy
     - Examples include CALGB 8811, Linker 4-drug regimen, hyper-CVAD, MRC UKALLXII/ECOG2993

3. **How are patients with relapsed/refractory ALL treated?**
   - Ph+ ALL: Consider ABL kinase domain mutation testing. Treatment options include
     - Chemotherapy ±TKI
     - TKI ± steroids
     - Blinatumomab (after failure of 2 TKIs). Blinatimumab can be used only if the ALL blasts express CD19
     - Inotuzumab ozogamicin (it is an option if the ALL blasts express CD22)
     - Tisagenlecleucel (chimeric antigen receptor [CAR] T cells, for age ≤25 years and refractory disease or ≥2 relapses and failure of 2 TKIs)
       - Allogeneic stem cell transplantation is considered if a morphological remission is obtained
   - Ph− ALL: Treatment options include
     - Multiagent chemotherapy
     - Blinatumomab for B-cell acute lymphoblastic leukemia (B-ALL)
     - Inotuzumab ozogamicin

   ○ Tisagenlecleucel (for age ≤25 years and refractory disease or ≥2 relapses)
   ○ Nelarabine for T-cell acute lymphoblastic leukemia (T-ALL)
      ■ Allogeneic stem cell transplantation is considered if a morphological re-
        mission is obtained.

QUESTIONS

1. A 43-year-old woman presents to the emergency room (ER) with progressive fatigue and frequent nose bleeds. A complete blood count
reveals a white blood cell (WBC) count of 78, hemoglobin (Hgb) of 9.3,
and platelet count of 17. Differential reveals 87% circulating blasts
with Aurer rods present. A bone marrow biopsy is performed and
confirms the diagnosis of acute myeloid leukemia. She begins induction chemotherapy with using daunorubicin 90 mg/m² and cytarabine
100 mg/m² in a standard 3 + 7 fashion. Human leukocyte antigen
(HLA) typing is sent on admission, and she is found to have a matched
related donor. Which of the following findings is considered favorable risk, indicating that the patient should proceed with consolidative
chemotherapy alone?
A. Normal female karyotype, *FLT3-ITD* mutation positive
B. Cytogenetics revealing t(6;9)
C. Cytogenetics revealing t(8;21), *c-KIT* mutation negative
D. Monosomal karyotype

2. A 25-year-old woman completed multiagent chemotherapy including
alkylating agents, etoposide, and radiation therapy for Ewing's sarcoma 2 years ago. She has been free of disease since, but on routine
blood work, she was noted to have a white blood cell (WBC) count of
51, hemoglobin (Hgb) of 8.6, and platelet count of 72. A bone marrow biopsy confirms the diagnosis of acute myeloid leukemia. Which
cytogenetic abnormality is she most likely to have?
A. 11q23 abnormality
B. t(8;21)
C. t(15;17)
D. Monosomy 7

3. A 57-year-old man is 10 days into therapy with all-trans retinoic acid
(ATRA) and arsenic trioxide for a diagnosis of low-risk acute promyelocytic leukemia (APL) when he begins to develop hypoxia, dyspnea,
and lower extremity edema. Chest x-ray reveals bilateral pulmonary
infiltrates. What is the most appropriate next step in management?
A. Obtain a nasopharyngeal swab for presumed viral lower respiratory
tract infection
B. Start dexamethasone 10 mg twice daily for presumed differentiation
syndrome
C. Order a stat high-resolution computed tomography scan and initiate
heparin drip
D. Perform a stat bedside transthoracic echocardiogram for suspected
therapy-induced cardiomyopathy

4. A 42-year-old man is diagnosed with Philadelphia chromosome–positive pre-B cell acute lymphoblastic leukemia (ALL). After undergoing intensive induction with multiagent chemotherapy and tyrosine kinase inhibitor (TKI), he achieves a complete morphologic remission. Minimal residual disease testing by quantitative polymerase chain reaction testing (qPCR) for the BCR-ABL translocation is also negative. He has a human leukocyte antigen (HLA)-matched related sibling. What is the best strategy for additional therapy?
   A. Consolidation with an allogeneic stem cell transplant
   B. Consolidation with chemotherapy and TKI
   C. Consolidation with chemotherapy followed by an autologous stem cell transplant
   D. Maintenance therapy with TKI indefinitely

5. A 37-year-old woman is diagnosed with acute myeloid leukemia (AML) after presenting with signs and symptoms of leukostasis due to a presenting white blood cell (WBC) of 175,000. She is appropriately treated for this medical emergency and then started on induction chemotherapy when her FLT3-ITD testing comes back positive. What additional therapy could you consider adding on day 8 of induction chemotherapy?
   A. Midostaurin
   B. Hydroxyurea
   C. Imatinib
   D. Ruxolitinib

6. A 43-year-old woman with standard-risk AML achieved a complete remission after undergoing induction chemotherapy with 3 + 7 chemotherapy. She proceeds with consolidation using high-dose cytarabine (HIDAC). During her second cycle of consolidation, she develops an acute onset of slurring of her speech, nystagmus, and ataxia. This is deemed to be cerebellar toxicity related to her cytarabine therapy. Fortunately, her symptoms resolve within 10 days. What further therapy should be recommended?
   A. Continue with HIDAC consolidation for two additional cycles at 50% dose reduction
   B. Continue with HIDAC consolidation for two additional cycles at same dose
   C. Discontinue any further HIDAC consolidation. Find an alternative consolidative therapy
   D. Discontinue all further therapy

7. A 32-year-old Hispanic man presents to the emergency room with a nosebleed that will not stop and a recent history of gum bleeding. He is not on any blood thinners. A complete blood count reveals a white blood cell (WBC) count of 3, hemoglobin of 7.9, and platelets of 71. A disseminated intravascular coagulation (DIC) panel demonstrates a fibrinogen of 47, prothrombin time (PT) of >16 seconds, and partial

thromboplastin time (PTT) of >72 seconds. A review of the peripheral blood smear shows rare WBCs that have irregular azurophilic granules and elongated needle-type structures in the cytoplasm. Peripheral blood flow cytometry and formal pathology review are pending. In addition to recommending an expedited bone marrow biopsy and cryoprecipitate for the patient's DIC, what else do you recommend?

A. Observation while you await the final pathology report
B. Start 3 + 7 chemotherapy immediately
C. Start all-trans retinoic acid (ATRA) immediately
D. Start hydroxyurea while you await the formal pathology report

ANSWERS

1. **C. Cytogenetics revealing t(8;21), *c-KIT* mutation negative.** The National Comprehensive Cancer Network (NCCN) recognizes a monosomal karyotype, t(6;9), and a normal female karyotype with *FLT3-ITD* mutation as well-validated poor-risk prognostic factors. As such, the recommendation for standard post-remission therapy would be an allogeneic stem cell transplant. Alternatively, the presence of a core binding factor leukemia, t(8;21), is a well-validated favorable-risk group. As such, the recommendation for standard post-remission therapy is high-dose cytarabine.

2. **A. 11q23 abnormality.** The multiagent chemotherapy this patient received in treatment for her Ewing's sarcoma has put her at risk for a treatment-related acute myeloid leukemia (AML), which occurs in about 10% to 20% of all cases of AML. The latency of 2 years between treatment and onset of AML favors topoisomerase II inhibitor (etoposide) as the culprit. T-AML caused by topoisomerase II inhibitors is often associated with translocation 11q23 (KMT2A, previously known as mixed lineage leukemia [MLL]). Alkylating agents, on the other hand, would be expected to have a longer latency period of 5 to 10 years, tend to be associated with antecedent treatment-related myelodysplastic syndrome (MDS), and are associated with complex cytogenetics as well as monosomy 5 or 7.

3. **B. Start dexamethasone 10 mg twice daily for presumed differentiation syndrome.** Differentiation symptom occurs in 2% to 30% of patients receiving ATRA or arsenic trioxide. Signs and symptoms include leukocytosis, dyspnea, fever, pulmonary edema or infiltrates, effusions, weight gain, and bone pain. Classically, it develops 10 to 12 days after initiation of therapy. Treatment includes prompt initiation of steroids as well as consideration of discontinuation of the differentiating agent (ATRA and/or arsenic trioxide), depending on the severity of symptoms.

4. **A. Consolidation with an allogeneic stem cell transplant.** The National Comprehensive Cancer Network (NCCN) continues to recommend allogeneic stem cell transplant in first complete remission (CR) due to lack of data on long-term survival with treatment involving a TKI with multiagent chemotherapy alone. Additionally, salvage therapy in the relapsed setting remains challenging and so stem cell transplant is recommended in first CR if available.

5. **A. Midostaurin.** Midostaurin is an oral tyrosine kinase inhibitor that was approved in April 2017 for the treatment of newly diagnosed AML harboring *FLT3* mutations. Approval was based on a randomized, double-blind trial of 717 patients with previously untreated FLT3+ AML. During this trial, patients received midostaurin 50 mg orally twice daily on days 8 to 21 of each cycle of induction and consolidation followed by continuous daily use for up to 12 cycles. The study demonstrated an improvement in overall survival for patients receiving midostaurin versus placebo (hazard ration [HR] 0.77, $p = 0.016$).

6. **C. Discontinue any further HIDAC consolidation. Find an alternative consolidative therapy.** Neurologic toxicity with HIDAC typically presents as ataxia, nystagmus, dysmetria, and dysarthria, whereas seizures, neuropathy, and cerebral dysfunction are far less common. Signs of cerebellar dysfunction usually appear between the 3rd and 8th day of treatment. With development of cerebellar toxicity, all further HIDAC should be stopped. Renal insufficiency is a risk factor for developing cerebellar toxicity with HIDAC chemotherapy. You should not rechallenge in the future, even with resolution of symptoms.

   However, after only two cycles of consolidative chemotherapy, you should also not completely stop consolidative chemotherapy. For these patients, you can consider an autologous transplant.

7. **C. Start ATRA immediately.** The description of the peripheral blood smear as well as the clinical presentation with low blood counts and DIC is highly suspicious for acute promyelocytic leukemia (APL). The high initial mortality rate from APL is predominantly related to DIC and bleeding complications. The potential risks of a single dose of ATRA, should the diagnosis NOT be APL, are low, whereas the risk of delaying administration of ATRA in the setting of true APL could be catastrophic.

- Fanconi's anemia (*FANCA, FANC, FANCG*)
- Dyskeratosis congenita (*DKC1, TERT, TERC*, others) and other disorders of short telomeres (termed telomeropathies)
- Severe congenital neutropenia aka Kostmann syndrome (*ELANE* and others)
- Neurofibromatosis (*NF1*)
- Ataxia-telangiectasia (*ATM*)
- Bloom syndrome (*BLM*)
- Noonan syndrome (*PTPN11* and others)
- Familial MDS with germline mutations in *GATA2, RUNX1, CEBPA, ETV6, ANKRD26, DDX41, SRP72*, and others

4. What is the pathogenesis of MDS?
- Exact pathogenesis is unknown.
- A hematopoietic stem cell is thought to acquire mutations resulting in clonal hematopoiesis, clonal expansion, morphologic dysplasia, and eventually ineffective hematopoiesis with cytopenias.

5. What is the hallmark of clonal hematopoiesis?
- Presence of a distinct population of hematopoietic cells (a clone) characterized by a somatic (i.e., acquired rather than inherited) genetic abnormality

6. What is clonal hematopoiesis of indeterminate potential (CHIP)?
- A precursor state for MDS. Similar precursor states are monoclonal gammopathy of undetermined significance (MGUS) for plasma cell neoplasms or monoclonal B-cell lymphocytosis (MBL) for chronic lymphocytic leukemia (CLL)
- Present in ~10% of people >65 years old
- Annual risk of progression to MDS is ~0.5% to 1%
- CHIP is characterized by age-related acquisition of somatic mutations in genes associated with myeloid neoplasia by normal hematopoietic cells. To diagnose CHIP, a somatic mutation has to be present at >2% variant allele frequency
- There are no cytopenias or morphologic dysplasia in CHIP

7. Besides CHIP, what other indolent myeloid hematopoietic disorders are recognized?

	ICUS	IDUS	CHIP	CCUS
Cytopenia	Yes	No	No	Yes
Dysplasia	No	Yes	No	No
Clonality	No	No	Yes	Yes

CCUS, clonal cytopenia of undetermined significance; ICUS, idiopathic cytopenia of undetermined significance; IDUS, idiopathic dysplasia of undetermined significance.

8. How common are karyotype abnormalities in MDS?
- A karyotype abnormality is detected in ~50% of MDS cases by standard cytogenetics.

9. **What is the most common chromosomal abnormality in MDS?**
   - del(5q): present in 10% to 15% of MDS patients

10. **What percentage of MDS patients has a somatic mutation in one or more recurrently mutated genes in this disease?**
    - Eighty to ninety percent of MDS patients have a somatic mutation in one or more recurrently mutated genes.

11. **What groups of genes are recurrently mutated in MDS and might indicate clonal hematopoiesis?**
    - Epigenetic regulators—*TET2, DNMT3A, ASXL1, EZH2, IDH1/IDH2, ATRX*
    - Splicing genes—*SF3B1, SRSF2*
    - Transcription factors—*RUNX1, GATA2*
    - Signaling—*NRAS/KRAS, CBL, JAK2*
    - Cohesins—*STAG2*
    - Others—*TP53*

12. **What are some clinical associations with the gene mutations already mentioned?**
    - *SF3B1*—presence of ringed sideroblasts
    - *ATRX*—acquired alpha-thalassemia
    - *RUNX1*—thrombocytopenia

SIGNS AND SYMPTOMS

1. **What are the common signs and symptoms of MDS?**
   - Incidental cytopenias
   - Infections (due to neutropenia)
   - Bleeding (due to thrombocytopenia)
   - Fatigue or other symptoms/signs of anemia

DIAGNOSIS

1. **What is the recommended workup for suspected MDS?**
   - History and physical exam (focus on family history, exposures, and additional features suggesting a congenital disorder)
   - Complete blood count with white blood cell differential
   - Peripheral blood smear
   - Serum ferritin level
   - Serum B12 and folic acid level (or red blood cell [RBC] folate), followed by homocysteine and methylmalonic acid (MMA) levels if necessary
   - Copper level (especially if patient has malabsorption, neuropathy, neutropenia, excess zinc intake)
   - Bone marrow aspiration and biopsy
   - Bone marrow cytogenetics (± fluorescence in situ hybridization [FISH] if classic karyotyping fails)

2. **What are some differential diagnoses for morphologic dysplasia in the bone marrow?**
   - Nutritional deficiencies (B12, folate, copper)
   - Heavy metal poisoning (zinc, lead, arsenic)
   - Excess alcohol consumption
   - Medications, including chemotherapy
   - HIV
   - Of note, ringed sideroblasts are common in the settings of excess alcohol consumption, heavy metal poisoning, and copper deficiency

3. **What are the diagnostic criteria for MDS?**
   - Persistent cytopenia(s)—hemoglobin <10, platelets <100,000, and absolute neutrophil count (ANC) <1,800
   - Presence of bone marrow morphologic dysplasia in >10% cells of at least one lineage or increased bone marrow blasts (>5%) or presence of >15% ringed sideroblasts (or >5% in the presence of *SF3B1* mutation)

4. **Can MDS be diagnosed without morphologic dysplasia?**
   - In the absence of dysplasia, MDS can be diagnosed if cytopenias are present in the setting of an MDS-defining karyotype abnormality (such as −7/del(7q), del(5q), del(13q), del(11q), del(17p), and many others). Of note, −Y, del 20q, and +8 are not MDS-defining karyotype abnormalities.

CLASSIFICATION

1. **What is taken into account when classifying MDS?**
   - Presence of dysplasia in single versus multiple lineages
   - Presence or absence of ringed sideroblasts (RSs)
   - Presence or absence of excess blasts, that is, >5% in bone marrow and >1% in peripheral blood
   - Presence of isolated del(5q) with no more than one additional abnormality except for del (7q)/−7

2. **What are the subtypes of MDS according to the World Health Organization (WHO) 2016 classification?**

MDS Subtype	Blood	Bone Marrow
MDS with single lineage dysplasia (MDS-SLD)	Single or bicytopenia, <1% blasts	<5% blasts, dysplasia in 1 cell line
MDS with multilineage dysplasia (MDS-MLD)	Bicytopenia or pancytopenia, <1% blasts	<5% blasts, dysplasia in 2 or 3 cell lines

(continued)

MDS Subtype	Blood	Bone Marrow
MDS with ringed sideroblasts with single lineage dysplasia (MDS-RS-SLD)	Single or bicytopenia, <1% blasts	<5% blasts, erythroid dysplasia only, ≥5%* or ≥15% ringed sideroblasts
MDS with ringed sideroblasts with multilineage dysplasia (MDS-RS-MLD)	Bicytopenia or pancytopenia, <1% blasts	<5% blasts, dysplasia in 2 or 3 cell lines, ≥5%* or ≥15% ringed sideroblasts
MDS associated with isolated del(5q)	Anemia, normal or elevated platelets, <1% blasts	<5% blasts, erythroid dysplasia only, isolated del(5q) or one additional abnormality other than del (7q) or monosomy 7
MDS with excess blasts-1 (MDS-EB-1)	<5% blasts, no Auer rods	5%–9% blasts, no Auer rods, dysplasia in 0–3 lineages
MDS with excess blasts-2 (MDS-EB-2)	Blasts 5%–19% or Auer rods	10%–19% blasts or presence of auer rods, dysplasia in 0–3 lineages
Myelodysplastic syndrome, unclassified (MDS-U)†	Cytopenias	<5% blasts, <15% ringed sideroblasts, dysplasia or no dysplasia with MDS characteristic cytogenetics

Note: Dysplasia is considered present if it involves at least 10% of a lineage.

Monocyte count is less than 1,000/microL in all subtypes of MDS.

*≥5% ringed sideroblasts is enough for diagnosis if *SF3B1* mutation is present

†Pancytopenia with dysplasia in one lineage is classified as MDS-U. Similarly, MDS in the setting of <5% bone marrow (BM) blasts (no Auer rods) and 1% peripheral blood (PB) blasts (documented on 2 occasions) is classified as MDS-U.

3. What is the only genetically defined MDS subtype?

- Del (5q) is the only genetic abnormality defining an MDS subtype.
- However, "MDS with isolated del(5q)" can be diagnosed with one additional cytogenetic abnormality as long as it is not del(7q) or monosomy 7.

PROGNOSTIC FACTORS

1. How are patients with MDS stratified into different risk groups?

- The International Prognostic Scoring System (IPSS) stratifies MDS into four risk groups: low risk (IPSS score 0), intermediate-1 risk (IPSS score 0.5–1), intermediate-2 risk (IPSS score 1.5–2), and high risk (IPSS score 2.5–3.5). Patients with low, intermediate-1-, intermediate-2-, and high-risk MDS by IPSS have median overall survivals of 5.7, 3.5, 1.2, and 0.4 years, respectively.
- The IPSS scoring system should only be used at diagnosis in nontherapy-related MDS.

IPSS Scores

	0	0.5	1	1.5	2
Percentage of bone marrow blasts	< 5	5–10	–	11–20	> 20
Karyotype*	Good	Intermediate	Poor	–	–
Number of cytopenias†	0–1	2–3	–	–	–

*Good karyotype risk: normal, –Y, del(5q), del(20q); poor karyotype risk: complex karyotype (≥ 3 abnormalities), chromosome 7 abnormalities; intermediate karyotype risk: all others.

†Neutropenia: absolute neutrophil count (ANC) <1,800; anemia: hemoglobin (Hgb) <10; thrombocytopenia: platelets <100,000.

- More recently, the IPSS has been refined (revised IPSS or IPSS-R) utilizing a larger patient cohort. This has allowed a further refinement of outcomes of patients, especially those with low-risk disease per IPSS. However, this still applies only to treatment-naïve patients with de novo disease.

Revised IPSS

	0	0.5	1	1.5	2	3	4
BM blasts	≤2		>2 to <5		5–10	>10	
Cytogenetics*	Very good		Good		Intermediate	Poor	Very poor
Hemoglobin	≥10		8 to <10	<8			
Platelets	≥100	50–100	<50				
Absolute neutrophil count	≥0.8	<0.8					

*Very good karyotype includes –Y or del(11q); good karyotype includes normal karyotype, del (5q), del(12p), del (20q), or a double abnormality including del(5q); intermediate karyotype includes del(7q), +8, +19, i(17q), and any other single or double independent clones; poor karyotype includes –7, inv(3)/t(3q)/del(3q), double abnormalities including –7/del(7q), or three abnormalities; very poor karyotype includes complex karyotype (≥3 abnormalities).

BM, bone marrow; IPSS, International Prognostic Scoring System.

- A third system, the World Health Organization (WHO) Classification–Based Prognostic Scoring System for MDS (WPSS) can be used throughout the MDS disease course. However, it is based on the 2008 WHO classification of MDS.

INDICATIONS FOR TREATMENT

1. What are the indications for therapy in MDS?

- Transfusion dependence or symptoms related to cytopenias
- Intermediate-2- or high-risk MDS (based on the International Prognostic Scoring System [IPSS])

TREATMENT

1. **What determines the initial treatment plan?**
   - Patient's risk based on the International Prognostic Scoring System (IPSS)—approach to low-/intermediate-1-risk disease is different than that to intermediate-2-/high-risk disease.

2. **What is the treatment of choice for patients with low-/intermediate-1-risk MDS with symptomatic/transfusion-dependent anemia and absence of del(5q)?**
   - The treatment of these patients is based on the erythropoietin level and the number of red blood cell transfusions per month. Erythropoietin-stimulating agents (ESAs) are the mainstay of treatment if erythropoietin (EPO) level is below 500. Of note, iron stores need to be replete before initiation of ESAs.
   - Patients with an EPO level <100 and <2 transfusions per month have a 74% chance of responding to ESAs. If EPO is 100 to 500 and/or they require more than two transfusions per month, the chance of response with ESA is 23%. If EPO >500, the chance of achieving an erythroid response with ESA is only 7%.
   - Most responses to ESAs occur within 8 weeks of treatment, though some patients might respond after 12 weeks of treatment. The median time of response is ~2 years.
   - In patients are not responding to ESAs, the addition of granulocyte colony-stimulating factor (G-CSF) should be considered. In patients who do not respond to ESAs ± G-CSF or who lose a response to this therapy, the addition of lenalidomide to the latter therapy should be strongly considered.
   - Patients predicted to have a low chance of responding to ESAs, that is, EPO level >500, are generally treated with DNA methyltransferase inhibitors (azacitidine or decitabine). Lenalidomide can be considered.

3. **Is lenalidomide indicated in patients with low-/intermediate-1-risk MDS with symptomatic or transfusion-dependent anemia in the absence of del(5q)?**
   - Lenalidomide results in an overall response rate of 26% in patients with low-/intermediate-1-risk MDS without del(5q). Lenalidomide, as a single agent, is therefore not generally recommended as frontline therapy for MDS patients without del(5q) and is only considered as an additional therapy to erythropoietin-stimulating agents (ESAs; ± G-CSF) after failure of the latter therapy (see preceding text).

4. **What is the treatment of choice for patients with low-/intermediate-1-risk MDS with symptomatic/transfusion-dependent anemia and isolated del(5q) abnormality?**
   - Lenalidomide (10 mg a day) is the treatment of choice for these patients.
   - Transfusion-dependent patients with low-/intermediate-1-risk MDS and del(5q) have ~67% chance of becoming transfusion independent (for medial duration of ~2–2.5 years) and ~62% chance of achieving complete cytogenetic response with lenalidomide.
   - Erythropoietin-stimulating agents (ESAs) are an alternative to lenalidomide in these patients (as in Question 2 in the preceding text) if EPO is <500.

5. **What is the treatment of choice for patients with low-/intermediate-1-risk MDS with thrombocytopenia and/or neutropenia?**
   - Observation, if the thrombocytopenia and/or neutropenia are not severe
   - Azacitidine or decitabine, if the thrombocytopenia and/or neutropenia are significant
   - Patients with low-/intermediate-1-risk MDS have better overall survival (according to retrospective data) if allogeneic hematopoietic stem cell transplantation (ASCT) is delayed until progression

6. **When is immunosuppressive therapy (antithymocyte globulin and cyclosporine) considered in MDS?**
   - Antithymocyte globulin and cyclosporine could be considered in a specific subgroup of younger patients (<60 years of age) with low-/intermediate-1-risk MDS with the following characteristics: hypocellular bone marrow, <5% blasts, presence of a paroxysmal nocturnal hemoglobinuria clone, presence of an HLA-DR15 haplotype, or the presence of *STAT3*-mutated T-cell clones.

7. **When should iron chelation be initiated in MDS?**
   - Currently, it is not recommended to routinely use iron chelation therapy in MDS and none of the iron chelating agents has been evaluated in a prospective clinical trial in MDS. Iron chelation may be considered in MDS patients undergoing curative intent therapy with allogeneic stem cell transplantation (ASCT). Therefore, ferritin should be monitored specifically in the latter patients.

8. **What are the treatment options for patients with intermediate-2-/high-risk MDS?**
   - Allogeneic stem cell transplantation (ASCT) is the only curative modality in MDS and is the treatment of choice in patients with intermediate-2-/high-risk disease. A retrospective analysis showed that patients with intermediate-2-/high-risk MDS have better overall survivals if they undergo ASCT. Administration of azacitidine or decitabine prior to ASCT is not routinely recommended because it has not been shown to add value in patients planning to proceed with ASCT; however, this should be considered in patients whose ASCT is expected to be delayed.
   - Patients who are not candidates for or who decline ASCT should be treated with azacitidine or decitabine. Azacitidine is the only one of these two drugs that was shown in a randomized control trial to confer a survival benefit compared to best supportive care. However, this is felt to be due to the different designs of the azacitidine and decitabine trials, and both drugs are considered to have equal value in MDS.

9. **For how many cycles should azacitidine or decitabine be given?**
   - Patients receiving azacitidine or decitabine who are not candidates for allogeneic stem cell transplantation (ASCT) should continue receiving these drugs until disease progression or if they develop side effects prohibiting their use. Patients should receive a minimum of 4 to 6 cycles of azacitidine or decitabine before declaring the patient nonresponsive to this therapy.

Myelodysplastic Syndromes

12

Jedrzej Wykretowicz and Rami N. Khoriaty

Mylodysplastic Syndromes

DEFINITION

1. **How are myelodysplastic syndromes (MDSs) defined?**
   - Clonal bone marrow neoplasms characterized by morphologic dysplasia and peripheral cytopenia(s) due to ineffective hematopoiesis

EPIDEMIOLOGY

1. **What is the usual age at diagnosis for MDS?**
   - Most patients are ≥65 years old (median age at diagnosis 70–75 years).
   - In younger patients (especially <50 years of age), consider the possibility of genetic predisposition, particularly if the MDS is not therapy related.

2. **How many new cases of MDSs are diagnosed every year in the United States?**
   - Per year, 10,000 to 15,000 new cases (likely an underestimate, with claims-based data suggesting ~30,000 new cases per year)

ETIOLOGY, RISK FACTORS, AND PATHOGENESIS

1. **What is the etiology of MDS?**
   - Exact etiology is uncertain.
   - Ninety percent of MDS cases arise de novo, 5% to 10% cases are therapy related, and 1% to 2% of cases have an inherited genetic predisposition.

2. **What are the common risk factors for MDS?**
   - Age (incidence rises exponentially with age)
   - Male sex
   - Chemotherapy exposure (most common culprits are alkylating agents and topoisomerase II inhibitors such as anthracyclines)
   - Radiation exposure
   - Benzene and other organic solvent exposure
   - Genetic predisposition (syndromic or nonsyndromic)

3. **What congenital syndromes predispose to MDS and what is (are) the commonly mutated gene(s) in each of these syndromes?**
   - Down syndrome (trisomy 21)

10. **Is there a role for combining a hypomethylating agent and lenalidomide in intermediate-2-/high-risk MDS?**
    - There is no role for this combination at this time (based on a randomized phase II trial).

CHRONIC MYELOMONOCYTIC LEUKEMIA

1. **What is chronic myelomonocytic leukemia (CMML)?**
   - CMML is an overlap syndrome between MDS and myeloproliferative neoplasms and has features of both
   - MDS features: dysplasia, anemia, and/or thrombocytopenia
   - Myeloproliferative features: leukocytosis, monocytosis, and splenomegaly

2. **What are the diagnostic criteria for CMML?**
   - CMML is characterized by absolute monocytosis (≥1,000), accounting for more than 10% of total white blood cell (WBC) count. The monocytosis should be persistent for more than 3 months with no other etiology identified.
   - CMML can only be diagnosed after ruling out other myeloid neoplasms (such as chronic myeloid leukemia [CML], polycythemia vera [PV], essential thrombocythemia [ET], or primary myelofibrosis [PMF]), and secondary causes of monocytosis.
   - In cases with eosinophilia, *PDGFRA*, *PDGFRB*, and *FGFR1* rearrangements or *PCM1-JAK2* fusion should be ruled out.
   - Bone marrow dysplasia is usually present.
   - Cytogenetic abnormalities are found in ~30% of patients with CMML.
   - In patients without cytogenetic abnormalities and without significant dysplasia on the bone marrow, other causes of monocytosis need to be carefully ruled out before a diagnosis of CMML can be made.

3. **What genetic changes are most often seen in CMML?**
   - Thirty percent of patients have clonal cytogenetic abnormalities. The most common ones are trisomy 8, abnormalities in chromosome 7 (−7 or del7q), −Y, and complex karyotypes.
   - More than ninety percent of patients have a recurrent mutation in one or more of the following genes: *SRSF2* (most common ~50%), *ASXL1*, *EZH2*, *TET2*, *RUNX1*, *JAK2*, *KRAS*, *NRAS*, and *CBL*.

4. **What are the two prognostic features for CMML?**
   - White blood cell (WBC) count >13,000 distinguishes myeloproliferative-CMML from myelodysplastic-CMML (WBC <13,000). The latter has a better prognosis.
   - Based on the number of blasts, CMML can be subdivided into CMML-0 (<1% peripheral blood blasts and <5% bone marrow blasts), CMML-1 (2%–4% peripheral blood blasts or 5%–9% bone marrow blasts), and CMML-2 (5%–19% peripheral blood blasts or 10%–19% bone marrow blasts) with progressively worse prognosis.

5. **How is CMML treated?**

- Asymptomatic patients with no significant anemia or thrombocytosis could be observed. Hydroxyurea could be utilized in these patients if they have a significantly increased leukocyte count or symptomatic splenomegaly.

- The only curative option for CMML is allogeneic stem cell transplantation (ASCT). Patients who require therapy should be directed toward ASCT if clinically appropriate. All patients should be evaluated for ASCT at diagnosis and a donor search should be initiated.

- Patients who require therapy but are not candidates for ASCT, or in whom ASCT has to be significantly delayed, should be treated with hypomethylating agents, azacitidine, or decitabine.

QUESTIONS

1. A 69-year-old female is evaluated for asymptomatic anemia found incidentally on a complete blood count (CBC) showing white blood cell (WBC) count 5,500/microL, hemoglobin (Hgb) 10.2 g/dL (mean corpuscular volume [MCV] 98), and platelet [PLT] count 240,000/microL. Comprehensive metabolic panel, iron studies, B12, and folic acid levels were all normal. A bone marrow biopsy showed 45% cellularity with normal trilineage hematopoiesis without evidence of dysplasia. Her karyotype was normal in all 20 cells examined. A myeloid molecular profile was sent and it showed a *DNMT3A* mutation with a 15% variant allele frequency. What best describes her condition?
   A. Idiopathic cytopenia of undetermined significance (ICUS)
   B. Clonal hematopoiesis of indeterminate potential (CHIP)
   C. Clonal cytopenia of undetermined significance (CCUS)
   D. Idiopathic dysplasia of undetermined significance (IDUS)
   E. Myelodysplastic syndrome (MDS)

2. A 62-year-old man was found to have an abnormal complete blood count (CBC) that showed white blood cells (WBCs) 4,000/μL (absolute neutrophil count [ANC] 1,500/microL), hemoglobin (Hgb) 8.5 g/dL (mean corpuscular volume [MCV] 102), and platelets 120,000/microL. He had normal laboratory studies including iron, Vitamin B12, folic acid levels, thyroid-stimulating hormone (TSH), and viral studies. He had a bone marrow biopsy that showed 3% blasts and dysplasia in all three lineages. He is inquiring about how quickly his disease will progress and about data on overall survival. Which of the following is NOT necessary to calculate his International Prognostic Scoring Systems-Revised (IPSS-R) score?
   A. Cytogenetics
   B. Peripheral blood blast count
   C. Bone marrow blast count
   D. Hemoglobin level
   E. Absolute neutrophil count

3. A 45-year-old woman is diagnosed with myelodysplastic syndrome (MDS) following routine blood work showing a white blood cell (WBC) count 3,700, hemoglobin (Hgb) 8.1 with mean corpuscular volume (MCV) 101, and platelets (PLT) 105,000. She has a normal physical exam without evidence of dysmorphic features and no prior radiation therapy or DNA-damaging drugs. Her laboratory studies including ferritin, B12, folate, HIV, and copper levels were normal and a bone marrow biopsy confirmed multilineage dysplasia with 2% blasts. No ringed sideroblasts were seen. Her bone marrow cytogenetics showed a complex karyotype: 46, XX, +1q, −7, del(11q) in 18 of 20 cells examined. The patient has no other medical problems, and her family history is positive for cytopenias in only one sibling (she has 6 siblings). Which of the following should be a part of her workup?
   A. Fluorescence in situ hybridization (FISH) panel looking for other common MDS abnormalities
   B. Diepoxybutane (DEB) test
   C. Assessing for mutations in *ALAS2*
   D. Assessing for mutations in *SF3B1*
   E. Assessing for mutations in *ATRX*

4. A 65-year-old woman had a complete blood count (CBC) performed for fatigue, which showed white blood cells (WBCs) 5,000 (absolute neutrophil count [ANC] 2,500), hemoglobin (Hgb) 8.5 (mean corpuscular volume [MCV] 104), and platelets 505,000. Iron, Vitamin B12, and folic acid levels were normal. EPO level was 200 mU/mL. The patient had a bone marrow biopsy, which showed a hypercellular marrow, with dysplasia in the erythroid lineage but normal myeloid and megakaryocytic lineages. There were 1.5% blasts seen in the aspirate smear. Cytogenetics showed del(5q) as the sole abnormality in 15 out of 20 cells examined. Which of the following is the best treatment option for the patient?
   A. Red blood cell transfusions only
   B. Lenalidomide single agent
   C. Azacitidine or decitabine
   D. Lenalidomide + a hypomethylating agent
   E. Allogeneic bone marrow transplantation

5. A 64-year-old man presents with a transfusion-dependent anemia (2 units of red cells every 6 weeks). Otherwise, he has a normal white blood cell (WBC) count at 6,000 with absolute neutrophil count (ANC) 4,000 as well as a normal platelet count at 250,000. A bone marrow aspirate and biopsy demonstrated myelodysplastic syndrome (MDS) with dysplasia in the erythroid lineage only. There were 1.8% blasts seen in the aspirate smear and no increased ringed sideroblasts. Cytogenetics showed del 20q. A serum erythropoietin level is 90 mU/mL. Which of the following is the best treatment option for this patient?

A. Red blood cell transfusions only
B. Erythropoietin-stimulating agent
C. Lenalidomide single agent
D. Hypomethylating agent
E. Allogeneic stem cell transplantation

6. A 62-year-old man with no other comorbidities and a good performance status was diagnosed with myelodysplastic syndrome (MDS) 2 years ago. He was on observation because he had mild cytopenias initially and he was asymptomatic. Over the recent few months, his counts started to drop, and his most recent complete blood count (CBC) showed white blood cells (WBCs) 1,000, absolute neutrophil count (ANC) 500, hemoglobin (Hb) 8.5, and platelets 40,000. A bone marrow biopsy was repeated and demonstrated a hypercellular marrow with dysplasia in all lineages, 12% blasts on the aspirate smear, and a complex karyotype. Which of the following is the best treatment option for this patient?
   A. Red blood cell transfusions only
   B. Lenalidomide
   C. Erythropoietin-stimulating agent in combination with thrombopoietin-stimulating agent
   D. Hypomethylating agent
   E. Allogeneic stem cell transplantation

7. A 78-year-old man with a history of coronary artery disease, severe chronic obstructive pulmonary disease (COPD), and hypertension has high-risk myelodysplastic syndrome (MDS) with pancytopenia (white blood cells [WBCs] 800, absolute neutrophil count (ANC) 300, hemoglobin [Hb] 8.5, and platelets 35,000). Bone marrow showed 11% blasts and cytogenetics demonstrated a complex karyotype. Which of the following is the best treatment option for this patient?
   A. Red blood cell transfusions only
   B. Lenalidomide
   C. Erythropoietin-stimulating agent in combination with thrombopoietin-stimulating agent
   D. Hypomethylating agent
   E. Allogeneic stem cell transplantation (ASCT)

8. A 59-year-old woman has a diagnosis of chronic myelomonocytic leukemia (CMML) with a most recent complete blood count (CBC) showing a white blood cell (WBC) count of 40,000 (ANC 25,000, absolute monocyte count 10,000), hemoglobin [Hb] 7.5, and platelets of 200,000. Her spleen is palpated 6 cm below the left costal margin. A recent bone marrow aspiration and biopsy showed 5% blasts. She has fatigue and shortness of breath on moderate exertion. The patient has no other comorbidities. Which of the following is the best treatment option for this patient?

A. Erythropoietin-stimulating agent in combination with a thrombopoietin-stimulating agent
B. Lenalidomide
C. Hypomethylating agent
D. High-dose cytarabine
E. Allogenic stem cell transplantation (ASCT)

9. A 64-year-old man was diagnosed with chronic myelomonocytic leukemia (CMML). His bone marrow biopsy demonstrated a hypercellular marrow with dysplasia in the myeloid lineage with 7% blasts on the aspirate smear. He had a normal karyotype. A myeloid mutational panel was sent. It is most likely to reveal a mutation in which of the following genes?
A. *SETBP1*
B. *FLT3*
C. *SF3B1*
D. *SRSF2*
E. *JAK2*

10. A 71-year-old man with chronic obstructive pulmonary disease (COPD) and coronary artery disease is evaluated for leukocytosis and splenomegaly. His most recent complete blood count (CBC) showed white blood cells (WBCs) 26,000, absolute neutrophil count (ANC) 13,000, monocytes 600, and no eosinophilia or basophilia. Hemoglobin (Hb) was 10.5 and platelets 120,000. Peripheral smear reviewed showed mild poikilocytosis with some teardrop cells and evidence of granulocytic dysplasia with a left shift (myelocytes and metamyelocytes account for ~20% of WBCs). His spleen is palpable 5 cm below the costal margin. He had normal laboratory studies including iron, Vitamin B12 and folic acid levels, thyroid-stimulating hormone (TSH), creatinine, and viral studies. Testing for *BCR-ABL* fusion, *JAK2*, *CALR*, and *MPL* mutations was negative, but a myeloid mutational panel showed a mutation in *SETBP1*. What is the most likely diagnosis?
A. Myelodysplastic syndrome (MDS)
B. Chronic myelomonocytic leukemia (CMML)
C. Chronic neutrophilic leukemia (CNL)
D. Chronic myeloid leukemia (CML)
E. Atypical chronic myeloid leukemia (aCML)

ANSWERS

1. **C. Clonal cytopenia of undetermined significance (CCUS).** CCUS, clonal cytopenia of undetermined significance, describes an indolent myeloid disorder characterized by unexplained cytopenias associated with a clonal abnormality, that is, a somatic mutation in one of the recurrently mutated genes in myeloid malignancy (present with >2% variant allele frequency). CCUS might declare itself/transform to MDS in the future.

2. **B. Peripheral blood blast count.** Peripheral blood blast count is used to classify myelodysplastic syndrome (MDS). For example, peripheral blood blasts ≥5% to 19% would classify MDS into MDS-EB-2 category. However, this parameter it is not part of the IPSS or IPSS-R.

3. **B. Diepoxybutane (DEB) test.** This patient is younger than 50 years and has MDS with several chromosomal abnormalities without previous radiation or chemical exposure. She also has a family history of cytopenia in her brother. She should have chromosomal breakage analysis with DEB or mitomycin C to screen for Fanconi anemia. A FISH panel does not provide additional value: Metaphase karyotyping was successful and showed a complex karyotype. Assessing for *ALAS2* mutations can help diagnose a congenital sideroblastic anemia; however, this patient does not have a microcytic anemia, and no ringed sideroblasts were seen on the bone marrow aspirate. *SF3B1* mutations are common in MDS with ringed sideroblasts, which are absent in this patient. *ATRX* mutations are seen in acquired alpha-thalassemia, which is characterized by a microcytic anemia (the MCV is not low here).

4. **B. Lenalidomide single agent.** This patient has low-risk myelodysplastic syndrome (MDS) with symptomatic anemia and del(5q) as the sole cytogenetic abnormality (5q syndrome). Lenalidomide 10 mg a day is the treatment of choice for this patient. Prior studies have shown that 67% of patients with the 5q syndrome treated with lenalidomide no longer needed transfusions. Erythropoietin-stimulating agents (ESAs; ± G-CSF) could be considered in this patient as well because EPO level was <500.

5. **B. Erythropoietin-stimulating agent.** This patient has low-risk MDS with transfusion-dependent anemia, no del (5q), and no other cytopenias. Because his erythropoietin level is low and he gets less than two units of red blood cell (RBC) transfusions a month, his chance of responding to erythropoietin-stimulating agents is ~74%.

6. **E. Allogeneic stem cell transplantation.** This is a patient with high-risk MDS. Allogeneic stem cell transplant (ASCT) is the only curative modality. A retrospective analysis showed that patients with intermediate-2-/high-risk MDS have better overall survival if they undergo ASCT. Hypomethylating agents prior to ASCT are not routinely recommended and have not been shown to add value in patients planning to proceed with ASCT; therefore, hypomethylating agents should be considered in patients whose ASCT is expected to be delayed. This patient has a good performance status and does not have other comorbidities, and would be a candidate for ASCT.

7. **D. Hypomethylating agent.** This is a patient with high-risk MDS. Though ASCT is the only curative modality, this patient is not a candidate for ASCT (comorbidities). Hypomethylating agents are the agents of choice. Studies have demonstrated that a hypomethylating agent (azacitidine) given to intermediate-2- or high-risk MDS patients delayed progression to acute myeloid leukemia (AML) and improved overall survival compared to supportive care alone.

8. **E. Allogenic stem cell transplantation (ASCT).** The patient has CMML-1 with symptomatic anemia. The only curative option is ASCT. This patient requires therapy for CMML, given the symptomatic anemia and should be directed toward ASCT. If ASCT has to be delayed, then a hypomethylating agent should be strongly considered as a bridge to curative intent therapy.

9. **C. SF3B1**. Mutations in *SRSF2*, a gene coding one of the splicing factors, have been described in ~50% of CMML cases. This is closely followed by mutations in *ASXL1* (40%–50%), which has been associated with inferior overall survival in patients with CMML. The remaining mutations listed as answers are infrequent in CMML and are encountered with higher frequency in other hematologic malignancies: *SETBP1* in chronic neutrophilic leukemia (CNL) and atypical chronic myeloid leukemia (aCML), *FLT3* in cytogenetically normal acute myeloid leukemia (AML), *SF3B1* in myelodysplastic syndrome (MDS) with ringed sideroblasts, and *JAK2* in myeloproliferative neoplasms (polycythemia vera, essential thrombocythemia, primary myelofibrosis).

10. **E. Atypical chronic myeloid leukemia (aCML).** This patient has atypical CML as characterized by leukocytosis with a left shift, where granulocytic precursors compromise >10% of the leukocytes. A *SETBP1* mutation is common in this disorder. Chronic neutrophilic leukemia is characterized by a predominance of neutrophils and bands with early precursors amounting to <10% of WBCs. A *CSF3R* mutation is characteristic for CNL; however, it can also be present in aCML. There is no monocytosis, ruling out CMML. Of note, the peripheral blood smear can resemble CML, but there is no eosinophilia or basophilia, and the patient had a negative *BCR-ABLPCR* testing. Also, granulocytic dysplasia on peripheral smear is common in aCML, which belongs to a category of myelodysplastic/myeloproliferative neoplasms in the 2016 World Health Organization (WHO) classification.

Non-Hodgkin Lymphoma— High Grade

13

John C. Reneau and Tycel J. Phillips

EPIDEMIOLOGY

1. **What is the most common subtype of non-Hodgkin lymphoma (NHL)?**
   - Diffuse large B-cell lymphoma (DLBCL) comprises approximately one third of all NHLs and is the most common aggressive NHL.

STAGING

1. **How are aggressive NHLs staged?**
   - The Lugano classification (based on the Ann Arbor staging system) is the current standard for staging NHL.

Stage	Involvement	Extranodal (E) Status
Limited		
I	One node or single nodal group on same side of the diaphragm	Single extranodal lesions without nodal involvement
II	Two or more nodal groups on the same side of the diaphragm	Stage I or II by nodal extent with limited contiguous extranodal involvement
II bulky	Same as above with "bulky"* disease	N/A
Advanced		
III	Nodes on both sides of the diaphragm or nodes above the diaphragm with splenic involvement	N/A
IV	Noncontiguous extralymphatic involvement	N/A

*Definition of "bulky" depends upon histology (≥10 cm for Hodgkin lymphoma, 6–10 cm suggested for diffuse large B-cell lymphoma, ≥7 cm suggested for follicular lymphoma).

DIAGNOSIS

1. **How is the diagnosis of high-grade NHL made?**
   - Excisional biopsy is preferred, except in cases where nodes are inaccessible, in which case, a core needle biopsy is acceptable. Fine needle aspiration should be

avoided since nodal architecture necessary for accurate diagnosis is difficult to fully assess.

2. What are the immunophenotypic markers of the aggressive NHLs?

NHL Subtype	sIg	CD5	CD10	CD20	Cyclin D1	Other
DLBCL	+	Rare	±	+	−	MUM-1±
						Bcl-6±
						C-Myc±
						BCL-2±
PMBCL	+	−	±	+	−	CD30±
						CD23±
						CD15−
Burkitt lymphoma	+	−	+	+	−	TdT−
Mantle cell lymphoma	++	+	−	+	+	CD23−
						FMC7+
						SOX11±

DLBCL, diffuse large B-cell lymphoma; NHL, non-Hodgkin lymphoma; PMBCL, primary mediastinal B-cell lymphoma.

3. What are the chromosomal translocations and their associated oncogene (and function) associated with aggressive NHL?

Non-Hodgkin Lymphoma Subtype	Cytogenetics	Oncogene	Function
DLBCL	t(14;18), t(3;14)	BCL2	Antiapoptosis
	t(3;v)	BCL6	Transcription factor
	t(2;8), t(8;14), t(8;22)	c-Myc	
PMBCL*	t(16;X)	CIITA	MHC class II transactivator
Burkitt lymphoma	t(8;14) most common t(2;8), t(8;22)	cMYC	Transcription factor
Mantle cell lymphoma	t(11;14)	Cyclin D1	Cell cycle regulator

DLBCL, diffuse large B-cell lymphoma; PMBCL, primary mediastinal B-cell lymphoma.

Diffuse Large B-Cell Lymphoma (DLBCL)

EPIDEMIOLOGY

1. **What is the median age of DLBCL patients?**
   - Median age at diagnosis is 65 years.

PATHOLOGY AND STAGING

1. **What is the cell of origin of DLBCL?**
   - Mature B lymphocyte
     - ○ GCB (60%): germinal center B cell, better 5-year survival at 75% (except "double hit" lymphomas, which have poor survival [see the following text])
     - ○ ABC/non-GCB (40%): activated B cell, inferior 5-year survival at 50%
   - Gene expression profiling (GEP) by DNA microarray classifies DLBCL into these distinct subgroups. GEP is not widely available, so most centers use the Hans algorithm (~80% concordance) as a surrogate:

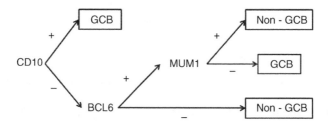

   - DLBCL may arise de novo or as a result of transformation from a more indolent form of lymphoma like follicular lymphoma, chronic lymphocytic leukemia, (Richter's transformation).

2. **What are the pathological characteristics of DLBCL?**
   - Hematoxylin and eosin (H&E) appearance
     - ○ There is effacement of the normal, follicular architecture of the lymph node.
     - ○ Tumor cells are large with abundant cytoplasm and often multiple nucleoli.
     - ○ The tumor cells are surrounded by nonmalignant cells.

3. **What studies are important in staging and workup of DLBCL?**
   - PET/CT
   - Complete blood count (CBC)
   - Liver function tests (LFT) and serum creatinine
   - Lactate dehydrogenase (LDH), uric acid, potassium, phosphorus, and calcium to evaluate for tumor lysis syndrome (TLS)
   - Bilateral bone marrow biopsy and aspirate if PET/CT scan was not performed or if there is concern for bone marrow involvement or other underlying bone marrow disorder based on presenting labs

- HIV testing
- Multigated acquisition scan (MUGA) or two-dimensional transthoracic echocardiography (TTE) prior to anthracycline-containing regimen (e.g., R-CHOP)
- Hepatitis B surface antigen (Hep B S Ag) and core antibody (Hep B C Ab) testing as regimens will contain rituximab, which can lead to hepatitis B reactivation
- Fertility counseling

PROGNOSTIC FACTORS

1. How is DLBCL risk stratified?

- Risk stratification is based on the International Prognostic Index (IPI) for non-Hodgkin lymphoma. Risk factors are given one point each in this model.

Risk Factors (1 Point Each)	IPI Score	IPI Risk Category	3-Year Overall Survival (%)
Age >60 years	0–1	Low	91
Serum LDH >upper limit of normal	2	Low intermediate	81
	3	High intermediate	65
ECOG performance status ≥2	4–5	High	59
Stage III–IV			
≥2 Extranodal sites			

ECOG, Eastern Cooperative Oncology Group; LDH, lactate dehydrogenase.

2. What are the risk factors for central nervous system (CNS) recurrence?

- Clinical risk factors: high or high intermediate IPI score, low albumin, retroperitoneal lymph node involvement, and particular extranodal sites (e.g., paranasal sinuses, orbit, breast, testes, kidney, adrenal gland, bone marrow)
- Molecular/cytogenetic risk factors: c-Myc positive and double hit lymphomas
- Presence of multiple risk factors confers increased risk compared with a single risk factor alone
- Check cell counts, protein, glucose, cytology, and flow cytometry on cerebrospinal fluid (CSF) examination if performed.

TREATMENT

1. What is the most commonly used chemotherapy regimen in DLBCL?

- R-CHOP (rituximab, cyclophosphamide, doxorubicin, vincristine, and prednisone) is the most commonly used regimen. R-CHOP should be given in 21-day cycles (R-CHOP-21). Monitor for signs of congestive heart failure (CHF), neuropathy, myelosuppression, and liver or renal dysfunction.
- Frontline treatment currently is not dependent on the DLBCL subtype (germinal center B cell [GCB] versus non-GCB), although clinical trials currently are being designed to determine if improvements to R-CHOP can be obtained.

- Response rate to R-CHOP is inferior in the non-GCB subtype compared to GCB based on historical data.
- If an anthracycline is contraindicated, regimens without doxorubicin such as R-CEOP (etoposide substituted for doxorubicin) can be used.

2. **What is the first-line treatment for different stages of DLBCL?**
   - Stages I to II, nonbulky (<7.5 cm): R-CHOP × 3 cycles, followed by involved field radiation therapy (IFRT), or R-CHOP × 6 cycles with or without IFRT
   - Stages I to II, bulky (≥7.5 cm): R-CHOP × 6 cycles followed by radiation to the "bulky" area
   - Stages III to IV: Clinical trial or R-CHOP × 6 cycles, consider IFRT to the "bulky" areas
     - If presentation includes systemic and parenchymal CNS disease, incorporate high-dose systemic methotrexate (3.5 g/m^2) on day 15 of R-CHOP cycles as well as intrathecal methotrexate by lumbar puncture.
     - If presentation includes concurrent leptomeningeal disease, then use R-CHOP plus high-dose systemic methotrexate (3.5 g/m^2) or intrathecal (IT) methotrexate.
     - If presentation includes testicular involvement, CNS prophylaxis would be recommended with intravenous (IV) or IT methotrexate, and scrotal radiation should be performed after completion of chemotherapy (risk of contralateral recurrence).
   - There is no definitive role for high-dose chemotherapy/autologous stem cell rescue (HDT/ASCR) in the first-line setting, although data suggests that high-risk patients might benefit

3. **How should TLS be monitored and prevented?**
   - Risk factors include stage III/IV disease, bulky disease, elevated lactate dehydrogenase (LDH) at baseline, evidence of spontaneous TLS, and decreased renal function at baseline.
   - Monitor uric acid, potassium, phosphorus, creatinine, calcium, and LDH if high risk and treat appropriately with fluids, allopurinol, or rasburicase.

4. **Should patients treated for DLBCL be placed on maintenance therapy?**
   - There is no role for maintenance rituximab for treatment of DLBCL.
   - There is some evidence that lenalidomide maintenance in patients 60 to 80 years old after response to R-CHOP may prolong progression-free survival.

5. **Who should receive CNS prophylaxis and what treatments are recommended?**
   - CNS relapse occurs in about 5% of high risk DLBCL patients and portends poor prognosis.
   - There is no consensus regarding which risk factors at diagnosis necessitate CNS prophylaxis (see preceding text for risk factors).
   - CNS prophylaxis can include intrathecal treatments with methotrexate or cytarabine. Depending upon age and renal function, can consider high-dose systemic methotrexate.

6. **How is response to therapy monitored (role of PET/CT)?**
   - Repeat PET/CT after three to four cycles to determine interval response to initial therapy (no consensus on utility), then 6 to 8 weeks after completion of chemotherapy, but before any planned radiation therapy (RT).
   - Frequent false-positive PET scans in this setting have been described. Therefore, a change in treatment plan should be backed up by a repeat biopsy of the PET-positive areas.
   - Surveillance imaging has not been shown to have any direct impact on patient outcomes in retrospective studies, but in select cases, imaging can be considered for surveillance for up to 2 years from completion of treatment.

7. **How is relapsed/refractory DLBCL commonly treated?**
   - Goal is to achieve complete remission (CR) or partial remission (PR) and proceed with autotransplant (if transplant eligible).
   - Options for transplant eligible patients include
     - Clinical trial (if designed to allow transition to transplant)
     - R-ICE (ifosfamide, carboplatin, etoposide)
     - R-GemOx (gemcitabine, oxaliplatin)
     - R-GDP (gemcitabine, dexamethasone, cisplatin)—efficacy does not seem to differ between germinal center B cell (GCB) and non-GCB subtypes, is well tolerated, and can be administered as an outpatient
     - R-DHAP (dexamethasone, high-dose cytarabine, cisplatin)—progression-free survival (PFS) benefit compared to ICE in patients with GCB subtype
   - Options for transplant ineligible patients include
     - Clinical trial
     - Regimens mentioned earlier if adequate functional status
     - Dose-adjusted (DA)-EPOCH (etoposide, prednisone, vincristine, cyclophosphamide, doxorubicin, +/- rituximab)
     - R^2 (lenalidomide, rituximab)—especially for non-GCB
     - Single agent rituximab

SPECIAL CONSIDERATIONS

1. **What is the role of hepatitis B prophylaxis in patients infected with hepatitis B during treatment with rituximab?**
   - Treatment with rituximab may cause hepatitis B reactivation.
   - Antiviral prophylaxis should be instituted in hepatitis B–infected patients who are planning to receive rituximab to prevent flares and related deaths.
   - Obtain baseline viral load before therapy; monitor viral loads monthly while on treatment and 3 months afterward.

2. **How is "double hit" lymphoma diagnosed and treated?**
   - "Double hit lymphoma" (also known as "DLBCL or HGB-NOS [intermediate between DLBCL and BL] with *MYC* rearrangement plus *BCL2* and/or *BCL6* rearrangements") is diagnosed by fluorescent in situ hybridization (FISH). These lymphomas have a rearrangement in the *MYC* gene combined with a

rearrangement in either *BCL2* or (less commonly) *BCL6*. If all three genes are rearranged, this is referred to as a "triple hit" lymphoma. The vast majority are germinal center B cell (GCB) subtype.

- Double hit lymphoma has a poor prognosis. Patients often present with elevated lactate dehydrogenase (LDH), extranodal disease, or central nervous system (CNS) involvement. They respond poorly to R-CHOP chemotherapy. Options for treatment include
  - ○ DA R-EPOCH
  - ○ R-HyperCVAD (rituximab, hyperfractionated cyclophosphamide, mesna, vincristine, doxorubicin, dexamethasone alternating with methotrexate, leucovorin, high-dose cytarabine, methylprednisolone)
  - ○ R-CODOX-M/R-IVAC (rituximab, cyclophosphamide, doxorubicin, vincristine, methotrexate, alternating with rituximab, ifosfamide, etoposide, cytarabine with intrathecal chemotherapy with all cycles)

3. **How is primary mediastinal large B-cell lymphoma (PMBL) diagnosed and treated?**
   - Derived from medullary thymic B cells and has unique molecular characteristics resembling nodular sclerosing Hodgkin lymphoma but is CD20+, CD30+/-, and CD15-.
   - Predominantly affects young (30s–40s) women with mediastinal (stage I/II) disease.
   - Commonly presents with superior vena cava (SVC) syndrome, pleural or pericardial effusion.
   - Widespread extranodal involvement is uncommon on initial presentation.
   - First-line treatment with DA-R-EPOCH is preferred. Recent data suggest no benefit to mediastinal radiation with this regimen. Alternatively, can use R-CHOP followed by involved field radiation therapy (IFRT).
   - At relapse, salvage regimens for DLBCL +/- radiation can be used followed by autologous hematopoietic stem cell transplantation (HSCT). 9q24 amplification is found in 70% of cases, which may predict response to PD-1/PD-L1 inhibition.

4. **How is "gray zone lymphoma" (B-cell lymphoma, unclassifiable, with features intermediate between DLBCL and Hodgkin lymphoma) diagnosed and treated?**
   - These are generally mediastinal (rarely non-mediastinal) tumors, which share features of both PMBL and Hodgkin lymphoma.
   - Diagnosis requires expert pathologic evaluation as there is a spectrum of morphologies and immunophenotypes with each tumor displaying unique features. Various tumors (or different parts within a single tumor) can display features resembling Hodgkin lymphoma, while others are more consistent with DLBCL.
   - Prognosis is poor. There is no consensus for treatment, but generally, treatments for other aggressive large cell lymphomas are preferred (R-CHOP, DA-R-EPOCH). Consolidative radiotherapy can also be considered for bulky or localized disease. Patients treated with Hodgkin-like regimens (ABVD) have inferior outcomes.

- At relapse, salvage regimens can be used followed by autologous HSCT. Other treatments like brentuximab vedotin should also be considered.

5. **What are special features of transformation of follicular lymphoma to DLBCL?**
   - Transformation happens at a rate of approximately 3% per year in the first 10 years; risk appears to plateau thereafter.
   - Prognosis is better in previously untreated patients with a localized area of transformation.
   - Transformation should be considered if there is a disproportionately rapid growth of a lymph node group with elevated lactate dehydrogenase (LDH; biopsy that lymph node group) or if an isolated area on a PET scan demonstrates higher fluorodeoxyglucose (FDG) avidity than the rest of the disease areas (biopsy the more intensely PET-avid lymph node).
   - Treat initially with R-CHOP. If the patient has previously received chemotherapy, then consolidation with autologous stem cell transplant should be performed in patients who obtain a complete remission or substantial partial remission. If the patient has previously received R-CHOP, then treatment should be given with salvage regimens such as R-ICE, R-DHAP, R-GemOX, and R-GDP followed by autologous stem cell transplant.

Burkitt Lymphoma (BL)

EPIDEMIOLOGY

1. **How common is BL?**
   - BL is rare, representing <1% of non-Hodgkin lymphoma (NHL) in adults.
   - There are three variants:
     - Endemic—most common childhood malignancy in equatorial Africa, associated with Epstein–Barr virus (EBV) infection.
     - Sporadic—1% to 2% of all lymphomas in American adults.
     - Immunodeficiency associated—seen in patients with HIV, organ transplant, and congenital immunodeficiency.

PRESENTATION

1. **What are the frequent clinical features of BL?**
   - Constitutional symptoms
   - Spontaneous TLS
   - Bone marrow involvement in up to 70% of patients at presentation
   - Leptomeningeal involvement in up to 40% of patients at presentation
   - Bulky abdominal (in adults) adenopathy

PATHOLOGY AND STAGING

1. **What is the classic pathologic description of BL?**
   - Described as a "starry sky" appearance

2. What studies are important in workup/staging of BL?
   - Same as DLBCL (see the section "Diffuse Large B-Cell Lymphoma (DLBCL)"), with the addition of lumbar puncture to evaluate for CNS involvement and unilateral bone marrow biopsy and aspirate in all patients

PROGNOSIS

3. What is the prognosis for adults diagnosed with BL?
   - With intensive, multiagent chemotherapy, 5-year survival is 40% to 90%.
   - Advanced age and stage at diagnosis is associated with inferior survival.

TREATMENT

1. What is the preferred initial treatment for BL?
   - One of the intensive, multiagent chemo regimens with CNS prophylaxis
     - CODOX-M (cyclophosphamide, vincristine, doxorubicin, high-dose methotrexate) alternating with IVAC (ifosfamide, etoposide, high-dose cytarabine), with intrathecal methotrexate or ara-C. Addition of rituximab may further improve outcomes in these patients. Difficult to tolerate for older patients or those with comorbidities
     - DA-R-EPOCH with intrathecal methotrexate
     - R-Hyper-CVAD (rituximab, hyperfractionated cyclophosphamide, vincristine, doxorubicin, dexamethasone, alternating with methotrexate and cytarabine) with intrathecal methotrexate gives similar outcomes
   - CNS prophylaxis is essential in BL
   - Limited staged patients (single abdominal site) can be treated with less intense regimens
   - R-CHOP is not adequate therapy

2. How is relapsed/refractory BL treated?
   - Relapse generally portends a poor prognosis.
   - Patients treated with inadequate initial therapy (e.g., R-CHOP) may respond to a more dose-intensive regimen (see preceding text).
   - No standard of care exists for relapsed BL.
   - Options for treatment include
     - Clinical trial
     - Alternate regimen (see question 1)
     - R-ICE, R-GDP, or high-dose cytarabine +/- rituximab
     - Best supportive care

Mantle Cell Lymphoma (MCL)

EPIDEMIOLOGY

1. How common is MCL?
   - Rare. Comprises 7% of non-Hodgkin lymphoma (NHL), but incidence is rising in the United States.

2. **What is the sex predominance of MCL?**
   - There is a striking male:female predominance of approximately 4:1.

PRESENTATION

1. **What are the frequent clinical features of MCL?**
   - Most cases present with advanced stage, extranodal involvement (commonly the gastrointestinal [GI] tract, liver, spleen, and bone marrow). CNS disease at presentation is rare, but relapse in the CNS occurs in up to 20% of cases.

PATHOLOGY AND STAGING

1. **What is the cell of origin inMCL?**
   - MCL likely has two distinct cellular origins:
     - ○ Classical MCL: naïve B cells that are SOX11+. These tend to behave more aggressively.
     - ○ Leukemic variant: antigen-experienced B cells that are SOX11-. These behave more indolently.

2. **What is the characteristic cytogenetic finding in MCL?**
   - Translocation (11;14) resulting in dysregulation of cyclin D1. Can also occur in some myelomas.

3. **What studies are important in workup/staging of MCL?**
   - Same as DLBCL (see section "Diffuse Large B-Cell Lymphoma [DLBCL]"), with the addition of bone marrow biopsy and immunophenotyping of peripheral blood and bone marrow by flow cytometry. Can consider omitting bone marrow biopsy if normal blood counts.
   - Lumbar puncture should be performed if neurologic symptoms and in patients with the blastic variant even if no other symptoms or risk factors for CNS involvement.
   - Given high prevalence of GI tract involvement, endoscopy should be performed in patients with symptoms.

PROGNOSTIC FACTORS

1. **Is mantle cell lymphoma (MCL) considered curable?**
   - Treatment for MCL is generally not considered curative, but frequently results in short (3–5 year) remissions.

2. **What are the known prognostic factors in MCL?**
   - MCL International *Prognostic Index* (MIPI) index is often used for prognosis. Incorporates age, performance status, lactate dehydrogenase (LDH), and white blood cell count
   - The blastoid variant is generally considered more clinically aggressive

TREATMENT

1. **What is the initial treatment for MCL?**
   - About 5–10% of patients with MCL display an indolent disease course and can be observed for a period of time prior to initiation of therapy. Unfortunately,

there are no well-validated means to identify these patients. Candidate markers for indolent behavior include low Ki-67 index, SOX11-negative disease, and IGVH-mutated status.

- Although rare, patients with limited-stage (stages I–II) disease could be treated with involved field radiation therapy (IFRT) and combination chemotherapy.
- For bulky stage II and for stages III/IV, optimal treatment is debatable.
- Patients who are candidates for autologous stem cell transplant should undergo induction chemotherapy, followed by high-dose therapy with autologous stem cell rescue. Recent data suggest maintenance rituximab has a survival benefit following autologous transplant (see the following).
  - Regimens that include high-dose cytarabine appear to be important in this setting (e.g., Nordic regimen, consisting of rituximab, cyclophosphamide, vincristine, doxorubicin, and prednisone, alternating with rituximab and high-dose cytarabine).
- Transplant ineligible patients can be treated with one of the following:
  - BR (bendamustine, rituximab)
  - R-HyperCVAD
  - R-CHOP—least optimal of these options; therefore, patients treated with R-CHOP should receive rituximab maintenance, typically every 2 months for 2 years.

2. What is the role of rituximab maintenance in MCL?

- Maintenance has demonstrated improvement in progression-free survival (PFS) after high-dose chemotherapy followed by autologous stem cell transplant and hints toward improvement in overall survival.
- The addition of R-maintenance to frontline R-CHOP has been shown to extend PFS in elderly patients with MCL. Current evidence does not indicate a benefit of rituximab maintenance after BR. R-CHOP + rituximab maintenance has similar outcomes to BR without maintenance.

QUESTIONS

1. A 59-year-old female presents with night sweats, weight loss, and palpable lymphadenopathy. On laboratory studies, she has a white blood cell (WBC) count of 12/mcL, hemoglobin of 12 g/dL, and platelet count of 120/mcL. Lactate dehydrogenase (LDH) is 450 U/L. A PET scan is performed, which demonstrates fluorodeoxyglucose (FDG) avid lymphadenopathy in cervical, axillary, mesenteric, and inguinal lymph nodes. An excisional lymph node biopsy is performed. Morphology reveals sheets of large atypical lymphocytes. Flow cytometry is positive for CD20, CD10, and surface immunoglobulin, negative for CD5 and cyclin D1. Fluorescence in situ hybridization (FISH) is performed, which is negative for BCL6 and MYC but positive for BCL2. What is the function of the BCL2 in her lymphoma?
   A. Overexpression of a transcription factor
   B. Overexpression of an antiapoptotic gene
   C. Overexpression of a cell cycle regulator
   D. Loss of function of a transcription factor
   E. Loss of function of an antiapoptotic gene

2. A 30-year-old female presents with shortness of breath and swelling in her neck. A CT of the thorax reveals a large mediastinal mass as well as axillary and cervical lymphadenopathy. PET scan redemonstrates activity in these areas. A lymph node biopsy is performed, which is consistent with a primary B-cell mediastinal lymphoma. A bone marrow biopsy is performed, which is unremarkable for involvement with lymphoma. Which of the following is the appropriate treatment regimen?
   A. Treatment with rituximab, cyclophosphamide, and fludarabine
   B. Treatment with R-HyperCVAD
   C. Treatment with dose-adjusted R-EPOCH
   D. Radiation therapy first to the mediastinum because of impending superior vena cava syndrome
   E. Treatment with rituximab and bendamustine

3. A 55-year-old man presents with 3 months of left testicle swelling. A mass is detected by ultrasound and he proceeds to an orchiectomy. Pathology returns consistent with diffuse large B-cell lymphoma (DLBCL). He has no other sites of disease on PET and diagnostic lumbar puncture (LP) revealed no evidence of central nervous system (CNS) involvement. What is the most appropriate management for this patient?
   A. No further therapy
   B. R-CHOP for 6 cycles
   C. R-CHOP for 6 cycles with intravenous (IV) or intrathecal (IT) methotrexate
   D. R-CHOP for 6 cycles followed by testicular radiation
   E. R-CHOP for 6 cycles with IV or IT methotrexate followed by testicular radiation

4. A 63-year-old woman with no past history and performance status of 1 presents with 3 months of weight loss, fatigue, night sweats, and growing axillary adenopathy. PET/CT shows widespread metabolically active adenopathy above and below the diaphragm. Malignant cells are positive for CD20, CD19, BCL6, and CD79a by immunohistochemistry. MUM1, CD10, and BCL2 are negative. Fluorescence in situ hybridization (FISH) shows MYC and BCL2 rearrangements, but no BCL6 rearrangement. What is the most appropriate treatment?
   A. R-CHOP x6
   B. Dose-adjusted R-EPOCH
   C. BR
   D. ABVD
   E. R-CEOP

5. A 69-year-old male presents with night sweats and weight loss. He is found to have diffuse lymphadenopathy above and below the diaphragm. He undergoes an excisional lymph node biopsy of an axillary node, which is consistent with diffuse large B-cell lymphoma. Which of the following tests are needed before considering initiating rituximab therapy?

A. Cytomegalovirus (CMV) serologies
B. Herpes simplex virus (HSV) serologies
C. Hepatitis B surface antigen, hepatitis B surface antibody
D. Respiratory virus panel
E. Epstein–Barr virus (EBV) serologies

6. A 25-year-old African male presents with a large palpable abdominal mass, which has been growing rapidly within the last 2 weeks. He has been experiencing night sweats, fevers, and weight loss. CT of the abdomen/pelvis demonstrates a large abdominal mass as well as diffuse mesenteric and retroperitoneal lymphadenopathy. His laboratory studies reveal a white blood cell (WBC) count of 20/mcL, hemoglobin of 9 g/dL, and platelet count of 90/mcL. A CT-guided core biopsy of the large mass reveals small monomorphic lymphocytes in a starry sky appearance. Ki67 staining is appreciated at 90%. By fluorescence in situ hybridization (FISH) he is found to have chromosomal translocation t(8;14). What is the main pathophysiology behind his lymphoma?
   A. A translocation causing overexpression of MYC
   B. A translocation causing overexpression of BCL 6
   C. A translocation causing overexpression of BCL2
   D. A translocation causing overexpression of cyclin D1
   E. A translocation causing overexpression of CIITA

7. A 68-year-old man presents with progressive lymphadenopathy, fevers, night sweats, and melena. Upper endoscopy reveals a fungating mass in the duodenum, which is biopsied. Pathology shows a lambda light chain restricted population, which is positive for CD5, CD20, and FMC7. CD23 and CD 10 are negative. What is the most likely cytogenetic abnormality?
   A. t(8;22)
   B. t(8;14)
   C. t(11;14)
   D. t(2;8)
   E. MYC amplification

ANSWERS

1. **B. Overexpression of an antiapoptotic gene.** BCL2 is an antiapoptotic gene that encodes one of the proteins involved in regulating cell death.

2. **C. Treatment with dose-adjusted EPOCH with rituximab.** Dose-adjusted EPOCH with rituximab has been shown to have a high cure rate and obviate the need for radiation therapy in patients with primary B-cell mediastinal lymphoma, and currently is a preferred regimen. The other treatment options are not appropriate or indicated in primary B-cell mediastinal lymphoma.

3. **E. R-CHOP for 6 cycles with IV or IT methotrexate followed by testicular radiation.** Testicular DLBCL indicates high risk for CNS involvement even with negative diagnostic lumbar puncture (LP) at diagnosis. Recommended treatment should include CNS prophylaxis and radiation to the contralateral testicle.

4. **B. Dose adjusted R-EPOCH.** This patient has a "double hit" lymphoma as evidenced by germinal center B cell (GCB) subtype diffuse large B-cell lymphoma (DLBCL) with MYC and BCL2 rearrangements by FISH. R-CHOP is inadequate therapy for these patients. Dose-adjusted R-EPOCH is the best choice.

5. **C. Hepatitis B surface antigen, hepatitis B surface antibody.** Rituximab has a risk of reactivating hepatitis B and therefore hepatitis B infection needs to be checked prior to therapy.

6. **A. A translocation causing overexpression of MYC.** Overexpression of cMYC is the major driver in the pathogenesis of Burkitt lymphoma/leukemia.

7. **C. t(11;14).** The presentation (gastrointestinal [GI] involvement) and immunophenotype are indicative of mantle cell lymphoma, which typically displays t(11;14) resulting in dysregulation of cyclin D1.

Non-Hodgkin Lymphoma— Low Grade

Melissa A. Reimers and Tycel J. Phillips

EPIDEMIOLOGY

1. Classify lymphomas into indolent or aggressive categories.

Indolent	Aggressive
Lymphoplasmacytic lymphoma/ Waldenström's macroglobulinemia	Diffuse large B-cell lymphoma
	Burkitt lymphoma
Chronic lymphocytic leukemias	Lymphoblastic lymphoma
Follicular lymphoma	Mantle cell lymphoma*
Marginal zone lymphoma	Primary mediastinal large B-cell lymphoma
MALT lymphoma	
Cutaneous T-cell lymphoma (mycosis fungoides and Sezary syndrome)*	Anaplastic large cell lymphoma
	Angioimmunoblastic T-cell lymphoma
Mantle cell lymphoma†	Extranodal NK/T-cell lymphoma
	Peripheral T-cell lymphoma not otherwise specified

*Discussed in Chapter 17.
†Can have indolent and aggressive presentations and is discussed in Chapter 13.
MALT, mucosa-associated lymphoid tissue.

ETIOLOGY AND RISK FACTORS

1. What risk factors are associated with the development of non-Hodgkin lymphoma (NHL)?

   - Farming (exposure to herbicides and pesticides, such as organochlorine, organophosphate, and phenoxyacid compounds)
   - Infections (see the following text)
   - Immunosuppressive drug use
   - Autoimmune diseases
   - Post–solid organ transplantation

2. What infections are associated with lymphoma, and what is the associated subtype of lymphoma?

   - HIV: AIDS-associated lymphoma

- Epstein-Barr virus (EBV): Burkitt's lymphoma in Africa, posttransplant lymphoproliferative disorders, NK/T-cell lymphoma, and diffuse large B-cell lymphoma (DLBCL) of the elderly
- HTLV-I: adult T-cell leukemia/lymphoma
- *Helicobacter pylori*: mucosa-associated lymphoid tissue (MALT) lymphoma
- Human herpesvirus-8: body cavity lymphoma
- Hepatitis C: splenic marginal zone lymphoma
- *Chlamydia psittaci*: orbital adnexal lymphoma
- *Campylobacter jejuni*: intestinal lymphoma
- *Borrelia burgdorferi*: cutaneous MALT lymphoma

STAGING

1. How is NHL staged?

Lugano Modification of Ann Arbor Staging System

Stage	Involvement	Extranodal (E) status
Stage I	One node or a group of adjacent nodes	Single extranodal lesions without nodal involvement
Stage II	Two or more nodal groups on the same side of the diaphragm	Stage I or II by nodal extent with limited contiguous extranodal involvement
Stage II bulky	Same as II with "bulky" disease (≥7.5 cm)	N/A
Stage III	• Nodes on both sides of the diaphragm • Nodes above the diaphragm with spleen involvement	N/A
Stage IV	Additional noncontiguous extralymphatic involvement	N/A

SIGNS AND SYMPTOMS

1. What are the common presenting signs and symptoms ofNHLs?
- Lymphadenopathy
- B symptoms
   - Fever (temperature >100.5°F)
   - Drenching night sweats
   - Unintentional weight loss (>10% loss within a 6-month period of time)
- Splenomegaly

DIAGNOSTIC FEATURES

1. What are the immunophenotypic markers of the indolent NHLs?

Non Hodgkin Lymphoma subtype	sIg	CD5	CD10	CD20	Other	Cyclin D1
CLL/SLL	Weak	+	−	Dim	CD23+ FMC− CD19+ CD20 dim	−
Follicular lymphoma	++	−	+	+	BCL-2+	−
Mantle cell lymphoma	++	+	−	+	CD23− FMC+	+
Marginal zone lymphoma/extranodal marginal zone lymphoma	+	±	−	+	MUM-1+ IRTA1+	−
Lymphoplasmacytic lymphoma/ Waldenström's macroglobulinemia	++	−	−	+	CD22+ CD25± CD38±	
Hairy cell leukemia		−	−		CD11c+ CD20+ (bright) CD22+ **CD25+*** CD103+ **CD123+*** **AnnexinA1+***	+

*Hairy cell variant CD25−, CD123−, annexinA1−

CLL, chronic lymphocytic leukemia; SLL, small lymphocytic leukemia.

2. What are the chromosomal translocations and their associated oncogene (and function) associated with indolent NHLs?

Non-Hodgkin Lymphoma subtype	Cytogenetics	Oncogene	Function
Follicular lymphoma	t(14;18)	*BCL2*	Antiapoptosis
Mantle cell lymphoma	t(11;14)	Cyclin D1	Cell cycle regulator
Marginal zone lymphoma/extranodal marginal zone lymphoma	t(11;18)	*API2*-MALT	Resistance to *Helicobacter pylori* treatment
Lymphoplasmacytic lymphoma	t(9;14)	*PAX-5*	Deregulation of *PAX-5* gene

Lymphoplasmacytic Lymphoma/Waldenström's Macroglobulinemia

SIGNS AND SYMPTOMS

1. **What is the clinical presentation of lymphoplasmacytic lymphomas?**
   - Monoclonal gammopathy, hyperviscosity syndrome (30%), neuropathy, amyloidosis, cryoglobulinemia, and cold agglutinin disease
   - Associated with hepatitis C infection

DIAGNOSIS

   - Serum immunoglobulin M (IgM) monoclonal gammopathy
   - Histologic evidence of lymphoplasmacytic cells in bone marrow
   - >90% of patients have a MYD88 mutation.

TREATMENT

1. **What are the indications for treatment of lymphoplasmacytic lymphoma?**
   Only treat symptomatic patients:
   - Hyperviscosity syndrome
   - Organomegaly
   - Cryoglobulinemia
   - Cold agglutinin disease
   - Cytopenias
   - Amyloidosis
   - Other disease-related symptoms (i.e., neuropathy, symptomatic adenopathy)

2. **What are some first-line treatment regimens for lymphoplasmacytic lymphoma/Waldenström's macroglobulinemia (WM)?**
   Non-stem cell toxic:
   - Proteasome inhibitor–based regimens (bortezomib/rituximab, bortezomib/dexamethasone (VD), bortezomib/dexamethasone/rituximab (RVD), carfilzomib/rituximab/dexamethasone (CRD))
   - Chemoimmunotherapy (rituximab monotherapy, rituximab/cyclophosphamide/dexamethasone, rituximab/cyclophosphamide/vincristine/prednisone [R-CVP], [R-CHOP])
   - Ibrutinib
   - Avoid single agent rituximab in patients with a markedly elevated serum immunoglobulin M (IgM)/serum viscosity without prior plasmapheresis due to concern for IgM flare, which can temporarily cause marked elevation in IgM and subsequent hyperviscosity

   Possible stem cell toxicity:
   - Bendamustine/rituximab (BR)
   - Cladribine ± rituximab
   - Fludarabine ± rituximab

3. **What is the treatment for hyperviscosity syndrome as related to Waldenström's macroglobulinemia?**
   - Plasmapheresis in emergent situations; then proceed with definitive therapy

Chronic Lymphocytic Leukemias

CHRONIC LYMPHOCYTIC LEUKEMIA/SMALL LYMPHOCYTIC LEUKEMIA DIAGNOSIS

1. **How is chronic lymphocytic leukemia (CLL) diagnosed?**
   - Usually by peripheral blood flow cytometry, less commonly biopsy. Requires $\geq 5 \times 10^9$/L monoclonal B lymphocytes

2. **How is small lymphocytic leukemia (SLL) diagnosed?**
   - Lymphadenopathy and/or splenomegaly; confirm by biopsy and $\leq 5 \times 10^9$/L peripheral blood monoclonal B lymphocytes

STAGING

Rai System

Stage	Description	Modified Risk Status
0	Lymphocytosis, lymphocytes in blood >5,000/mcL and >40% lymphocytes in bone marrow	Low
I	Stage 0 with enlarged node(s)	Intermediate
II	Stage 0–I with splenomegaly, hepatomegaly, or both	Intermediate
III*	Stage 0–II with hemoglobin <11.0 g/dL or hematocrit <33%	High
IV*	Stage 0–III with platelets <100,000/mcL	High

*Excludes immune-mediated cytopenias.

Binet System

Stage	Description
A	Hemoglobin $\geq$10 g/dL and platelets >100,000/mm^3 and <3 enlarged areas
B	Hemoglobin $\geq$10 g/dL and platelets $\geq$100,000/mm^3 and $\geq$3 enlarged areas
C	Hemoglobin <10 g/dL and/or platelets <100,000 mm^3 and any number of enlarged areas

TREATMENT

1. **What are the indications for treating CLL/SLL?**
   - Low-risk (Rai stage 0) or intermediate-risk (Rai stage I–II) asymptomatic CLL is treated with observation only.

- Symptomatic or high-risk (Rai stage III–IV) CLL requires treatment, with regimen choice based on comorbidities and functional status.
- Indications for treatment:
  - Disease-related symptoms: severe fatigue, night sweats, weight loss, fever (without infection), threatened end-organ function, progressive bulky disease (spleen >6 cm below costal margin, lymph nodes >10 cm), progressive anemia or thrombocytopenia

2. What are first-line therapies for treating CLL/SLL?

- Without 17p deletion/*TP53* mutation:
  - ≥65 years or significant comorbidities: ibrutinib, obinutuzumab + chlorambucil, ofatumumab + chlorambucil, bendamustine ± rituximab
  - <65 years without significant comorbidities: chemoimmunotherapy with fludarabine, cyclophosphamide, rituximab (FCR), fludarabine and rituximab (FR), bendamustine ± rituximab, ibrutinib
- With 17p deletion/*TP53* mutation:
  - First line: ibrutinib, high-dose methylprednisolone (HDMP) + rituximab, alemtuzumab
  - Relapsed/refractory: ibrutinib, venetoclax + rituximab, idelalisib ± rituximab

3. How is transformed CLL managed?

- Treat CLL that has transformed to diffuse large B-cell lymphoma or Hodgkin lymphoma according to standard regimens for aggressive lymphoma.

PROGNOSIS

1. How is prognosis determined in CLL?

- Serum markers: thymidine kinase, beta-2 microglobulin
- Flow cytometry:
  - CD38: favorable if <30%, ≥30% unfavorable
  - ZAP-70: favorable if <20%, ≥20% unfavorable
  - IGHV: favorable if >2% mutation, ≤2% mutation unfavorable
- Fluorescence in situ hybridization (FISH):

Unfavorable	Neutral	Favorable
del(11q)	Normal	**del(13q)**
~18%, associated with extensive adenopathy, disease progression, and shorter survival	+12	Most common (55%)
del(17p)		
Associated with *TP53* gene loss and worst outcomes: short treatment-free survival, short median survival, and poor response to chemotherapy		

MONOCLONAL B-CELL LYMPHOCYTOSIS

Defined as absolute monoclonal B lymphocyte count $<5,000$ mm^3, all lymph nodes <1.5 cm, no anemia or thrombocytopenia

What is the management of monoclonal B-cell lymphocytosis (MBL)?

Observation only

Hairy Cell Leukemia

1. How is hairy cell leukemia diagnosed?
- Characteristic hairy cells on peripheral blood smear and on bone marrow examination, with increased bone marrow reticulin

TREATMENT

2. What are hairy cell leukemia treatment indications?
- Systemic symptoms: splenic discomfort, recurrent infections, hemoglobin <12 g/dL, platelets $<100,000$/mcL, ANC $<1,000$/mcL
- Otherwise observation only

3. What is the first-line treatment?
- Cladribine (do not administer if active life-threatening or chronic infection)
- Pentostatin

4. How is relapse treated?
- If complete response: observation until indication for treatment
  - Relapse at <1 year: clinical trial, alternate purine analog ± rituximab, interferon alpha
  - Relapse at ≥1 year: retreat with initial purine analog (or alternative) ± rituximab
- If less than complete response:
  - Same treatment as if relapse at <1 year
- At disease progression, vemurafenib ± rituximab (BRAF mutation only) or ibrutinib

Follicular Lymphoma

GRADE AND PROGNOSTIC FACTORS

1. How do we determine the grade of follicular lymphoma (FL)?
- Grade 1 to grade 2: less than 15 centroblasts per high-power field
- Grade 3: more than 15 centroblasts per high-power field

2. What are the components of the Follicular Lymphoma International Prognostic Index (FLIPI)?

Criteria (one point for each)	Risk group (number of factors)
Age ≥60 years	Low (0–1)
Number of nodal sites ≥5	Intermediate (2)
LDH >ULN (upper limit of normal)	High (≥3)
Hemoglobin level <12 g/dL	
Ann Arbor Stage III or IV	

LDH, lactate dehydrogenase.

3. **What is the 5-year and 10-year overall survival (OS) rate of low-, intermediate-, and high-risk FL by the FLIPI?**

Risk	5-Year OS (%)	10-Year OS (%)
Low	86	71
Intermediate	71	40
High	51	37

4. **What are the poor risk factors associated with FL?**
   - According to the Group d'Etude des Lymphomes Folliculaire (GELF) criteria, the poor prognostic factors are
     ○ Involvement of three or more nodal sites, each with diameter of at least 3 cm
     ○ Any nodal/extranodal mass with diameter of at least 7 cm
     ○ Presence of B symptoms
     ○ Splenomegaly
     ○ Pleural effusion or ascites
     ○ Cytopenias (white blood cells [WBCs] <1.0 × 10/L and/or platelets <100 × 10/L)
     ○ Circulating tumor cells (>5.0 × 10/L malignant cells)
   - Strongest predictor of long-term outcomes is duration of first remission after frontline chemoimmunotherapy, with worse prognosis if relapse <2 years after initial treatment

TREATMENT

1. **What are the indications for treatment of FL?**
   - Symptomatic (B symptoms present)
   - Threatened end-organ function
   - Cytopenia secondary to lymphoma marrow involvement
   - Bulky disease (as defined by the GELF criteria)
   - Steady progression

2. **How do you treat asymptomatic advance stage follicular lymphoma?**
   - Observation

3. **How do you treat grade 3 follicular lymphoma or an aggressive presentation of follicular lymphoma?**
   - Same management as diffuse large B-cell lymphoma, treat with rituximab, cyclophosphamide, vincristine, adriamycin, prednisone (R-CHOP). (Note that grade 3a follicular lymphoma typically follows a more indolent course and should be observed, while grade 3b follicular lymphoma is more aggressive and will likely need systemic therapy as indicated.)

4. **What are the treatment options for limited stage (I–II) grade 1/2 FL?**
   - Potentially curative local radiotherapy for stage I or contiguous stage II
   - Rituximab monotherapy
   - Observation

5. **What are some first-line treatment regimens for stage III/IV grade 1/2 FL?**
   - Bendamustine + rituximab
   - Rituximab, cyclophosphamide, vincristine, prednisone (R-CVP), R-CHOP
   - Rituximab monotherapy

6. **What is the role of maintenance rituximab?**
   - The role for maintenance is controversial. It has been demonstrated to improve progression-free survival but has not demonstrated any survival benefit in any of the studies conducted to date. As currently indicated, this can be considered in all patients with follicular lymphoma after initial therapy.

7. **What are some second-line treatment regimens for relapsed/refractory low-grade FL?**
   - First-line chemoimmunotherapy regimen not used previously can be administered as second-line therapy. Recent data indicates benefit of second-generation CD20 antibody, obinutuzumab, in combination with bendamustine over bendamustine + rituximab with caveat of increased infection risk. Has not been evaluated in combination with CHOP in this setting
   - Radioactive monoclonal antibody (radioimmunotherapy)
   - Idelalisib
   - Lenalidomide
   - Clinical trials

8. **How should we treat histological transformation of FL to aggressive lymphoma (such as diffuse large B-cell lymphoma [DLBCL])?**
   - Transformed FL should be treated the same way as a DLBCL (please see details in Chapter 13) with exception that patients previously exposed to chemotherapy should be referred for autologous stem cell transplantation if responsive to therapy.

Marginal Zone Lymphoma

SIGNS AND SYMPTOMS

1. **What is the clinical presentation of extranodal marginal zone MALT lymphoma?**
   - Signs and symptoms from involvement of the gastrointestinal (GI) tract, respiratory tract, salivary gland, kidney, prostate, lung, eye (conjunctiva), and other organs
   - Associated with autoimmune disease, such as Sjögren syndrome or Hashimoto thyroiditis

2. **What is the clinical presentation of splenic marginal zone lymphoma?**
   - Splenomegaly, circulating lymphocytosis, cytopenias
   - Peripheral circulating malignant lymphocytes may display villous cytoplasmic projections

TREATMENT

1. **What is the initial treatment for stage I or II gastric MALT lymphoma with positive *Helicobacter pylori*?**
   - Treatment of *H. pylori* with antibiotics

2. **What are the initial treatment options for stage I or II gastric MALT lymphoma without *Helicobacter pylori* infection?**
   - Local radiation
   - Single agent rituximab (if radiation is contraindicated)

3. **What is the treatment of stage III/IV MALT lymphoma that involves the stomach?**
   - Rare. Should confirm diagnosis. If confirmed, can consider rituximab + focal radiation to stomach or systemic chemoimmunotherapy

4. **What is the treatment for nodal marginal zone lymphoma?**
   - Same as for follicular lymphoma

5. **What is the initial treatment for symptomatic, splenic marginal zone lymphoma without hepatitis C infection?**
   - Splenectomy or single-agent rituximab

6. **What is the treatment for symptomatic, splenic marginal zone lymphoma with hepatitis C infection?**
   - Treat hepatitis C infection first. If resolution of the lymphoma does not occur, then treat similar to splenic marginal zone without hepatitis C.

7. **What is the treatment for asymptomatic, splenic marginal zone lymphoma?**
   - Observation

QUESTIONS

1. A 70-year-old man is referred for an elevated white blood cell count of 35,000/mcL discovered during a routine evaluation. Peripheral blood flow cytometry shows 20×10^9/L monoclonal B lymphocytes. The patient is asymptomatic. Physical exam is notable for palpable but non-bothersome cervical and bilateral axillary lymphadenopathy. Hemoglobin and platelets are normal. What is the appropriate treatment recommendation?
    A. Start ibrutinib
    B. Start bendamustine 70 mg/m² + rituximab
    C. Start bendamustine 90 mg/m² + rituximab
    D. Observation only

2. The patient in question 1 returns 2 years later with progressive fatigue and increasingly bothersome cervical lymphadenopathy. He also notes abdominal distension and early satiety. White blood cell (WBC) count is now 60,000/mcL, and his peripheral monoclonal B cell lymphocyte count has increased to 45,000/mcL. His hemoglobin is 10.8 g/dL, and his platelet count is 95,000/mcL. Fluorescence in situ hybridization (FISH) analysis shows a 13q deletion. The patient is otherwise feeling well and has a performance status of 1. How should the patient be managed?
    A. Start ibrutinib
    B. Start bendamustine 70 mg/m² + rituximab
    C. Fludarabine 25 mg/m² and rituximab 375 mg/m²
    D. Fludarabine 25 mg/m², cyclophosphamide 250 mg/m², and rituximab 375 mg/m²
    E. Observation only

3. The following clinical vignette is a two-part question:
    A 65-year-old female presents with enlarged lymph nodes in her axillary and inguinal regions. She undergoes an excisional lymph node biopsy, which is consistent with follicular lymphoma, grade 2. She denies any fevers, night sweats, or weight loss. She has no other symptoms associated with her enlarged lymph nodes. She otherwise continues to work full-time, with an Eastern Cooperative Oncology Group (ECOG) performance score of 0. A PET scan reveals uptake in her cervical, axillary, and inguinal lymph nodes, and all nodes are less than 3 cm. She does not demonstrate any splenomegaly. Her lactate dehydrogenase (LDH) is 180 U/L. Her complete blood counts reveal a white blood cell (WBC) count of 7.7/microL, hemoglobin of 13.5 g/dL, and platelet count of 165/microL. Her bone marrow biopsy is negative for involvement of her follicular lymphoma.
    A. What is her Follicular Lymphoma International Prognostic Index (FLIPI) risk?
        A. Low risk
        B. Intermediate risk
        C. High risk
        D. Very high risk

    B. **What is the appropriate initial step in management?**
      A. Treatment with rituximab and bendamustine
      B. Treatment with rituximab, cyclophosphamide, vincristine, and prednisone (R-CHOP)
      C. Observation only
      D. Treatment with rituximab monotherapy × 4 doses

4. **A 60-year-old female was treated with 6 cycles of rituximab, cyclophosphamide, vincristine, and prednisone (R-CHOP) for symptomatic follicular lymphoma. Her follow-up PET scan reveals a complete remission. She has come to your clinic today and asks about the role of maintenance rituximab after chemotherapy.**
What is the benefit of maintenance rituximab in follicular lymphoma patients treated with chemotherapy?
    A. Decreased risk of infection
    B. Increased overall survival
    C. Increased progression-free survival
    D. Increased quality of life
    E. Decreased risk of transformation

5. **A 66-year-old female is evaluated for palpable lymph nodes, which she noted in her axillary regions. She undergoes a CT scan of her chest, abdomen, and pelvis, which demonstrates axillary, retroperitoneal, and mesenteric lymphadenopathy. An excisional lymph node biopsy is performed of an axillary node. The flow cytometry is positive for CD20, CD5, surface immunoglobulin, and cyclin D1 and negative for CD10 and CD23.**
What is the associated chromosomal translocation with her lymphoma?
    A. t(14;18)
    B. t(11;18)
    C. t(11;14)
    D. t(9;14)
    E. t(9;22)

6. **A 56-year-old female presents with worsening abdominal discomfort and weight loss. She was evaluated by her gastroenterologist and underwent an upper endoscopy, which revealed a gastric ulcer and mild mucosal erythema of her gastric wall. Her ulcer is biopsied and is remarkable for gastric mucosa-associated lymphoid tissue (MALT) lymphoma. Her *Helicobacter pylori* testing is positive. Her complete blood counts and comprehensive metabolic panel are all within normal range. She does not exhibit any lymphadenopathy on physical exam or on her recent CT scan of the abdomen and pelvis.**
What is the next appropriate step in treatment?
    A. Referral for radiation therapy
    B. Start proton pump inhibitor therapy and repeat an endoscopy in 3 months
    C. Treat her *H. pylori* with antibiotics and a proton pump inhibitor
    D. Treat with rituximab monotherapy
    E. Treat her *H. pylori* with antibiotics and a proton pump inhibitor with concurrent radiation therapy

7. A 72-year-old otherwise healthy man presents with 4 months of gradually worsening fatigue, night sweats, decreased appetite, occasional headaches, and recent onset of numbness and tingling of the hands. His laboratory evaluation is notable for a hemoglobin of 10.5 g/dL, platelet count of 100, an M-protein of 0.5 g/dL, and serum immunoglobulin G (IgG) 650 mg/dL (620–1,520 mg/dL), serum IgM 4,621 mg/dL (50–370 mg/dL), and serum IgA 35 mg/dL (40–350 mg/dL). Which additional finding is necessary to confirm a diagnosis of Waldenström's macroglobulinemia (WM)?
   A. Presence of a *MYD88 L265P* gene mutation
   B. Serum viscosity of >4 centipoise (CP)
   C. ≥10% bone marrow involvement by small lymphocytes with plasmacytoid or plasma cell differentiation
   D. Elevated serum kappa free light chain level

8. The patient in the preceding question is deemed to require therapy for his Waldenström's macroglobulinemia. Which of the following would NOT be considered an appropriate initial treatment for this patient?
   A. Ibrutinib
   B. Single agent bortezomib
   C. Plasmapheresis
   D. Dexamethasone, rituximab, cyclophosphamide (DRC)

9. Which of the following infections and lymphoma associations is incorrect?
   A. HTLV—adult T-cell leukemia/lymphoma
   B. Human herpesvirus-8—body cavity lymphoma
   C. *Campylobacter jejuni*—intestinal lymphoma
   D. *Borrelia burgdorferi*—orbital adnexal lymphoma
   E. Epstein-Barr virus (EBV)—NK/T-cell lymphoma

10. A 55-year-old man presents with mild pancytopenia: white blood cells (WBCs) 3,200/mcL (absolute neutrophil count [ANC] 2000, absolute lymphocyte count [ALC] 1,200, absolute monocyte count 0), hemoglobin (Hb) 12.1, platelets 110,000. He is asymptomatic and does not have recurrent infections. Bone marrow biopsy demonstrates mild reticulin fibrosis, no dysplasia, no hyperplasia in any of the lineages, and normal blast count. Flow cytometry shows a monoclonal lymphocytic population with the following profile: CD5(-), CD(10(-), CD11c(+), CD20(+), CD103(+). His exam demonstrates normal spleen size and no enlarged lymphadenopathy. His renal and liver functions are normal. How should this patient be treated?
    A. Cladribine
    B. Pentostatin
    C. Rituximab
    D. Vemurafenib
    E. Observation

ANSWERS

1. **D. Observation only.** The patient has Rai stage I (intermediate-risk) chronic lymphocytic leukemia (CLL) and remains asymptomatic; he does not require systemic treatment at this time.

2. **A. Start ibrutinib.** The patient has now progressed, with symptomatic Rai stage IV disease with constitutional symptoms, anemia, and thrombocytopenia. Given his age >65 years, systemic therapy with ibrutinib rather than chemoimmunotherapy is appropriate.

3. **A. B. Intermediate risk.** Her FLIPI score is 2 because she has one point for age >60 years and one point for stage III disease.
   B. C. Observation only. She has asymptomatic grade 2 follicular lymphoma; observation is appropriate at this time.

4. **C. Increased progression free survival.** The PRIMA trial (*Lancet* 2011; 377(9759):43–51) demonstrated increased progression-free survival after using maintenance rituximab for 2 years after the completion of chemotherapy for follicular lymphoma. It did not demonstrate increased overall survival, decreased risk of transformation, or improved quality of life. It demonstrated an increased risk of infection in the maintenance rituximab arm.

5. **C. t(11;14)** is associated with cyclin D1 which is associated with mantle cell lymphoma; t(14;18) is associated with BCL2 and follicular lymphoma; t(11;18) is associated with marginal zone lymphoma; t(9;14) is associated with lymphoplasmacytic lymphoma; and t(9;22) is associated with the BCR/ABL and chronic myeloid leukemia.

6. **C. Treat her *H. pylori* with antibiotics and a proton pump inhibitor.** After therapy is complete, a repeat endoscopy should confirm eradication of her gastric MALT lymphoma and *H. pylori*. If eradicated, she can be observed. If her disease is still persistent, other treatment modalities could be considered.

7. **C. ≥10% bone marrow involvement by small lymphocytes with plasmacytoid or plasma cell differentiation** with a typical immunophenotype (surface IgM+, CD5−, CD10−, CD11c−, CD19+, CD20+, CD22+, CD23−, CD25+, CD27+, FMC7+, CD103−, CD138−) is required to make a diagnosis of WM in addition to the presence of an IgM monoclonal gammopathy. The *MYD88 L265P* gene mutation is observed in about 90% of WM cases, but is not a diagnostic criterion. Elevated serum viscosity and abnormalities in the free serum kappa and lambda light chains may be present but are not required for diagnosis.

8. **D. Dexamethasone, rituximab, cyclophosphamide (DRC).** Rituximab-containing regimens should not be administered to patients with serum immunoglobulin M (IgM) levels greater than 4,000 mg/dL due to the risk of IgM flare in patients with such high levels, given the attendant risk of hyperviscosity syndrome. Non-rituximab-containing regimens or initial plasmapheresis to decrease the circulating IgM burden would be appropriate management approaches.

9. **D. *Borrelia burgdorferi*—orbital adnexal lymphoma.** *B. burgdorferi* is associated with cutaneous mucosa-associated lymphoid tissue (MALT) lymphoma, while *Chlamydia psittaci* is associated with orbital adnexal lymphoma. All the other answer options in this question are correct.

10. **E. Observation.** This patient has hairy cell leukemia. Given his peripheral blood counts are in a reasonable range (ANC >1,000, Hb >12, platelets >100,000) and that he is asymptomatic with no splenic discomfort or recurrent infections, he should be observed (no indication for therapy).

Multiple Myeloma and Plasma Cell Dyscrasias

15

Maryann Shango and Erica Campagnaro

EPIDEMIOLOGY

1. What are the plasma cell dyscrasias?

- Plasma cell myeloma (aka multiple myeloma [MM])
- Monoclonal gammopathy of undetermined significance (MGUS)
- Solitary plasmacytoma
- Light and heavy chain deposition diseases
- Primary amyloidosis (aka AL amyloidosis, light-chain amyloidosis)
- Polyneuropathy, organomegaly, endocrinopathy, M-spike, skin changes (POEMS)

2. How common is MM?

- MM represents approximately 10% of hematologic malignancies and 1% of all cancers

3. What is the significance of MM?

- MM is conventionally considered incurable; accounts for 20% of deaths from hematologic malignancy and 2% of all cancer deaths

ETIOLOGY AND RISK FACTORS

1. What is the etiology of MM?

- MM is a cancer of plasma cells that arises from the premalignant plasma cell dyscrasia, MGUS

2. What are the risk factors of MM?

- Risk factors for MM include advanced age, male gender, Black race, obesity, immunosuppression, and certain environmental exposures, including radiation and benzene

SCREENING AND DIAGNOSTIC CRITERIA

1. Who should be screened for MM?

- Routine screening for MGUS and MM is not recommended. Testing should occur when there are clinical features consistent with myeloma or other plasma cell dyscrasia, such as otherwise unexplained hypercalcemia, renal failure, anemia, bone pain, or lytic bone lesions on imaging
- Other potential signs and symptoms of myeloma include frequent infections, high or low serum total protein, hyperviscosity, neuropathy, and generalized

symptoms of advanced malignancy such as weight loss, fevers, and drenching night sweats

2. **What tests are important for assessing plasma cell dyscrasias, including MM?**
   - Complete blood count with differential and peripheral blood smear
   - Comprehensive metabolic panel to assess calcium, albumin, renal, and liver function
   - Serum beta-2 microglobulin ($\beta2M$) and lactate dehydrogenase (LDH) - (prognostic)
   - Serum quantitative immunoglobulins IgG, IgA, and IgM (IgD and IgE only if suspected)
   - Serum and 24-hour urine protein electrophoresis with immunofixation
   - Serum free light chain (FLC) quantification
   - Serum viscosity if: monoclonal immunoglobulin level is 5 g/dL or presence of symptoms suggestive of hyperviscosity
   - Skeletal survey to screen for lytic bone lesions
     - Must include humeri and femoral bones
     - Bone lesions in POEMS (polyneuropathy, organomegaly, endocrinopathy, M-spike, skin changes) are typically sclerotic
   - More sensitive imaging with CT, whole body MRI (total spine and pelvis if whole body unavailable), or PET/CT (correlates lytic lesions with metabolic activity) is recommended for patients with bone pain that is unexplained by plain radiographs. Other indications for more sensitive bone imaging include compression fractures, neurological deficit, uncertainty of presence or burden of bone disease, or ruling out other sites of disease in suspected solitary plasmacytoma
   - Bone marrow aspirate and core biopsy
     - Core biopsy is commonly used to assess bone marrow architecture and percentage of clonal plasma cells and is needed if amyloid testing is planned.
     - Aspirate is commonly used to assess cell surface markers by flow cytometry, myeloma risk/staging by conventional cytogenetics, and fluorescence in situ hybridization (FISH) for commonly acquired genetic mutations in myeloma.
       - Bone marrow aspirate commonly underestimates marrow plasma cell percentage.
   - If AL amyloidosis is suspected, confirm diagnosis with Congo red staining and amyloid protein identification by immunohistochemistry and mass spectrometry on affected tissue (e.g., bone marrow biopsy, fat pad aspirate, other affected organs)

3. **What are the diagnostic criteria for active MM (requiring treatment)?**
   - Confirmation of a clonal plasma cell disorder—can be plasmacytoma of bone or soft tissue (extramedullary) and/or ≥10% clonal bone marrow plasma cells with at least one of the following:

- Any plasma cell dyscrasia-related end-organ damage:
  - Anemia (hemoglobin <10 g/dL or >2 g/dL below lower normal limit)
  - Renal insufficiency (creatinine >2 mg/dL or creatinine clearance <40 mL/min)
  - Elevated serum calcium level (calcium >11 mg/dL or >1mg/dL above upper limit normal)
  - ≥1 osteolytic bone lesions on skeletal survey, CT, or PET/CT (1 lesion is sufficient if marrow plasmacytosis ≥10%)
- Clonal plasma cells ≥60% of bone marrow cellularity
- Involved to uninvolved free light chain (FLC) ratio ≥100
- MRI with >one focal bone lesion measuring ≥5 mm
- CT or PET/CT

4. **What are the diagnostic criteria and characteristics of other plasma cell dyscrasias?**
   - MGUS
     - Serum monoclonal (M) protein ≤3 g/dL
     - Clonal plasma cells <10% of bone marrow
     - Absence of end-organ damage attributed to plasma cell dyscrasia
     - Treatment: monitor for progression, or intervention on clinical trial
   - Smoldering multiple myeloma (SMM)
     - Serum M protein ≥3g/dL or Bence-Jones protein ≥500 mg/24 hours
     - ≥10% and <60% marrow clonal plasma cells
     - No end-organ damage or other myeloma defining events
     - No amyloidosis
     - Treatment: monitor for progression, or intervention on clinical trial
   - Solitary plasmacytoma
     - Single clonal plasma cell tumor without evidence of end-organ damage attributable to monoclonal plasma cells
     - Perform PET/CT or whole body MRI and bone marrow biopsy to look for systemic disease
       - Scans negative, no marrow plasmacytosis = solitary plasmacytoma
         - Treatment: involved field radiation, typical dose 40–50 Gy, monitor for progression
         - Up to 90% cure
       - Scans negative, <10% clonal marrow plasma cells = solitary plasmacytoma with minimal marrow involvement
         - Treatment: involved field radiation, typical dose 40–50 Gy, monitor for progression
         - 50% or more progress to MM in the next 5 years
       - Scans positive or ≥10% clonal marrow plasma cells = MM
         - Treatment: treat as MM. If the patient's systemic disease is SMM, could treat with radiation followed by monitoring for progression

- POEMS (osteosclerotic myeloma)
  - A clonal plasma cell-driven syndrome associated with
    - <u>P</u>olyneuropathy—symmetric ascending peripheral neuropathy involving sensory or motor neurons, typically painful
    - <u>O</u>rganomegaly—enlargement of spleen, lymph nodes, and/or liver. Association with concurrent Castleman's disease
    - <u>E</u>ndocrinopathy
    - <u>M</u>onoclonal gammopathy—typically λ-restricted
    - <u>S</u>kin changes—hyperpigmentation, hypertrichosis, telangiectasias
    - Typically high serum vascular endothelial growth factor (VEGF) levels
    - Treatment: alkylator-based chemotherapy, high-dose melphalan with autologous hematopoietic stem cell support
- Light and heavy chain deposition diseases (aka Randall disease)
  - Typically a low-burden clonal plasma cell disorder that secretes a "malignant protein," which is an immunoglobulin (light or heavy chain) with a propensity to deposit in tissues causing tissue damage and organ dysfunction
  - Nonfibrillary, amorphous eosinophilic material that is Congo red stain negative
  - Majority will have a serum M protein (~85%)
  - Diagnosis of exclusion—must rule out more common diseases such as lymphoplasmacytic lymphoma with immunoglobulin G (IgG) deposition, chronic lymphocytic leukemia/small lymphocytic lymphoma (CLL/SLL) with IgM deposition, extranodal marginal zone lymphoma with IgA deposition
  - Treatment: varies, directly at the underlying clonal cells
- AL amyloidosis (light chain amyloidosis, primary amyloidosis)
  - Characterized by systemic deposition of an amyloid protein that is composed of immunoglobulin light chains folded into a *beta*-pleated sheet
  - Amyloid protein deposition damages the affected organ(s), resulting in problems such as neuropathy, heart failure, pulmonary infiltrates, malabsorption and bowel dysmotility, nephrotic syndrome, skin lesions, and easy bruising
  - Treatment: similar to treatment for MM; since this is a typically a low-burden disease, maintenance therapy is less common in amyloidosis compared to MM

PATHOLOGY

1. What is the cell of origin for the malignant plasma cells of MM?
   - MM cells are post-germinal center plasma cells identifiable by somatic mutations in the variable region of the immunoglobulin heavy chain gene

SIGNS AND SYMPTOMS

1. What are the most common symptoms of MM?
   - Anemia (73%)

- Bone pain due to lytic lesions (58%)
- Increased creatinine (48%)
- Fatigue (32%)
- Hypercalcemia (28%)
- Weight loss (24%)

2. **What are less common but important signs and symptoms?**
   - Plasmacytoma
   - Neuropathy
   - Spinal cord compression (5%—due to plasmacytoma or vertebral body fracture)
   - Hyperviscosity

RISK STRATIFICATION

Categorization of mutation risk can vary between publications

1. **Which features are associated with high-risk disease?**
   - (FISH showing t(14;16), t(14;20), or del(17p13)
   - LDH >upper limit normal (ULN)
   - Primary plasma cell leukemia (≥20% plasma cells on manual differential or ≥2,000 plasma cells/microL)
   - ~15% of multiple MM are high risk with median survival 2 to 3 years despite standard therapy

2. **Which features are associated with intermediate-risk disease?**
   - FISH showing t(4;14), 1q, deletion 13 by karyotype, or hypodiploidy by conventional cytogenetics

3. **Which features are associated with standard-risk disease?**
   - Everyone who does not fit high- or intermediate-risk disease is considered to have standard-risk disease. Median survival is 8 to 10 years

4. **Do any genetic features predict response to specific therapies?**
   - Poor outcome previously associated with t(4;14) and monosomy 13/deletion 13 (by karyotype) or hypodiploidy is abrogated at least partially with early use of bortezomib-based therapy. This is why they are now classified as intermediate risk

5. **What are favorable prognostic factors?**
   - Hyperdiploidy, typically affecting the odd-numbered chromosomes, Eastern Cooperative Oncology Group Performance Status (ECOG PS) 0 to 2, age less than 70 years, and normal albumin

STAGING

1. **Which staging system is preferred for MM?**
   - The Revised International Staging System (R-ISS)

2. How is MM staged according to the R-ISS?

- The R-ISS uses serum beta-2 microglobulin (β2M), serum albumin, lactate dehydrogenase (LDH), and cytogenetics
- Stage I: β2M <3.5 mg/L, albumin $\geq$3.5 g/dL, LDH within normal limits, no del(17p), t(4;14), or t(14;16)—5-year progression-free survival (PFS) and overall survival (OS) 55% and 82%, respectively
- Stage II: neither stage I nor stage III (5-year PFS and OS 36% and 62%, respectively)
- Stage III: β2M $\geq$5.5 mg/L, LDH >ULN, and/or del(17p), t(4;14), or t(14;16) by FISH (5-year PFS and OS 24% and 40%, respectively)

TREATMENT

General Treatment Principles

1. Which plasma cell dyscrasias should be treated?

- Treating MGUS or SMM with standard chemotherapy has not shown improvement in survival; observation to monitor for progression to active MM is the standard of care
- Patients with high-risk MGUS or SMM are encouraged to participate in clinical trials to evaluate the possible utility of newer agents earlier in the disease course
- Patients with active MM should be treated since end-organ damage from MM is present or imminent

2. What are the main factors in determining best frontline therapy for patients with newly diagnosed MM?

- Disease risk
- Eligibility for high-dose chemotherapy followed by autologous hematopoietic cell transplantation (HCT)

3. Which MM patients receive induction therapy?

- All

4. Is there a standard induction therapy?

- No, but in general, triplet regimens are preferred over doublets if tolerated by patients.

5. How do you decide what induction therapy to use?

- Disease risk stratification, patient factors (performance status, comorbidities, psychosocial support), institutional resources (e.g., infusion availability, clinical trial availability), eligibility for autologous HCT

6. What happens after induction therapy?

- Post-induction therapy is dependent on eligibility and timing of autologous HCT. Generally, if HCT is not pursued, patients continue therapy, which may be the same or a modified version of their induction regimen, until progression or therapy intolerance occurs

7. **What are some key agents used in *first-line* MM treatment and what are their common toxicities?**
   - Bortezomib
     - Mechanism: proteasome inhibition
     - Side effects: peripheral (sensory) neuropathy, thrombocytopenia, herpes zoster reactivation
     - Hepatic metabolism: Liver dysfunction requires dose adjustment (useful in renal failure or chronic kidney disease [CKD] patients)
     - Herpes zoster prophylaxis with acyclovir or valacyclovir is required
   - Thalidomide
     - Mechanism: immunomodulation (drugs in this class are also known as IMiDs—immunomodulatory drugs)
     - Side effects: peripheral neuropathy, constipation, fatigue, edema, somnolence, and venous thrombotic events (VTEs)
     - If used in combination with high-dose dexamethasone, and/or patient is at high risk for thrombosis (i.e., history of VTE, diabetes mellitus, coronary artery disease), VTE prophylaxis with warfarin to achieve international normalized ratio (INR) 2–3 or prophylactic or full-dose low-molecular-weight heparin (LMWH) is recommended
     - If used in combination with bortezomib or low-dose dexamethasone, and patient is without high baseline risk of VTE, prophylactic LMWH, fixed and low-dose warfarin, or low-dose aspirin are acceptable options for VTE prophylaxis
   - Lenalidomide
     - Mechanism: immunomodulation
     - Side effects: myelosuppression, venous thromboembolism, and fatigue
     - Renal metabolism: significant renal dysfunction requires dose adjustment
     - VTE prophylaxis same as that with thalidomide
     - This is a preferred agent in patients with preexisting peripheral neuropathy

8. **What is the role of bisphosphonates in MM?**
   - Bisphosphonates decrease the risk of skeletal fractures and improve bone-related pain
   - Recommended for patients with active MM, with or without known bone disease
   - The drugs approved for this use in the United States are pamidronate and zoledronic acid, both dosed by intravenous infusion monthly
     - Intravenous zoledronic acid has been shown to reduce mortality by about 16% compared to oral clodronic acid with extension of median overall survival by 5.5 month (*Lancet* 2010; 376:1989–1999)
   - Optimal treatment duration is unknown, but current recommendations are to administer an intravenous bisphosphonate monthly for 2 years. At that point,

could consider stopping or increasing the interval between infusions, depending on how well the MM is controlled

- Side effects can include hypocalcemia, renal insufficiency, and osteonecrosis of the jaw. Dental exam is recommended prior to initiation of bisphosphonates

Principles of Autologous HCT in MM

1. **What is the role of autologous HCT in MM therapy?**
   - Autologous HCT results in higher response rates and prolonged PFS compared to standard therapies; survival data from phase 3 studies are mixed
   - Autologous HCT should be considered in all eligible MM patients, regardless of disease risk

2. **Who is eligible for an autologous HCT?**
   - The eligibility criteria for autologous HCT are not standardized; the decision for HCT is often individualized
   - Age 75 years, Eastern Cooperative Oncology Group Performance Status (ECOG PS) ≥ 3, or other significant comorbidities (e.g., heart failure, significant pulmonary disease) are generally considered too risky for autologous HCT

3. **When are autologous hematopoietic stem cells collected?**
   - Usually after 2 to 4 months of induction therapy and/or after cytoreduction by at least 50% (partial remission [PR])

4. **When is the best time to complete an autologous HCT?**
   - Autologous HCT can be completed "early" (after first remission) or "late" (at the time of first relapse, after second remission). Studies investigating the differences between early and late HCT are ongoing

5. **Can a patient undergo a second autologous HCT?**
   - Yes. Usually, enough hematopoietic stem cells are collected to perform two autologous HCTs. These can be used in the setting of "tandem" HCT for patients with suboptimal response (very good partial response [VGPR; cytoreduction by at least 90%] or better not reached after first HCT), usually within 3 to 6 months of the first HCT or at the time of relapse if it occurs at least 18 months after first HCT

Principles of First-Line Therapy

1. **Are doublet or triplet regimens preferred as induction therapy for newly diagnosed MM patients?**
   - In younger and/or fit patients, triplet regimens generally improve overall response rate, progression-free survival, and overall survival and are preferred over doublet regimens in patients who can tolerate them

2. **What are the initial treatment options for MM patients who are autologous HCT candidates?**
   - Key point: Avoid prolonged treatment with alkylating agents (cyclophosphamide or melphalan) or lenalidomide, which can prevent successful stem cell collection

- Standard-risk MM:
  - Induction therapy can be followed by autologous stem cell transplant (SCT) immediately ("early") or after first relapse ("late")
  - The most commonly used induction regimen for standard-risk and fit myeloma patients is bortezomib, lenalidomide, and dexamethasone (VRD). Two-drug combinations, such as bortezomib or lenalidomide with dexamethasone (Vd or Rd), may be used in frail patients
- Intermediate or high-risk MM:
  - Use bortezomib-based regimens for frontline treatment if a clinical trial is not available or not preferred by the patient
  - The most commonly used induction regimen for high-risk myeloma is also VRD
  - Induction therapy should be followed by HCT in most patients
  - Bortezomib should remain part of maintenance therapy after induction and HCT (most important in t(4;14))

3. **What are the initial treatment options for MM patients who are not candidates for autologous HCT?**
   - In general, the same induction regimens used for patients who are eligible for HCT are used for those ineligible for HCT. Prolonged use of alkylating agents and/or lenalidomide is acceptable as first-line therapy in patients who are not candidates for HCT
   - For intermediate- or high-risk patients, a bortezomib-based regimen should be used, generally in a triplet combination, for example, bortezomib, lenalidomide, and dexamethasone (VRD) or bortezomib, melphalan, and prednisone (VMP)

4. **How long should treatment for multiple myeloma be continued after patient has had a maximal response to therapy?**
   - Optimal duration of therapy remains unknown. Because of substantial improvement in progression-free survival with prolonged therapy, maintenance therapy (low dose, usually single agent) is usually continued after initial treatment until progression of disease or development of unmanageable toxicity

Maintenance Therapy

1. **What is the goal of maintenance therapy?**
   - To increase the duration of response to induction therapy. The Food and Drug Administration (FDA) approved lenalidomide in 2017 for maintenance therapy after autologous stem cell transplant due to substantial improvement in progression-free survival based on two randomized, phase 3 trials, CALGB 100104 and IFM 2005-02

2. **What drugs are recommended as maintenance therapy?**
   - The NCCN recommends both lenalidomide and bortezomib as potential maintenance therapies; lenalidomide is FDA approved for maintenance therapy after autologous SCT

3. **What is the appropriate duration of maintenance therapy?**
   - Optimal duration of therapy remains unknown. Because of substantial improvement in progression-free survival with prolonged therapy, maintenance therapy (low dose, usually single agent) is usually continued after initial treatment until progression of disease or development of unmanageable toxicity
     - ○ When considering duration of maintenance therapy, complications associated with prolonged treatment with lenalidomide, such as increased risk of secondary malignancies, increased risk of infection, and impact on quality of life should be considered along with disease risk

Relapsed or Refractory Disease

1. **What is the definition of progressive disease after initial treatment?**
   - Twenty-five percent increase in any of the following on at least two separate lab draws:
     - ○ Serum or urine monoclonal immunoglobulin
     - ○ Bone marrow clonal plasma cell percentage
     - ○ Change in the kappa/lambda serum FLC ratio
   - Increase in size of a preexisting bony lesion or plasmacytoma
   - The appearance of new bony lesions or plasmacytomas
   - New and otherwise unexplained serum calcium >11.5 mg/dL

2. **What treatment strategies are available for relapsed disease?**
   - If it has been 1 year or more since initial therapy, repeating initial therapy is reasonable
   - Combination therapy using agents of a different class should be considered, for example, using a bortezomib-based regimen if a lenalidomide-based regimen was given first line
   - Autologous HCT should be considered in suitable patients including previously transplanted patients relapsing more than 18 months after initial transplant
   - Allogeneic stem cell transplantation is not a standard recommendation due to high treatment-related morbidity and mortality, but can be considered in the context of a clinical trial in a high-risk patient
   - In general, it is expected that subsequent treatments will result in less tumor reduction for a shorter period of time than previous treatments. Exceptions to this can happen, especially when changing drug classes

3. **How is relapsed disease risk-stratified?**
   - If relapse is ≤12 months since initial therapy, the disease is classified as high risk regardless of initial risk stratification
   - For high-risk patients at diagnosis, if relapse is >2 years after initial therapy, disease is considered standard risk at time of relapse in the absence of any new high-risk cytogenetic findings

4. **What additional drugs are available for *relapsed/refractory* disease?**
- Immunomodulators:
  - Pomalidomide: approved for relapse within 60 days of third-line therapy after lenalidomide and bortezomib
- Proteasome inhibitors:
  - Carfilzomib: approved for relapse within 60 days of first-line therapy if given alone after immunomodulatory therapy and bortezomib, or after one to three lines of therapy if given in combination with RD. Available as intravenous infusion only, less peripheral neuropathy than bortezomib
  - Ixazomib: approved in combination with RD after failure of first-line therapy. Oral drug, causes less peripheral neuropathy, but more gastrointestinal (GI) toxicity (e.g., nausea and diarrhea) than bortezomib
- Monoclonal antibodies:
  - Daratumumab: anti-CD38 antibody, a protein densely expressed on the surface of plasma cells. It is approved in combination with lenalidomide/dexamethasone or bortezomib/dexamethasone in patients who have received at least one prior therapy for MM, or as a third-line option in patients who have received at least two prior MM therapies, including lenalidomide, in combination with pomalidomide/dexamethasone. It is also approved as a single agent in patients who have received at least three prior MM therapies, which include a proteasome inhibitor and immunomodulatory drug (IMiD). Available as intravenous infusion only, infusion reactions common with first dose
  - Elotuzumab: anti-SLAMF7 antibody, which is a glycoprotein expressed on both natural killer (NK) and MM cells. It is approved after one to three lines of therapy in combination with RD. Available as intravenous infusion only, infusion reactions common with first dose
- Histone deacetylase inhibitors:
  - Panobinostat: approved with Vd after two prior therapies that must have included bortezomib and an immunomodulatory drug. Oral, associated with GI toxicity (e.g., nausea and diarrhea)

QUESTIONS

1. A 65-year-old man was referred to you after workup of anemia revealed an M protein of 5 g/dL with several lytic lesions on skeletal survey. Bone marrow biopsy showed 35% clonal plasma cells, with fluorescence in situ hybridization (FISH) showing t(4;14) and deletion 13. He is working full-time as a construction manager and runs about 5 miles per week. What is your treatment recommendation?
   A. Bortezomib, lenalidomide, and dexamethasone (VRD), with stem cell collection after four cycles and plan for early autologous hematopoietic cell transplantation (HCT)
   B. Carfilzomib, pomalidomide, and dexamethasone (KPD), with stem cell collection after four cycles and plan for early autologous HCT
   C. VRD without stem cell collection
   D. Lenalidomide and dexamethasone (RD) with stem cell collection after four cycles and plan for early autologous HCT

2. A 79-year-old woman was recently diagnosed with multiple myeloma and presents to you to start therapy with lenalidomide and low-dose dexamethasone. She lives independently, and participates in a twice-weekly swimming class. She has no history of peptic ulcer disease (PUD), gastritis, or gastrointestinal (GI) bleed. She has no other comorbidities. What is the best way to reduce her risk of venous thrombotic events (VTE)?
   A. Dose-adjusted warfarin for international normalized ratio (INR) goal 2 to 3
   B. Fixed, low-dose warfarin, 1 to 2 mg daily
   C. Low-dose aspirin (81 or 100 mg daily)
   D. Enoxaparin 40 mg daily

3. Bisphosphonates in multiple myeloma patients do which of the following?
   A. Reduce skeletal-related events
   B. Improve bone pain
   C. Reduce risk of myeloma-related renal dysfunction
   D. A and B

4. A 55-year-old woman presents with left upper arm pain and was found to have a 3-cm humeral mass on imaging. Humeral biopsy confirmed a monoclonal plasma cell population. Bone marrow biopsy showed 5% monoclonal plasma cells, and serum blood tests were negative for anemia, hypercalcemia, and renal dysfunction. No bone lesions were identified on skeletal survey or PET/CT. How would you treat this patient?
   A. Definitive radiation to the humeral plasmacytoma followed by observation
   B. Palliative radiation to the humeral plasmacytoma followed by bortezomib, lenalidomide, and dexamethasone (VRD) and autologous hematopoietic cell transplantation (HCT)
   C. Surgical resection
   D. VRD and autologous HCT followed by maintenance therapy as guided by her risk stratification

5. Which of the following characterize high-risk multiple myeloma (MM)?
   A. Relapse at 14 months after autologous hematopoietic cell transplantation (HCT)
   B. 1q amplification
   C. Trisomy 15
   D. t(14;20)

6. A 65-year old woman was referred to you after her primary care physician found an M protein of 3.3 g/dL during a workup for unexplained mild normocytic anemia, hemoglobin (Hg) 11.2 g/dL. She has normal calcium levels, negative Bence-Jones protein, normal renal function, and negative skeletal survey for lytic lesions. Bone marrow biopsy

shows 35% monoclonal plasma cells. She owns a bookstore and runs a dessert catering service on the side. What is your next step in management?

A. Obtain fluorescence in situ hybridization (FISH) studies from bone marrow aspirate to risk stratify and determine therapy
B. Start bortezomib, lenalidomide, and dexamethasone and refer to bone marrow transplant (BMT) in preparation for autologous stem cell transplant
C. Continue observation and recheck complete blood count (CBC), serum creatinine, serum calcium, urine protein electrophoresis (UPEP) with immunofixation, serum protein electrophoresis (SPEP), and free light chain ratio in 6 to 8 weeks
D. Obtain an MRI of the spine and pelvis or PET/CT to rule out bone lesions missed by routine skeletal survey

7. A 56-year-old woman undergoes autologous stem cell transplant (SCT) after she achieves a complete remission with bortezomib, lenalidomide, and dexamethasone for multiple myeloma (MM) with t(4;14). Her most recent bone marrow biopsy showed no evidence of disease, and blood work looking for M protein or serum free light chains has remained negative. What would you recommend she do to help increase the amount of time she is in remission?

A. Start lenalidomide maintenance therapy
B. Start bortezomib maintenance therapy
C. Proceed with second autologous SCT ("tandem" SCT)
D. Observation

8. A 75-year-old man presents with newly diagnosed multiple myeloma (MM) after he suffered a pathologic hip fracture. He is overall active and independent in his activities of daily living (ADLs), but reports grade 2 peripheral neuropathy. He is currently living with his sister, who reports that the patient sleeps on the couch all day and uses a cane to help transport himself into the bathroom or kitchen. He is otherwise independent in all of his ADLs, but get up and go test is delayed. In addition to starting him on a bisphosphonate, what regimen would be most appropriate for him?

A. Bortezomib, lenalidomide, dexamethasone
B. Carfilzomib, lenalidomide, dexamethasone
C. Bortezomib and dexamethasone
D. Lenalidomide and dexamethasone

9. A 69-year-old woman presents to your clinic for an incidental finding of M protein of 3.5 g/dL, found on serum protein electrophoresis (SPEP) completed for an elevated protein gap on routine blood work. Her primary care physician completed her workup and found no substantial anemia, renal dysfunction, or bone lesions on skeletal survey. She denied symptoms of bone pain and only complained of fatigue. You complete a bone marrow biopsy, which reveals about 65%

involvement of her marrow by monoclonal plasma cells. Cytogenetics reveal chromosome 13 deletion; t(4;14) is noted on fluorescence in situ hybridization (FISH). Which of the following is the strongest predictor of her progression to active multiple myeloma?

A. t(4;14)

B. M protein ≥3g/dL

C. >60% monoclonal plasma cell involvement of bone marrow

D. Chromosome 13 deletion on karyotype

10. A 61-year-old man presents to you for a second opinion for therapy recommendations in the setting of progressive multiple myeloma (MM) defined by an increase in his serum free light chains by over 25% of his nadir. He received RVD about 3 years ago with very good partial response (VGPR), followed by autologous stem cell transplantation. He did not receive any maintenance therapy and he has been on observation since. He owns a business and continues to work fulltime. He denies any neuropathy and has no history of blood clots. What treatment regimen would be best suited for him?

A. RVD

B. Bortezomib, pomalidomide, dexamethasone

C. Carfilzomib, pomalidomide, dexamethasone

D. Panobinostat, bortezomib, dexamethasone

ANSWERS

1. **A. Bortezomib, lenalidomide, and dexamethasone (VRD), with stem cell collection after four cycles and plan for early autologous hematopoietic cell transplantation (HCT).** This patient has intermediate-risk disease by FISH analysis due to t(4;14) and deletion 13. These were classified as high risk until bortezomib-containing regimens brought their outcomes closer to that of standard-risk patients. He should therefore receive a bortezomib-containing regimen. This patient has a good performance status and should be considered for an autologous HCT, and therefore his stem cells should be collected after approximately the fourth cycle of induction therapy. KPD has not yet been approved in the frontline setting. Prolonged treatment with lenalidomide (generally, eight cycles or more) can interfere with the ability to mobilize and collect stem cells.

2. **C. Low-dose aspirin (81 or 100 mg daily).** This is a standard-risk patient for VTE on lenalidomide therapy as she is active without other VTE risk factors. For these patients, low-dose aspirin is sufficient for VTE prophylaxis.

3. **D. A and B.** Bisphosphonates have been shown in several studies to reduce risk of new skeletal events and reduce myeloma-related bone pain. Bisphosphonates may cause renal toxicity, so renal function must be monitored and doses adjusted as needed with treatment.

4. **A. Definitive radiation to the humeral plasmacytoma followed by observation.** This patient has a solitary plasmacytoma of bone (SPB) with minimal (<10%) bone marrow involvement. Definitive radiation (total dose 40–50 Gy) is the standard of care for SPB, and after completing this, she would undergo surveillance to monitor for progression of her underlying monoclonal gammopathy of undetermined significance (MGUS). PET/CT is important to rule out other possible bone lesions to confirm the diagnosis of SPB with minimal marrow involvement rather than multiple myeloma (MM).

5. **D. t(14;20).** Relapse within 1 year of HCT qualifies as high-risk MM. Trisomies and 1q amplification qualify as low- and intermediate-risk disease, respectively. t(14;20), t(14;16), and del17p are cytogenetic markers of high-risk MM, as is evidence of plasma cell leukemia.

6. **D. Obtain an MRI of the spine and pelvis or PET/CT to rule out bone lesions missed by routine skeletal survey.** This patient has smoldering multiple myeloma based on her monoclonal serum protein of 3 g/dL and >10% clonal plasma cells in her bone marrow, but she has no evidence of end-organ damage. Prior to diagnosing her with smoldering myeloma and considering observation or clinical trial for smoldering myeloma, however, she needs to be assessed for bone lesions that may have been missed by skeletal survey. This can be completed with whole body MRI, MRI total spine and pelvis (if whole body MRI is not available), or PET/CT. Up to 50% of patients without lytic lesions on skeletal survey will have bone lesions on more sensitive imaging.

7. **B. Start bortezomib maintenance therapy.** This patient is fit and has achieved a complete remission after autologous SCT and therefore will unlikely benefit from tandem transplant. Lenalidomide is Food and Drug Administration (FDA) approved for maintenance therapy after autologous SCT. Bortezomib-based maintenance therapy should be chosen over lenalidomide in this patient's case due to the presence of t(4;14), and studies showing that treatment with bortezomib abrogates the risk of this mutation.

8. **D. Lenalidomide and dexamethasone.** Lenalidomide and dexamethasone are standard therapy for older and/or frail MM patients. Bortezomib and dexamethasone would also be reasonable in this patient population, but is a less good choice for this patient who has preexisting neuropathy.

9. **C. >60% monoclonal plasma cell involvement of bone marrow.** Having ≥60% bone marrow clonal plasma cells and an involved-to-uninvolved serum free light chain ratio >100 are "biomarkers of active disease" and are associated with an approximately 80% risk of progression to active multiple myeloma (MM) with elevated calcium, renal insufficiency, anemia, bone abnormalities (CRAB) criteria within 2 years. It is recommended that she start treatment to prevent the high probability of end-organ damage by MM.

10. **A. RVD.** RVD is a reasonable treatment for this fit man with minimal comorbidities and disease-related symptoms who relapsed after 3 years of remission without maintenance therapy. It is expected to be effective, with a known side effect profile in this patient, and the other drugs can be reserved for later lines of treatment.

Andy Nguyen and Catherine Lee

Immunodeficiency-Associated Lymphoproliferative Disorders

DEFINITION

Immunodeficiency-associated lymphoproliferative disorders are a group of lymphoid neoplasms that are associated with an immunosuppressed state, that is, after solid organ or allogeneic hematopoietic cell transplant (HCT) period, on immunosuppressive medications for autoimmune or rheumatologic disorders, with primary immune disorders, or with HIV infection.

Posttransplant Lymphoproliferative Disorders

EPIDEMIOLOGY

1. **What is the incidence of posttransplant lymphoproliferative disorders (PTLDs)?**
   - Most common malignancy seen after solid organ transplant (up to 20%) and uncommon after allogeneic HCT
   - Incidence varies by type of transplant but estimated to be 1% at 10 years
   - Eighty percent occur within the first year post-transplant

ETIOLOGY AND RISK FACTORS

1. **What is the etiology of PTLD?**
   - In the majority of patients, it is related to B-cell expansion induced by infection with *Epstein-Barr virus* (EBV) in the setting of chronic immunosuppression and decreased T-cell surveillance.
   - Seventy percent or more are EBV related.
   - EBV is a common pathogen and 90% to 95% of adults are seropositive.
   - EBV-infected B cells can originate from either the host or donor.
   - Host-derived PTLD is most common in solid organ transplantation.
   - Donor-derived PTLD is more common in allogeneic HCT.

2. **What are the common risk factors for PTLD?**
   - Degree of T-cell immunosuppression (most common immunosuppressive treatments are calcineurin inhibitors [tacrolimus, cyclosporine])

- Highest in those with multiorgan transplant > lung transplant > liver, stem cell, and heart > is renal transplant (least common)
- Increased risk for PTLD EBV–negative recipients of EBV-positive donor organs

CLASSIFICATION

1. **Types of PTLD; World Health Organization classification**
   - Early lesions: Polyclonal B cells without signs of transformation
     - Plasmacytic hyperplasia
     - Infectious mononucleosis-like lesions
   - Polymorphic PTLD: polyclonal or monoclonal B cells with malignant transformation but does not meet criteria for B-cell or NK-/T-cell lymphoma
   - Monomorphic PTLD: monoclonal malignant cells that meet criteria for B-cell or NK-/T-cell lymphoma
     - *B-cell neoplasms*
       - Diffuse large B-cell lymphoma
       - Burkitt lymphoma
       - Plasma cell myeloma
       - Plasmacytoma-like lesion
       - Other
     - *T-cell neoplasms*
       - Peripheral T-cell lymphoma
       - Hepatosplenic T-cell lymphoma
       - Other
     - *Classical Hodgkin lymphoma-type PTLD*

SIGNS AND SYMPTOMS

1. **What are the signs and symptoms of PTLD?**
   - B symptoms such as fevers, weight loss, night sweats, failure to thrive, and fatigue
   - Lymphadenopathy
   - Fifty percent present with extranodal masses, such as gastrointestinal (GI) tract, lung, liver, and the allografted organ itself

DIAGNOSIS

1. **How is this diagnosed?**
   - Tissue biopsy and histologic evaluation

TREATMENT

1. **How is PTLD treated?**
   - Options include reduction in immunosuppression, rituximab, radiation, or a combination of therapies. Initial management is dependent on the type of PTLD.
   - Early lesions are less aggressive than polymorphic PTLD, and both are less aggressive than monomorphic PTLD

○ Early lesions: Consider reduction in immunosuppression alone

○ Polymorphic PTLD: If CD20 positive, consider rituximab with reduction in immunosuppression ± chemotherapy. If CD20 negative, consider chemotherapy plus reduction in immunosuppression

○ Monomorphic PTLD: reduction in immunosuppression plus chemotherapy used for non-Hodgkin lymphoma (cyclophosphamide, doxorubicin, vincristine, and prednisone). If CD20⁺ PTLD, add rituximab

○ Classical Hodgkin lymphoma–like PTLD: Use similar protocols as those used to treat classical Hodgkin Lymphoma, that is, ABVD ± radiation therapy

2. **Is antiviral therapy effective for treatment of PTLD?**

● Antiviral prophylaxis may decrease the incidence of PTLD; however, there is no convincing data to show it has efficacy in the treatment of PTLD

AIDS-Related Lymphoma

DEFINITION

AIDS-related lymphoma includes non-Hodgkin lymphoma (NHL), Hodgkin lymphoma (HL), primary effusion lymphoma (PEL), and central nervous system (CNS) lymphoma.

EPIDEMIOLOGY

1. **What is the incidence of NHL and (HL in HIV-positive patients?**

● Incidence of NHL is 1.2% per year

● A 25% to 40% risk of malignancy in HIV patients, with 10% of those being NHL

● AIDS-related lymphoma is more common in males than in females

● NHL is an AIDS-defining malignancy

● HL is not an AIDS-defining malignancy

● There is a 15- to 30-fold increase in HL found in the HIV population

2. **What is the incidence of primary effusion lymphoma?**

● Least common NHL, accounting for 1% to 4% of all AIDS-related lymphomas

3. **What is the incidence of CNS lymphoma?**

● Accounts for 15% of NHL in HIV-positive patients

● Incidence is 2% to 6% in HIV-positive patients

ETIOLOGY AND RISK FACTORS

1. **What are the risk factors for NHL in HIV-positive patients?**

● Low CD4 count

● High HIV viral load

- Combination antiretroviral therapy decreases the incidence of NHL and primary central nervous system (CNS) lymphoma

CLASSIFICATION

1. **What are the subtypes of AIDS-related lymphoma?**
   - Systemic non-Hodgkin lymphoma
     - Diffuse large B-cell lymphoma (75%)
     - Burkitt lymphoma (25%)
     - Plasmablastic lymphoma (<5%)
     - T-cell lymphoma (1%–3%)
     - Indolent B-cell lymphoma (<10%)
   - Primary effusion lymphoma (PEL)
   - CNS lymphoma
   - Hodgkin lymphoma

SIGNS AND SYMPTOMS

1. **What are the signs and symptoms?**
   - Systemic NHL and HL present with B symptoms (fever, weight loss, night sweats) and extranodal disease. Also consider cytopenias, hypercalcemia, and labs consistent with tumor lysis syndrome as a presentation.
   - Most commonly involved extranodal sites are the gastrointestinal (GI) tract, bone marrow, liver, lung, and CNS.
   - PEL involves pleura and pericardium or presents as ascites. Patients can have dyspnea or chest pain.
   - CNS lymphoma presents with headaches, confusion, seizures, visual changes, or focal neurological deficits.

STAGING

1. **How are patients with AIDS-related lymphoma staged?**
   - The same system used for NHL/HL in the HIV-negative population is used.

DIAGNOSIS

1. **How do you diagnose a patient with AIDS-related lymphoma?**
   - Must have HIV infection
   - Biopsy of tissue and histological confirmation
   - PEL: Effusion will contain malignant cells with HHV-8 virus in the nuclei of these cells
   - CNS lymphoma: either by biopsy of brain mass or cerebral spinal fluid evaluation

TREATMENT

1. **What are the treatments for AIDS-related lymphomas?**
   - All patients should be started on combination antiretroviral therapy if not already on treatment

- AIDS-related NHL and HL are treated similarly like non-AIDS-related lymphoma counterpart
- Diffuse large B-cell lymphoma (DLBCL) treated with rituximab, cyclophosphamide, doxorubicin, vincristine, and prednisone (R-CHOP) with CNS prophylaxis
- Burkitt lymphoma treated with R-CODOX-M-IVAC or DA-R-EPOCH
- HL is treated with ABVD
- CNS lymphoma treated with high-dose intravenous methotrexate. Radiation may play a role in palliation of symptoms
- PEL carries a poor prognosis. Chemotherapy is the mainstay of treatment, that is, CHOP, DA-EPOCH, and CODOX-M-IVAC. Most PEL cases do not express CD20; therefore, rituximab is excluded. However, it can be considered for treatment of rare cases of CD20-positive PEL

Iatrogenic Immunodeficiency Lymphoproliferative Disorders in Nontransplant Settings

DEFINITION

Iatrogenic immunodeficiency lymphoproliferative disorders are a group of lymphoid neoplasms associated with those in an immunocompromised state, such as patients with autoimmune/rheumatic disorders or in the posttransplant period being treated with immunosuppression (see preceding text for posttransplant lymphoproliferative disorders [PTLDs]).

ETIOLOGY

1. **What types of immunosuppressive treatment (IST) are related to iatrogenic lymphoproliferative disorders?**
   - Methotrexate, infliximab (TNF alpha-blocker), and mycophenolate mofetil are agents used in autoimmune/rheumatic disorders, which are commonly associated with PTLD.

EPIDEMIOLOGY AND RISK FACTORS

1. **What are the risk factors for developing iatrogenic immunodeficiency lymphoproliferative disorders?**
   - Underlying autoimmune disorders, such as rheumatoid arthritis, psoriasis, and inflammatory bowel disease requiring treatment with immunosuppressive therapy
   - There is a high association between hepatosplenic T-cell lymphoma and patients on infliximab for Crohn's disease

PATHOLOGY

- Immunosuppressive treatment (IST), such as MTX, can impair T-cell-mediated immune surveillance and allow expansion of clonal B-cell population

- ○ Forty percent of MTX-related lymphoproliferative disorders (LPDs) are EBV positive
- ○ Can develop into NHL or HL

TREATMENT

1. What are the treatments for IST-related lymphoproliferative disorders?

- Stop underlying IST.
- Discontinuing MTX in MTX-associated LPD can lead to regression in one out of three cases.
- Regression is rare in those related to infliximab.
- Treatment is similar to that in PTLD—use chemotherapy appropriate to the lymphoma subtype.

QUESTIONS

1. A 60-year old Caucasian male with newly diagnosed AIDS is referred to oncology for a newly diagnosed stage IV high-grade diffuse large B-cell lymphoma (DLBCL) with bone marrow involvement. He has not started combination antiretroviral therapy yet. He denies headache, confusion, vision changes, or other focal neurological changes. His Eastern Cooperative Oncology Group (ECOG) performance status score is 2. What is the optimal treatment regimen?
   A. The patient's disease is very advanced and the best supportive care with a hospice should be pursued
   B. Combination antiretroviral therapy, chemotherapy, and prophylactic intrathecal chemotherapy
   C. Chemotherapy alone
   D. Combination antiretroviral therapy alone

2. Which of the following is not considered an AIDS-defining malignancy?
   A. Hodgkin lymphoma
   B. High-grade diffuse large B-cell lymphoma (DLBCL)
   C. Cervical cancer
   D. Burkitt lymphoma

3. A 52-year-old female presents to clinic on day 72 following allogeneic bone marrow transplantation for acute myeloid leukemia (AML). She is on tacrolimus to prevent graft rejection and graft-versus-host disease. She reports one day of high fevers, night sweats, and feeling unwell. She is Epstein-Barr virus (EBV) seronegative. On physical exam, a 2-cm cervical lymph node is palpated. She undergoes excisional biopsy of the node and pathology shows histologic features of a monomorphic CD20-positive diffuse large B-cell lymphoma (DLBCL). What is the next best step in management?
   A. Radiation therapy
   B. PET/CT scan
   C. Taper immunosuppression
   D. Chemotherapy plus rituximab

4. A 56-year-old Caucasian male with a 10-year history of Crohn's disease presents with abdominal pain, bloating, nausea, and vomiting. He has had loss of appetite over the past 3 months and has lost 15 pounds. During your interview, you are told by the patient that his Crohn's disease has been treated with mesalamine, steroids, and methotrexate for many years. He has been off all treatment for the past 2 months due to progressive cytopenias. What is your next step in management?
   A. Resume treatment with methotrexate
   B. Obtain a CT scan of the abdomen and pelvis
   C. Perform an esophagogastroduodenoscopy (EGD)
   D. Check lactate dehydrogenase (LDH)

5. A 45-year-old woman with AIDS presents with shortness of breath and cough. She had not been taking her antiretroviral therapy and her CD4 count is <100. A chest x-ray (CXR) reveals a large right-sided effusion. She undergoes thoracentesis and the fluid is positive for malignant cells consistent with B-cell non-Hodgkin lymphoma (NHL). Polymerase chain reaction (PCR) is positive for HHV-8. What is the best treatment? Her Eastern Cooperative Oncology Group (ECOG) performance status score is 2.
   A. Combination antiretroviral therapy
   B. Best supportive care and hospice
   C. Cyclophosphamide, doxorubicin, vincristine, and prednisone (CHOP) plus rituximab plus combination antiretroviral therapy
   D. Cyclophosphamide, doxorubicin, vincristine, and prednisone (CHOP) plus combination antiretroviral therapy

ANSWERS

1. **B. Combination antiretroviral therapy, chemotherapy, and prophylactic intrathecal chemotherapy.** This patient has an AIDS-defining lymphoma. Most non-Hodgkin lymphomas in HIV-infected individuals are most frequently of B-cell origin and are frequently associated with Epstein-Barr virus (EBV) infection. The optimal initial therapy for lymphomas in the setting of HIV has yet to be defined. However, current recommendations include the following: (a) combination antiretroviral therapy to help control the HIV infection and allow for the administration of chemotherapy; (b) chemotherapy that is specific to the type of lymphoma—if CD20 positive, rituximab should be given; and (c) patients with AIDS-related NHL are at increased risk of central nervous system involvement and therefore, administration of prophylactic intrathecal chemotherapy is reasonable.

2. **A. Hodgkin lymphoma.** The three cancers considered as AIDS-defining cancers or malignancies are Kaposi sarcoma, aggressive B-cell non-Hodgkin lymphoma, and cervical cancer.

3. **C. Taper immunosuppression.** This patient has posttransplant lymphoproliferative disorder (PTLD). Most cases of PTLD in the setting of allogeneic hematopoietic cell transplantation are due to donor EBV–infected B cells passed to the host (recipient). Owing to suppressed T-cell activity from tacrolimus, these EBV-infected B cells may proliferate at a high rate and lead to a lymphoproliferative disorder. Patients can present with constitutional symptoms. If PTLD is suspected, the patient should undergo workup, including CT scans or PET/CT followed by tissue biopsy. In this case, the patient had a palpable lymph node and an excisional biopsy was performed immediately. Pathology was consistent with CD20-positive DLBCL. Withdrawal of immunosuppression should be performed immediately when PTLD is suspected or diagnosed in a patient. Systemic therapy with chemoimmunotherapy should then be considered for appropriate patients.

4. **B. Obtain a CT scan of the abdomen and pelvis.** This patient likely has an iatrogenic lymphoproliferative disorder due to immune suppression therapy (IST) for his Crohn's disease. The most common ISTs associated with iatrogenic lymphoproliferative disorders are methotrexate, infliximab, calcineurin inhibitors, and mycophenolate mofetil. Patients often present with B symptoms (i.e., fever, night sweats, anorexia, weight loss). This patient requires imaging tests to evaluate for the presence of lymphadenopathy or extranodal masses. If present, an excisional biopsy should be performed for histologic evaluation. If positive for lymphoma, the next step in management includes withdrawal of immunosuppressive medications ± chemotherapy or radiation therapy.

5. **D. Cyclophosphamide, doxorubicin, vincristine, and prednisone (CHOP) plus combination antiretroviral therapy.** This patient has a primary effusion lymphoma (PEL). PEL is a rare and aggressive B-cell

non-Hodgkin and is an AIDS-defining cancer. It is a lymphoma that usually presents with malignant effusions without tumor masses. HHV-8 virus is pathognomonic for PEL. More than 70% of cases occur with concurrent Epstein-Barr virus (EBV) infection. It is associated with a poor prognosis. Although PEL is a B-cell NHL, in most cases, these cells do not express CD20. In appropriate patients, optimal treatment consists of combination antiretroviral therapy and chemotherapy (CHOP) without rituximab.

T-Cell and NK-Cell Neoplasms

Sumana Devata and Ryan A. Wilcox

EPIDEMIOLOGY

1. How common are the different T-cell lymphoma (TCL) subtypes?

- Peripheral T-cell lymphomas (PTCLs) are a heterogeneous group of diseases that account for <15% of all non-Hodgkin lymphomas (NHLs) in Western countries, and 15% to 20% in Asia.
- Cutaneous T-cell lymphomas (CTCLs) account for approximately 75% of cutaneous lymphomas.

2. What are the most common PTCL subtypes?

- There are many PTCL subtypes, and the most common subtypes of nodal PTCL are:
  - Peripheral T-cell lymphoma, not otherwise specified (PTCL-NOS; 26%)
  - Angioimmunoblastic T-cell lymphoma (AITL; 19%)
  - Anaplastic large cell lymphoma, anaplastic lymphoma kinase (ALK±) (ALCL; 12%)
    - ALK(+) (6.6%): median age of onset 34 years
    - ALK(−) (5.5%): median age of onset 58 years
  - Other subtypes include: extranodal NK/T-cell lymphoma (ENKL), nasal type; hepatosplenic T-cell lymphoma (HSTCL); subcutaneous panniculitis-like T-cell lymphoma (SPTCL); enteropathy-associated T-cell lymphoma (EATL); adult T-cell leukemia/lymphoma (ATLL)

3. What are the most common CTCL subtypes?

- There are also many CTCL subtypes, and the most common subtypes are:
  - Mycosis Fungoides (MF; 38%)
  - CD30+ T-cell lymphoproliferative disorders (10.2%) (Differential diagnosis: primary cutaneous ALCL, Lymphomatoid papulosis, MF with large cell transformation)
  - Sézary Syndrome (SS; 0.8%)

RISK FACTORS

1. What are the risk factors and associations for various subtypes of PTCL and CTCL?

- Variable depending on the subtype:
  - HSTCL: chronic immunosuppression
  - ATLL: human T-cell leukemia virus type 1 (HTLV-1) infection, most common in Caribbean islands and southern Japan

○ EATL: celiac disease

○ ENKL: Epstein–Barr virus (EBV) infection, most common in Asia

○ ALK(−), ALCL: breast implants, lymphoma involving the fibrous capsule around the implant without invasion of underlying breast tissue

SIGNS AND SYMPTOMS

1. What are the signs and symptoms of patients with PTCL?

- Lymphadenopathy (LAD), cytopenias, elevated lactate dehydrogenase (LDH), and advanced-stage disease at presentation are commonly seen. Unique features are as follows:
  ○ PTCL-NOS: 50% with concurrent extranodal disease (liver, bone marrow, skin, and GI tract)
  ○ AITL: Acute onset LAD, B-symptoms, organomegaly, also associated with eosinophilia, pruritic rash, autoimmune events (rheumatoid arthritis, thyroid disease, vasculitis), polyarthritis, effusions/ascites, polyclonal hypergammaglobulinemia, elevated erythrocyte sedimentation rate (ESR), hypoalbuminemia, positive Coombs test

2. What are the signs and symptoms of patients with CTCL?

- MF: Patch/plaque, pruritic, multifocal lesions typically appearing in non-sun–exposed skin
- SS: Generalized erythroderma, scaling of the hands and feet, ectropion

3. Is there standard diagnostic criteria for MF and SS?

- The International Society for Cutaneous Lymphomas (ISCL) has an algorithm to standardize the approach for these diseases, which is based on clinical, histopathologic, molecular, and immunopathologic criteria.

STAGING

1. How are T-cell lymphomas staged?

- Most subtypes of PTCL are staged according to the Ann Arbor lymphoma staging system (see Chapter 13).
- CTCL employs a modified tumor, nodes, metastasis, and blood (TNMB)-based staging approach (Table 17.1).

PATHOLOGY

1. Are there any common genetic mutations seen in nodal PTCL?

- ALK(−) ALCL: *DUSP22* (prevalence 30%, favorable prognosis) and *TP63* (prevalence 8%, unfavorable prognosis) rearrangements have been described.
- ALK(+) ALCL: t(2;5), *ALK* rearranged with *NPM*

2. What are the lymph node histopathological features of nodal PTCL?

- PTCL-NOS
  ○ Effacement of lymph nodes with cells of variable size; sheets of atypical lymphocytes in a paracortical or diffuse pattern; mixture of plasma calls and eosinophils; high mitotic rate

TABLE 17.1 ■ MF/SS TNMB Classification and Survival

TNMB Classification					Median OS (years)	10-Year		
Stage	T	N	M	B		OS (%)	DSS (%)	RDP (%)
IA	1	0	0	0,1	35.5	88	95	12
IB	2	0	0	0,1	21.5	70	77	38
IIA	1,2	1,2	0	0,1	15.8	52	67	33
IIB	3	0–2	0	0,1	4.7	34	42	58
IIIA	4	0–2	0	0	4.7	37	45	62
IIIB	4	0–2	0	1	3.4	25	45	73
IVA1	1–4	0–2	0	2	3.8	18	20	83
IVA2	1–4	3	0	0–2	2.1	15	20	80
IVB	1–4	0–3	1	0–2	1.4	18 (5 year)	18 (5 year)	82 (5 year)

Note: T1 – patches or plaques, <10% body surface area (BSA); T2 – patches or plaques, >10% BSA; T3 – cutaneous tumors >1cm; T4 – erythroderma, >80% BSA; N1 – NCI LN 0–2; N2 – NCI LN 3; N3 – NCI LN 4; M1 – visceral involvement; B0 – no significant amount of atypical circulating cells, <5%; B1 – atypical circulating cells, >5%; B2 – Absolute Sézary count ≥ 1000 cells/mm, positive clone

The above table was adapted with permission from Wilcox RA. Cutaneous T-cell lymphoma: 2014 update on diagnosis, risk-stratification, and management. *Am J Hematol.* 2014;89(8):837–851.

BSA, body surface area; DSS, disease-specific survival; NCI, National Cancer Institute; OS, overall survival; RDP, risk of disease progression; TNMB, tumor, node, metastasis, and blood.

- ALCL
  - Sinusoidal growth pattern (and may mimic metastatic carcinoma)
  - Classical variant: large blastic cells with prominent nucleoli and abundant cytoplasm
    - Hallmark cells: eccentric nuclei, eosinophilic paranuclear hof (Figure 17.1)
  - Immunophenotypic markers: CD30+
- AITL
  - Partial or complete effacement of lymph nodes; neovascularization or arborizing endothelial venules. AITL are derived from follicular helper T cells (explaining the B-cell and follicular dendritic cell expansion observed). Typified by a mixture of plasma cells, B-cell immunoblasts, small lymphocytes, eosinophils, follicular dendritic cells, and medium-sized malignant cells with abundant cytoplasm.

3. What are the common histopathological features of CTCL?

- MF
  - Band-like infiltrate small-intermediate mononuclear cells with cerebriform nuclei in upper dermis and epidermal keratinocytes (also known

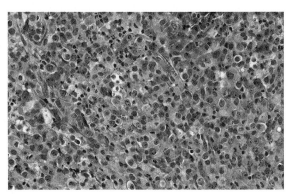

FIGURE 17.1 ■ Hallmark cells with eccentric nuclei and eosinophilic paranuclear hof as seen in ALCL. (Courtesy of the University of Michigan Department of Pathology)
ALCL, anaplastic large cell lymphoma.

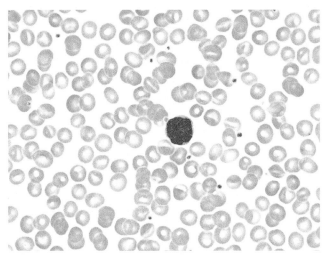

FIGURE 17.2 ■ Peripheral blood smear with cerebriform (Sézary) cell. (Courtesy of the University of Michigan Department of Pathology)

      as epidermotropism) or in intraepidermal aggregates (Pautrier microabscesses) cerebriform (indented nuclei) with surrounding clear cytoplasm

- SS
  - ○ Circulating large lymphocytes with cerebriform nuclei in the peripheral blood (Figure 17.2)
  - ○ T-cell gene rearrangement (TGR): positive
  - ○ CD4/CD8 ratio ≥10; loss of CD7

PROGNOSTIC FACTORS

1. How are patients with PTCL risk stratified?

- In general, the International Prognostic Index (IPI) is applicable to PTCL.
- A similar Prognostic Index for T-cell lymphoma (PIT) can also be used.

IPI Prognostic Factors	PIT Prognostic Factors
Age > 60	Age > 60
LDH > ULN	LDH > ULN
ECOG PS ≥ 2	ECOG PS ≥ 2
Ann Arbor stage ≥ 3	Bone marrow involvement
Number of extranodal sites > 2	

Number of IPI factors determine prognostic group: Low = 0–1; low-intermediate = 2; high-intermediate = 3; high = 4–5

2. **How does the prognosis of PTCL compare with aggressive B-cell NHL?**
   - Stage for stage outcomes are inferior for patients with PTCL compared to those with aggressive B-cell NHL.

3. **What is an additional important prognostic factor for ALCL?**
   - The presence or absence of an ALK fusion protein significantly affects ALCL prognosis.
   - ALK(+) ALCL has a 5-year overall survival (OS) rate of 70%, while ALK(−) ALCL has a 5-year OS rate of 49%.

4. **What prognostic factor is associated with CTCL?**
   - Median survival is linked to stage at diagnosis (see Table 17.1).

TREATMENT

Indications for Treatment

1. **When should treatment be initiated for PTCL?**
   - Overall, the survival for patients with untreated PTCL is measured in months; treatment should be initiated once diagnosis is established.

2. **How are the different stages of CTCL managed?**
   - Limited stage (I-IIA): skin-directed therapies
   - Advanced stage (IIB-IVB): systemic therapies

First-Line Therapy

1. **What is standard first-line therapy for the common PTCL subtypes?**
   - ALK(+) ALCL
     - Multiagent, anthracycline-based therapy ± etoposide x 6 cycles, ± radiation therapy (RT)
       - Age > 60 years, CHOP (cyclophosphamide, doxorubicin, vincristine, prednisone)
       - Age < 60 years, CHOEP (CHOP plus etoposide) or CHOP
     - Stage I-II disease: Consider 3–4 cycles of chemotherapy followed by RT
   - PTCL-NOS, ALK(−) ALCL, AITL
     - Consider clinical trial participation.

○ Multiagent chemotherapy (CHOP or CHOEP) x 6 cycles. Abbreviated chemotherapy (3–4 cycles) followed by RT (as in limited-stage diffuse large B-cell lymphoma [DLBCL]) may be considered in selected patients.

2. **What is the role of consolidative autologous stem cell transplant (ASCT) after complete response with first-line therapy?**

- Stage III/IV disease: In contrast to DLBCL, most transplant-eligible patients with stage III/IV PTCL-NOS, ALK(−) ALCL, and AITL achieving a complete remission with induction first-line therapy (CHOP or CHOEP) undergo consolidation with high-dose therapy and ASCT, as this approach appears to be associated with improved progression-free survival/OS.

- Stage I/II disease: ASCT is considered for stage I-II (high-intermediate/high IPI) PTCL-NOS, ALK(−) ALCL, and AITL in first remission. Favorable outcomes have been reported in DUSP22 rearranged ALK(−) ALCL without ASCT in first remission.

- Young patients with ALK(+) ALCL do not typically receive consolidative treatment in first remission due to favorable 5-year OS with chemotherapy.

3. **What treatment is given for CTCL?**

- Treatment includes a variety of agents (used as single agent or in combination) such as:
  ○ Skin directed: UV light phototherapy, topical corticosteroids, topical nitrogen mustard, bexarotene (low dose), local XRT, total skin electron beam therapy (TSEBT)
  ○ Systemic: Retinoids, histone deacetylase (HDAC) inhibitors, interferon alfa, pralatrexate, brentuximab (e.g., in transformed MF), clinical trial participation

Second-Line Therapy

1. **What treatment options exist for relapsed or refractory PTCL?**

- Consider clinical trial participation.
- Elderly AITL patients unable to tolerate chemotherapy: Consider corticosteroids or immunosuppressive therapy with cyclosporine.
- No standard second-line treatment. Overall response rates in relapsed/refractory PTCL are ~20% to 50%; however, responses are not typically durable.
  ○ Single-agent regimens: Brentuximab (ORR ~85% in ALCL), romidepsin, belinostat, pralatrexate (limited activity in AITL)
  ○ Multiagent chemotherapy is similar to aggressive B-cell lymphoma regimens without rituximab (e.g., ICE, DHAP, GemOx)
- Stem cell transplantation
  ○ ASCT can be considered for patients who did not undergo transplant in first complete remission.
  ○ Allogeneic stem cell transplantation can lead to durable responses in up to 60% of relapsed/refractory cases but is associated with up to a 30% rate of treatment-related mortality.

SPECIAL CONSIDERATIONS

1. **What are notable aspects of other, less common subtypes of PTCL?**
   - Extranodal NK/T cell lymphoma, nasal type. EBV associated (EBER positive)
     - ○ Typically present with nasal obstruction or invasion of nose, palate, and sinuses
     - ○ Multimodality treatment with concurrent chemotherapy and RT for patients with stage I/IIE disease. CHOP alone is ineffective.
       - ■ RT with cisplatin followed by VIPD (etoposide, ifosfamide, cisplatin, dexamethasone) x 3 cycles, or RT with DeVIC (dexamethasone, etoposide, ifosfamide, carboplatin) x 3 cycles, or asparaginase-containing regimens prior to and following RT (in "sandwich" approach).
       - ■ High response rates are seen with checkpoint blockade in relapsed/refractory setting.
   - Adult T-cell leukemia/lymphoma, HTLV-1 associated
     - ○ Clinically variable with acute, smoldering, lymphomatous and chronic types
     - ○ Peripheral blood lymphocytes have hyperlobated nuclei with condensed chromatin appearing as a clover leaf or flower.

QUESTIONS

1. **Which of the following peripheral T-cell lymphoma (PTCL) subtypes has the best prognosis?**
   A. Angioimmunoblastic T-cell lymphoma (AITL)
   B. Anaplastic large cell lymphoma (ALCL), ALK +
   C. Extranodal NK/T cell lymphoma
   D. ALCL, ALK −

2. **A 47-year-old Jamaican man presents with an elevated lymphocyte count and peripheral blood shows some cells with hyperlobated nuclei appearing like clovers. Which pathogen is typically associated with this PTCL subtype?**
   A. *H. pylori*
   B. Epstein–Barr Virus (EBV)
   C. Human T-cell leukemia virus type 1 (HTLV-1)
   D. Cytomegalovirus (CMV)

3. **A 60-year-old man presents with years of pruritus with large scattered pink/erythematous patches on his chest, back, upper arms, and thighs. Past biopsies have showed eczema and folliculitis, and topical treatments have not resulted in improvement. Repeat biopsy shows mononuclear cells with cerebriform nuclei in upper dermis and epidermal keratinocytes with intraepidermal aggregates forming microabscess-like structures. What is the most likely diagnosis?**
   A. Sézary syndrome (SS)
   B. Atopic dermatitis
   C. Psoriasis
   D. Mycosis fungoides
   E. Infection

4. A 68-year-old man develops joint pain and swelling, fatigue, short-ness of breath, night sweats, lower extremity erythematous rash, and enlarged neck lymph nodes. Labs show a white blood cell count of 10 K/microL with an absolute lymphocyte count of 0.5 K/microL, hemoglobin of 6.5 g/dL, platelet count of 130 K/microL, total bilirubin 4.5 mg/dL, and lactate dehydrogenase (LDH) > 2x the upper limit of normal. Chest x-ray shows bilateral pleural effusions. What is the most likely diagnosis?
   A. Angioimmunoblastic T-cell lymphoma (AITL)
   B. Mycosis fungoides
   C. Peripheral T-cell lymphoma, not otherwise specified (PTCL-NOS)
   D. Follicular lymphoma

5. A woman without a significant past medical history and only surgical history of bilateral breast implants presents with right-sided breast fullness. In addition to a primary breast carcinoma, which of the fol-lowing is in the differential diagnosis?
   A. Angioimmunoblastic T-cell lymphoma (AITL)
   B. Peripheral T-cell lymphoma, not otherwise specified (PTCL-NOS)
   C. Metastatic disease
   D. Anaplastic large cell lymphoma (ALCL), ALK (−)

6. Which virus is commonly associated with NK T-cell lymphoma?
   A. Human T-cell leukemia virus type 1 (HTLV-1)
   B. Epstein–Barr Virus (EBV)
   C. Cytomegalovirus (CMV)
   D. Human herpesvirus 8 (HHV 8)

7. True or false: All T-cell lymphomas are staged using the Ann Arbor Staging System?
   A. True
   B. False

ANSWERS

1. **B. Anaplastic large cell lymphoma (ALCL), ALK +.** ALK + ALCL has the best overall prognosis of the above PTCL subtypes with a 5-year overall survival rate of 70%. Note, International Prognostic Index (IPI) risk group should also be taken into account and is still prognostic.

2. **C. Human T-cell leukemia virus type 1 (HTLV-1).** This man most likely has ATLL given his heritage and peripheral blood features; this is associated with HTLV-1 infection.

3. **D. Mycosis fungoides.** The clinical history and pathology results with epidermotropism and Pautrier microabscess formation are consistent with mycosis fungoides.

4. **A. Angioimmunoblastic T-cell lymphoma (AITL).** AITL is the most likely diagnosis given the systemic symptoms of arthritis, effusions, B-symptoms, and lymphadenopathy, as well as likely hemolytic anemia with an elevated bilirubin and LDH.

5. **D. Anaplastic large cell lymphoma (ALCL), ALK (–).** ALK(–) ALCL has been associated with breast implants. Implant removal and capsulectomy followed by observation is associated with favorable long-term disease-free survival for patients without an associated mass.

6. **B. Epstein–Barr Virus (EBV).** NK T-cell lymphoma is associated with EBV infections.

7. **B. False.** Cutaneous T-cell lymphoma (CTCL) staging is different from other non-Hodgkin lymphomas and staging uses a tumor, nodes, metastasis, and blood (TNMB) classification system.

Hodgkin Lymphoma

Darren King and Shannon Carty

DEFINITION/CLASSIFICATION

1. **What is Hodgkin lymphoma (HL)?**
   - HL is a lymphoid neoplasm characterized by malignant cells with a unique morphology/immunophenotype surrounded by extensive inflammatory infiltrate, consisting of histiocytes, T lymphocytes, B lymphocytes, plasma cells, and eosinophils. The actual malignant cells of HL may make up as little as 1% of the total cellularity of a given nodal tumor, with the remainder consisting of inflammatory background.

2. **How is HL classified?**
   - HL comprises two entities with distinct pathobiology and prognosis, classical Hodgkin lymphoma (cHL) and nodular lymphocyte predominant Hodgkin lymphoma (NLPHL).

EPIDEMIOLOGY

1. **How common is HL?**
   - HL accounts for approximately 12% of all lymphomas in the United States (about 8,260 new cases in 2017). Worldwide, HL comprises approximately 8% of lymphomas per World Health Organization (WHO) estimates.

2. **How common are the histologic subtypes of HL?**
   - cHL makes up 95% of cases. Its histologic subtypes are nodular sclerosing (70%), mixed cellularity (25%), lymphocyte rich (5%), and lymphocyte depleted (<1%).
   - NLPHL makes up 5% of HL cases. It is characterized by an indolent course and late relapses and is clinically managed like an indolent NHL; see the following text.

3. **What are the demographics of HL?**
   - Bimodal age distribution with the first peak around age 20 years and the second near age 65 years
   - In cHL there is a slight male predominance, whereas 75% of patients with NLPHL are male.

ETIOLOGY AND RISK FACTORS

1. **What are risk factors for HL?**
   - Socioeconomic status is directly associated with the nodular sclerosing subtype and inversely associated with the mixed cellularity variant

- Immunosuppression (e.g., solid organ or hematopoietic transplants)
- Autoimmune diseases (e.g., rheumatoid arthritis)
- HIV/AIDS is associated with Epstein-Barr virus (EBV)-positive, lymphocyte-depleted subtype
- There is an increased incidence in patients with affected family members, but no known genetic predisposition

STAGING

1. Define the staging for HL.

Ann Arbor Staging

Stage	Description
I	Involvement of single lymph node region or structure (e.g., spleen, thymus, Waldeyer's ring) or a single extranodal site
II	Involvement of two or more lymph nodes or lymphoid structures on the same side of the diaphragm
III	Involvement of lymph nodes or lymphoid structures on both sides of the diaphragm
IV	Diffuse or disseminated involvement of one or more extranodal organs beyond I_E[a] including any liver or bone marrow involvement, with or without associated lymph node involvement

- *a = Contiguous extranodal extension indicated by "E"*
- *B symptoms (significant unexplained fever, night sweats, or unexplained weight loss exceeding 10% of body weight during the 6 months prior to diagnosis) indicated by "A" (absence) or "B" (presence)*
- *Bulky disease (mediastinal mass >1/3 diameter of thorax or any mass >10 cm) indicated by "X"*

SIGNS AND SYMPTOMS

1. What are the common signs and symptoms of HL?
    - Most patients present with asymptomatic lymphadenopathy or an incidentally discovered mediastinal mass.
    - B symptoms include fevers (unexplained, persistent/recurring temperature >38°C), drenching night sweats, and weight loss (>10% over preceding 6 months), seen in 20% of early and 50% of advanced stage disease. B symptoms are very rare in NLPHL.

2. What is the pattern of disease involvement in HL?
    - Cervical nodes are most commonly affected, followed by mediastinal nodes.
    - Spread is generally to adjacent lymph nodes.
    - Bone marrow involvement is observed in fewer than 5% of cases.

DIAGNOSTIC CRITERIA

1. **What is the optimal approach to the diagnosis of HL?**
   - Excisional lymph node biopsy. Tumor in HL has a very small component of malignant cells, with a surrounding reactive milieu of lymphocytes, eosinophils, and fibrosis (sclerosis). Excisional lymph node biopsy is far better at documenting this architecture than core biopsy
   - Clinical staging done using PET/CT scans
   - Bone marrow biopsy is no longer required for staging if PET/CT is consistent with marrow involvement. Bone marrow biopsy should be performed in the presence of cytopenias and a negative PET/CT

2. **How is the diagnosis of cHL made?**
   - Presence of mononuclear Hodgkin cells or multinucleate Hodgkin/Reed-Sternberg (HRS) cells in an inflammatory background (see Figure 18.1)
   - Typical immunophenotype of cHL is CD15 and CD30 positive with absence of the usual B-cell markers CD20, CD79a, and the common leukocyte antigen CD45. PD-L1 is often expressed.

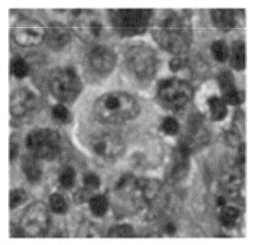

FIGURE 18.1 ■ Reed–Sternberg cell surrounded by inflammatory infiltrate.

3. **How is nodular lymphocyte predominant HL diagnosed?**
   - Presence of LP cells (formerly called lymphocytic and histiocytic, or L&H cells) with "popcorn" appearance
   - Typical immunophenotype is CD15 and CD30 negative with positivity for the B-cell markers CD20, CD79a, and the common leukocyte antigen CD45

4. **What is the cell of origin of HL?**
   - Determining the cell of origin of the HRS cells of cHL took many years to clarify due to the unique immunophenotype of these cells as well as the paucity of actual HRS cells in any given tumor specimen, which is primarily comprised of inflammatory infiltrate. Through the use of single-cell microdissection, it was

ultimately determined that although HRS cells do not express immunoglobulin or other typical B-cell makers, they do show immunoglobulin g (Ig) variable region (V) rearrangement. This indicates that the HRS cells of cHL derive from a preapoptotic germinal center B lymphocyte. The LP cells of NLPHL have also been shown to derive from a germinal center B lymphocyte and have also undergone somatic Ig V rearrangement. Unlike cHL, the LP cells of NLPHL do express immunoglobulin.

5. **What other disease is often confused with NLPHL on the basis of histology/immunophenotype?**
   - NLPHL must be carefully distinguished from the T-cell-/histiocyte-rich variant of diffuse large B-cell lymphoma (DLBCL).

INDICATIONS FOR TREATMENT

1. **Who requires treatment for HL?**
   - All patients with cHL should be considered for initial treatment with curative intent.
   - Likewise, all patients with NLPHL should be considered for therapy at the time of diagnosis (e.g., radiation with nonbulky stage IA/IIA disease, immunochemotherapy—e.g., rituximab, cyclophosphamide, doxorubicin, vincristine and prednisone [R-CHOP]—in bulky limited stage or advanced stage disease; however, observation alone may be considered for some patients, e.g., excised stage I disease).

PROGNOSTIC FACTORS

1. **What are unfavorable factors in early stage (I–IIA) cHL?**
   - Large mediastinal mass (greater than 1/3 of mediastinal diameter), extranodal disease, erythrocyte sedimentation rate (ESR) $\geq$ 50 mm/hour without or $\geq$30 mm/hour with B symptoms, greater than or equal to three nodal sites, and/or bulky disease.

2. **What are unfavorable prognostic factors in advanced stage (IIB–IV) cHL? How does the International Prognostic Factor score impact outcome?**
   - Factors include age > 45 years, male sex, stage IV, albumin < 4 g/dL, hemoglobin < 10.5 g/dL, white blood cell count > 15,000/mm^3, lymphopenia (one point for each).

Score	5-Year FFP (%)	5-Year OS (%)
0	84	89
1	77	90
2	67	81
3	60	78
4	51	61
5–7	42	56

FFP, freedom from progression; OS, overall survival.

3. **What are other poor prognostic factors for HL?**
   - Positive PET scan after two cycles of ABVD (adriamycin, bleomycin, vinblastine, dacarbazine) strongly associated with inferior 2-year progression-free survival
   - Increased density of lymphoma-associated macrophages (CD68-positive cells)

4. **How are interim PET scans interpreted?**
   - The 5-Point Deauville scoring system has been developed for interim PET reporting in lymphoma patients undergoing treatment. Scores are assigned as follows (with interim PET compared to baseline PET):
     - 1: No residual uptake above background level
     - 2: Residual uptake less than or equal to mediastinum
     - 3: Residual uptake greater than mediastinum but not greater than liver
     - 4: Residual uptake moderately increased compared to liver
     - 5: Residual uptake markedly increased compared to liver OR with new sites of disease
   - A Deauville score of 1 to 3 is considered PET negative, a score of 4 to 5 is considered PET positive

5. **What is the prognosis for HL?**
   - Cure is obtained in over 80% of all patients.
   - Five-year survival is >90% in early and >75% in advanced stage disease.

TREATMENT

1. **What is the initial treatment for early stage (I–IIA) cHL?**
   - In limited stage, favorable risk disease, a standard approach is combined modality therapy with two cycles of ABVD (doxorubicin/bleomycin/vinblastine/dacarbazine) with restaging PET/CT followed by 20 Gy of involved site radiation therapy (ISRT). Limited stage, unfavorable risk disease may be treated with four cycles of ABVD followed by 30 Gy of ISRT. An alternative approach, sparing radiation therapy and its potential risks, is three to six cycles of ABVD alone, in a risk-adapted fashion (i.e., depending upon the quality of response observed on interim PET/CT).
   - The Stanford V regimen (doxorubicin, vinblastine, mechlorethamine, etoposide, vincristine, bleomycin, prednisone) is an alternative to ABVD.

2. **How is advanced stage (IIB–IV) cHL managed?**
   - Chemotherapy alone with ABVD (doxorubicin/bleomycin/vinblastine/dacarbazine) for six cycles. Outcome appears to be optimized if treatment delays and dose reductions are avoided.
   - BEACOPP (bleomycin, etoposide, adriamycin, cyclophosphamide, vincristine [Oncovin], procarbazine, prednisone) and Stanford V (doxorubicin, vinblastine, mechlorethamine, etoposide, vincristine, bleomycin, prednisone) are alternative regimens.
   - Consolidative radiation therapy is an option for patients with bulky disease.

3. **What are treatment options for relapsed/refractory HL?**

- First relapse or progression following initial standard treatment (e.g., ABVD [doxorubicin/bleomycin/vinblastine/dacarbazine] +/- radiation) can be treated with brentuximab vedotin or salvage chemotherapy, such as ICE (ifosfamide/carboplatin/etoposide) or a gemcitabine-containing regimen. Those patients who achieve a remission are candidates for high-dose chemotherapy followed by autologous stem cell transplant, with consideration of posttransplant brentuximab.

- Patients who relapse or progress following these salvage regimens can be considered for therapy with brentuximab, immune checkpoint blockade, or further chemotherapy (e.g., bendamustine). Those achieving a response are candidates for allogeneic stem cell transplant.

- Relapse or progression following allogeneic stem cell transplant may be treated with observation alone, a clinical trial, single-agent therapy (e.g. mTOR inhibitor, HDAC inhibitor), or radiation therapy, depending on the patient's disease and performance status.

4. **What is brentuximab vedotin? What are its usual toxicities?**

- Brentuximab vedotin is an anti-CD30 monoclonal antibody conjugated to a mitotic spindle inhibitor. Its use has been approved in patients who relapse following autologous hematopoietic stem cell transplantation (auto-HSCT) or who are not deemed candidates for transplant. Its main toxicity as a single agent is peripheral neuropathy. Its use in combination with bleomycin is contraindicated, given the risk for potentiating pulmonary toxicity.

5. **How is nodular lymphocyte predominant disease managed?**

- Radiation therapy alone for stages IA and IIA
- Chemotherapy ± radiation for stages IB and IIB
- Observation may be appropriate for asymptomatic patients with advanced stage disease that is nonbulky and slowly progressive
- Immunochemotherapy (e.g., R-CHOP) for symptomatic advanced disease
- Single-agent rituximab has also shown disease activity in both the frontline and relapsed settings

SPECIAL CONSIDERATIONS

1. **What are the significant toxicities from treatment?**

- Pulmonary toxicity from bleomycin. Bleomycin can be safely omitted from cycles #3-6 of ABVD (doxorubicin/bleomycin/vinblastine/dacarbazine) in patients with advanced stage disease

- Myelosuppression with ABVD. Less than 10% of patients develop febrile neutropenia. It is important (and safe) to maintain dose intensity through cytopenias

- Infertility (much more common with BEACOPP [bleomycin, etoposide, adriamycin, cyclophosphamide, vincristine {Oncovin}, procarbazine, prednisone] regimen than ABVD)

- Cardiac dysfunction from radiation (e.g., pericarditis, coronary artery disease, and valvular disease) or chemotherapy (e.g., heart failure due to anthracyclines)
- Secondary malignancies (e.g., breast cancer in females who have received thoracic radiation) Therapy-related myelodysplastic syndrome (MDS) and acute myelogenous leukemia (AML) are less common in patients receiving ABVD than in patients who receive MOPP (mechlorethamine/vincristine/procarbazine/prednisone) or BEACOPP regimens

QUESTIONS

1. A 30-year-old female smoker has begun treatment for stage IIIA Hodgkin lymphoma. She is receiving ABVD (doxorubicin/bleomycin/vinblastine/dacarbazine). She has read about bleomycin-induced pulmonary toxicity and is very anxious about this potential side effect. Which of the following does *not* increase the risk of bleomycin-induced pulmonary toxicity?
   A. Renal insufficiency
   B. Concomitant use of brentuximab
   C. Smoking
   D. Younger age

2. An otherwise healthy 45-year-old male completed six cycles of ABVD (doxorubicin/bleomycin/vinblastine/dacarbazine) for stage IV classical Hodgkin lymphoma (cHL). Six months following completion of treatment, he noticed an enlarging cervical lymph node. Biopsy was performed, which confirmed relapse. PET/CT shows diffuse disease. Which of the following is the most appropriate next step in management?
   A. Initiate BEACOPP (bleomycin, etoposide, adriamycin, cyclophosphamide, vincristine [Oncovin], procarbazine, prednisone)
   B. Initiate brentuximab
   C. Initiate salvage chemotherapy with ICE (ifosfamide/carboplatin/etoposide) and plan for autologous stem cell transplant (auto-SCT)
   D. Proceed to nonmyeloablative allogeneic stem cell transplant

3. A 35-year-old female is receiving treatment for stage IIA classical Hodgkin lymphoma with ABVD (doxorubicin/bleomycin/vinblastine/dacarbazine). Following her first two cycles of ABVD, which of the following is most predictive of a worse progression-free survival (PFS)?
   A. Unchanged size of mediastinal mass per interim CT
   B. No change in fluorodeoxyglucose (FDG) avidity of mediastinal mass per interim PET
   C. Elevation of erythrocyte sedimentation rate (ESR)
   D. Persistence of B symptoms

4. A 24-year-old female was diagnosed with stage IIIB classical Hodgkin lymphoma (cHL) with a bulky mediastinal mass. Her treatment comprised six cycles of ABVD (doxorubicin/bleomycin/vinblastine/

dacarbazine) and radiation to the mediastinum. She completed treatment 4 years ago. Long-term surveillance does *not* include which of the following?

A. Breast MRI or early mammogram
B. Thyroid function testing
C. Yearly history and physical exam
D. Annual PET scan

5. A 20-year-old male undergoes biopsy of an enlarged left cervical lymph node and is diagnosed with classical Hodgkin lymphoma, nodular sclerosing subtype. PET/CT is performed, which shows fluorodeoxyglucose (FDG) uptake in the left cervical lymph node region, but no other areas of pathologic uptake. Complete blood count (CBC) and lactate dehydrogenase (LDH) are normal. The patient has no B symptoms. The patient is very hesitant about undergoing bone marrow biopsy as part of his staging workup. Which of the following staging steps/results can best reassure his hematologist that a bone marrow biopsy is not essential?

A. Normal CBC
B. Normal LDH
C. Lack of B symptoms
D. PET/CT

6. A 75-year-old male was diagnosed with stage IA nodular lymphocyte predominant Hodgkin lymphoma (NLPHL) of the mediastinum. He underwent radiation therapy to the mediastinum and did well for 5 years. Now, at age 80 years, he has a biopsy-proven recurrence in the right cervical lymph node chain, outside his prior radiation field. He is asymptomatic. PET/CT staging is consistent with stage III disease. The patient has an Eastern Cooperative Oncology Group (ECOG) performance status of 1 to 2, but desires further treatment. Which of the following would *NOT* be a reasonable treatment strategy?

A. Observation
B. Single-agent rituximab
C. R-CHOP
D. BEACOPP (bleomycin, etoposide, adriamycin, cyclophosphamide, vincristine [Oncovin], procarbazine, prednisone)

7. Which of the following is NOT an unfavorable risk factor in early stage (I–IIA) classical Hodgkin lymphoma?

A. A mediastinal mass that is 25% the mediastinal diameter
B. Extranodal disease
C. Erythrocyte sedimentation rate (ESR) ≥ 50 mm/hour without or ≥30 mm/hour with B symptoms
D. Three or more nodal sites
E. Bulky disease

8. **Which of the following is NOT an unfavorable risk factor in advanced stage (IIB–IV) classical Hodgkin lymphoma?**
   A. Age > 35 years
   B. Male sex
   C. Stage IV
   D. Albumin <4 g/dL
   E. Hemoglobin <10.5
   F. White blood cell (WBC) >15,000/mm^3
   G. Lymphopenia

ANSWERS

1. **D. Younger age.** Older age is associated with increased risk of bleomycin-induced pulmonary toxicity, and, as a result, this drug is usually removed from treatment in elderly patients. Renal insufficiency, concomitant use of brentuximab, and smoking have all been associated with increased risk of bleomycin-induced pulmonary toxicity. It remains unclear whether granulocyte colony-stimulating factor (G-CSF) may potentiate bleomycin-induced pulmonary toxicity; however, many clinicians avoid its use.

2. **C. Initiate salvage chemotherapy with ICE (ifosfamide/carboplatin/ etoposide) and plan for autologous stem cell transplant (auto-SCT).** Standard initial treatment for relapsed cHL is salvage chemotherapy (such as ICE) followed by auto-SCT. Retreating with a combination chemotherapy regimen without auto-SCT would not be indicated with a relapse this early. Brentuximab and allogeneic stem cell transplant are indicated in patients relapsing following autologous hematopoietic stem cell transplant (auto-HSCT).

3. **B. No change in FDG avidity of mediastinal mass per interim PET.** Interim PET scan following two cycles of ABVD has been shown to be the most powerful predictor of PFS. Its prognostic significance is superior to the International Prognostic Score (IPS). PET scans are interpreted according to the Deauville 5-Point scoring system.

4. **D. Annual PET scan.** Because of its high cure rates, long-term follow-up for cHL requires monitoring of a number of possible late complications. Women who received radiation therapy to the chest are at a higher risk of developing (often bilateral) breast cancer and require close monitoring with breast MRI or early mammogram. Thyroid function should be monitored, as the gland may be affected by mediastinal radiation. After completion of treatment, National Comprehensive Cancer Network (NCCN) guidelines recommend history and physical should be performed every 3 to 6 months for the first 1 to 2 years, then every 6 to 12 months until year 3, and then yearly. Surveillance with PET scan is **NOT** indicated in the absence of clinical concern for relapse.

5. **D. PET/CT.** Bone marrow biopsy is no longer always considered an essential part of the staging workup for Hodgkin lymphoma given the sensitivity/specificity of PET scan for marrow involvement.

6. **D. BEACOPP (bleomycin, etoposide, adriamycin, cyclophosphamide, vincristine [Oncovin], procarbazine, prednisone).** NLPHL typically follows an indolent course, but often with late relapses. Given its distinct clinical course and immunophenotype, the decision to treat should be approached in a way similar to the indolent non-Hodgkin lymphomas. Observation in an asymptomatic patient, single-agent rituximab, and combination therapy with R-CHOP are reasonable options in a patient with advanced age and borderline performance status. BEACOPP would not be appropriate.

7. **A. A mediastinal mass that is 25% the mediastinal diameter.** A mediastinal mass that is greater than one third of mediastinal diameter is not considered an unfavorable risk factor in early stage classical Hodgkin lymphoma. All the other answers are unfavorable risk factors in early stage classical Hodgkin lymphoma.

8. **A. Age > 35 years.** Age > 45 years (and not age >35 years) is not considered an unfavorable risk factor in advanced stage classical Hodgkin lymphoma. All the other answers are unfavorable risk factors in advanced stage classical Hodgkin lymphoma.

Darren King and Patrick Burke

HISTIOCYTIC DISORDERS

1. **What is a histiocyte?**
   - Histiocyte is a somewhat archaic morphologic term used to describe tissue-resident, monocyte-derived macrophages. Histiocytic disorders may be benign or malignant, and span a broad range of clinical presentations and pathobiology.

2. **How are the histiocytic disorders classified?**
   - An updated classification of histiocytic disorders has been recommended by the Histiocyte Society as follows:

Histiocytosis Group	Diseases
"L" Group ("Langerhans")	• LCH
	• ICH
	• ECD
	• Mixed LCH/ECD
"C" Group ("Cutaneous/ Mucocutaneous")	• XG Family: JXG, AXG, SRH, BCH, GEH, PNH
	• Non-XG Family: Cutaneous RDD
	• Cutaneous non-LCH with a major systemic component
"R" Group ("Rosai-Dorfman")	• Familial RDD
	• Sporadic Rosai-Dorfman disease
"M" Group ("Malignant Histiocytoses")	• Primary malignant histiocytoses
	• Secondary malignant histiocytoses associated with another hematologic neoplasm
"H" Group ("Hemophagocytic Lymphohistiocytosis")	• Primary (Inherited) HLH
	• Secondary HLH

(continued)

Histiocytosis Group	Diseases
	• HLH of Unknown Origin

AXG, adult xanthogranuloma; BCH, benign cephalic histiocytosis; ECD, Erdheim-Chester disease; GEH, generalized eruptive histiocytosis; HLH, hemophagocytic lymphohistiocytosis; ICH, indeterminate cell histiocytosis; JXG, juvenile xanthogranuloma; LCH, Langerhans cell histiocytosis; PNH, progressive nodular histiocytosis; RDD, Rosai-Dorfman disease; SRH, solitary reticulohistiocytoma.

Source: Emile JF et al. Revised classification of histiocytoses and neoplasms of the macrophage-dendritic cell lineages. *Blood* 2016 127:2672–2681.

3. **What is a Langerhans cell?**
   - Langerhans cells are a subset of dendritic cells localized to the skin and other epithelial mucosa. They are antigen presenting cells and are morphologically characterized by the presence of "tennis-racket"-shaped Birbeck granules. They proliferate/replenish locally in response to inflammation.

4. **What is Langerhans cell histiocytosis (LCH)?**
   - LCH is a spectrum of disorders ranging from localized, self-resolving lesions to highly morbid/fatal disseminated disease. The disease is characterized by the clonal proliferation and accumulation of a cell population morphologically resembling Langerhans cells (including presence of Birbeck granules); however, LCH is **not** thought to derive from normal Langerhans cell populations. The cells of LCH are phenotypically characterized as CD14+, which is a **monocytic** marker **not** found on Langerhans cells, which are of the **dendritic** cell lineage.

5. **What is the epidemiology of LCH?**
   - LCH is a rare disease, with case series and epidemiological studies suggesting a childhood incidence of 3–5 cases per million and an adult incidence of 1–2 cases per million. Males may be at higher risk of developing LCH. LCH of the lung is strongly associated with smoking.

6. **What are the clinical features of LCH?**
   - LCH typically presents as single or multiple lytic bone lesions, with proliferating histiocytes (and reactive lymphocytes, eosinophils, and macrophages) which can infiltrate any organ, including the central nervous system (CNS). Approximately 55% of patients present with disease limited to a single organ (or bone), with the remainder showing multisystem involvement.

LCH Organ Site	Clinical Features
Bone	• Lytic lesions
	• Base of skull lesions may lead to cranial nerve palsies, exophthalmos, or diabetes insipidus

(continued)

LCH Organ Site	Clinical Features
Skin	• Brown/purple papules
	• Eczematous rash
	• Oral lesions/ulcers/gingivitis
Lymph nodes (approximately 20% of patients)	• Lymphadenopathy
Bone Marrow	• Cytopenias
Liver/Spleen	• Organomegaly
	• Hypersplenism
	• LFT abnormalities
CNS	• Central diabetes insipidus (posterior pituitary infiltration)
	• Neurodegeneration (ataxia, cognitive decline)
Gastrointestinal Tract	• Diarrhea
	• Malabsorption
Lung	• Dyspnea
	• Abnormalities
	• Spontaneous pneumothorax

7. **What are "risk organs" in LCH?**
   - Involvement of the disease in several organs is thought to convey a worse prognosis. These "risk organs" are the bone marrow, liver, spleen, and possibly lung.

8. **What endocrinopathies may be seen in patients with LCH?**
   - The most common endocrinopathy associated with LCH is central diabetes insipidus (DI) due to infiltration of the posterior pituitary gland. Other endocrinopathies reported include hypogonadism, glucose intolerance, growth retardation, and thyroid enlargement.

9. **What other names is LCH known by?**
   - Historically, LCH has been known by a number of names, including Hand-Schüller-Christian disease (clinical triad of exophthalmos, diabetes insipidus, and skull lesions), histiocytosis X, Letterer-Siwe disease (presenting with lymphadenopathy, rash, hepatosplenomegaly, fever, anemia, and thrombocytopenia), and eosinophilic granuloma of the bone.

10. **How is LCH diagnosed?**
    - Biopsy of a suspected lesion (preferably skin or bone) should show presence of cells positive for CD1a, S100 and CD207, and/or presence of Birbeck granules.

11. **What is the risk stratification of LCH?**
    - LCH is risk-stratified based on single-organ versus multi-organ involvement, and presence of disease in "risk organs."
        - Single system LCH: Unifocal or multifocal disease within a single organ/system, no involvement of "risk organs"
        - Multisystem LCH: Disease presence in 2 or more organ systems or involvement of "risk organs"

12. **How is LCH treated?**
    - Multiple treatment regimens for LCH exist, with chemotherapy regimens including use of such cytotoxics as cytarabine, vinblastine, and cladribine. LCH of the bone may be treated by local resection/curettage with or without steroid therapy, external beam radiation therapy, bisphosphonates, or chemotherapy. LCH of the skin may be treated by resection, steroids, ultraviolet B (UVB) radiation therapy/photodynamic therapy, or chemotherapy. Multisystem disease in adults is typically treated with chemotherapy. Patients whose disease fails to respond to treatment within 6 weeks have a poor prognosis. End-organ damage (e.g., lung, liver) may warrant solid organ transplant if systemic disease is otherwise well-controlled. Allogeneic hematopoietic cell transplant may be curative; however, its role in LCH has not yet been firmly established. Participation in clinical trials, especially for multisystem or relapsed/refractory disease, is encouraged.

13. **What other diseases make up the "L" (Langerhans-like) category of histiocytoses?**
    - In addition to LCH, the "L" group of histiocytoses includes indeterminate cell histiocytosis (ICH) and Erdheim-Chester disease (ECD).
        - ICH resembles LCH both clinically and morphologically; however the clonal cells in ICH show absent CD207 expression, unlike LCH.
        - ECD occurs at a mean age of 55–60 years old (3:1 male to female ratio). PET/CT is highly indicative of disease, with the finding of bilateral symmetric cortical osteosclerosis of the diaphyseal and metaphyseal regions. Cardiac involvement and retroperitoneal fibrosis is common. MRI of the brain and MR or CT of the aorta, cardiac MRI, and transthoracic echocardiogram are recommended to complete evaluation for extent of disease.
        - The histologic pattern of ECD on biopsy are foamy histiocytes infiltrating tissue, typically with fibrosis present and abundant reactive lymphocytes and neutrophils. The histiocytes of ECD can be distinguished from LCH based on CD1a negativity in the former; however, cases of mixed ECD/LCH components have been described.

14. **What is the role of BRAF mutations in the "L" group of histiocytsoses?**
    - The *BRAF* V600E mutation has been found to be highly characteristic of "L" group histiocytoses, with case series reporting more than half of LCH cases positive for the mutation, and approximately 50% of ECD cases. Patients who are *BRAF* wild-type may have mutations in *MAP2K1* (*MEK1*), downstream of *BRAF*. These mutations are mutually exclusive. The presence of a *BRAF*

mutation may aid in diagnosis of a morphologically challenging case. LCH and ECD patients have shown major responses to oral *BRAF* and/or *MEK*-inhibitor therapy, and testing for this mutation is recommended after failure of frontline treatment.

15. **What are the diseases in the "C" (Cutaneous/Mucocutaneous) group of histiocytoses?**
    - The "C" group is comprised of the following diseases:
      o Xanthogranuloma (XG) Family: Juvenile xanthogranuloma (JXG), adult xanthogranuloma (AXG), and solitary reticulohistiocytoma (SRH) are characterized by well-circumscribed dermal nodules sparing the epidermis containing macrophages, foamy cells, lymphocytes, and eosinophils. JXG appears within the first few years as one or several yellow skin nodules, which usually spontaneously resolve. Disease may be extracutaneous or disseminated, however. AXG is typically a persistent, single lesion. SRH lesions are show infiltration by oncocytic macrophages and ground-glass giant cells.
      o Non-XG Family: Skin-localized Rosai-Dorfman disease (RDD, see the following), necrobiotic xanthogranuloma (NXG, characterized by paraproteinemia, large ulcerated plaques commonly in the periorbital and thoracic regions, with associated cardiomyopathy and underlying hematologic malignancies), multicentric reticulohistiocytosis (MRH, typically affects 50–60-year-old women with polyarthritis, association with malignancy/autoimmune disease, and pathognomonic periungual "coral bead" papules).

16. **What are the diseases in the "M" (Malignant) group of histiocytoses?**
    - The "M" group of histiocytoses are anaplastic tumors with phenotypic features characteristic of histiocytes (e.g., CD1a and CD207 expression). Malignancy is determined based on mitotic activity and cellular atypia on biopsy. These tumors may be primary (involving the skin, lymph nodes, GI tract, or widely disseminated) or secondary and associated with another underlying hematologic malignancy. Response to conventional cytotoxic chemotherapy is typically poor.

17. **What are the diseases in the "R" (Rosai-Dorfman) group of histiocytoses?**
    - The "R" group of histiocytoses are comprised of RDD in its sporadic and familial forms.
      o Classical sporadic RDD involves the lymph nodes, is usually diagnosed in children, and clinically presents with massive cervical lymphadenopathy, fever, sweats, fatigue, and weight loss. Extranodal disease may involve the skin, bone, CNS soft tissue, and retro-orbital tissue.
      o Diagnosis is based on biopsy showing histiocytes, which are negative for CD1a and CD207 (unlike LCH).
      o Patients may demonstrate autoimmune hemolytic anemia, hyperferritinemia, hypergammaglobulinemia, and leukocytosis.
      o Sporadic RDD usually resolves spontaneously and with good prognosis but with 5% to 11% mortality rate.

○ Familial RDD may be diagnosed in H Syndrome (an inherited condition due to *SLC29A3* mutation associated with hyperpigmentation, hypertrichosis, hepatosplenomegaly, hearing loss, heart abnormalities, hypogonadism, short height, hyperglycemia, and hallux valgus) or autoimmune lymphoproliferative syndrome (ALPS) associated with germline *TNFRSF6* mutation.

18. What are the diseases in the "H" group of histiocytoses?

● The "H" group of histiocytoses comprises hemophagocytic lymphohistiocytosis (HLH) in its primary and secondary forms.

19. What is HLH?

● HLH is a rare, highly morbid syndrome characterized by multi-organ system failure in the setting of hyperactivation of the immune system with accumulation of activated macrophages.

20. How is HLH diagnosed?

● The diagnosis of HLH is clinical, based on meeting five of the eight criteria below OR presence of a defined molecular mutation:

○ Fever >38.0 °C

○ Splenomegaly

○ Cytopenias involving at least two lineages (Hgb <9 g/dL, platelets <100,000, or absolute neutrophil count <1,000)

○ Hypertriglyceridemia (fasting triglycerides ≥ 265 mg/dL) OR fibrinogen <150 mg/dL

○ Ferritin ≥ 500 ng/mL

○ Hemophagocytosis noted in bone marrow, spleen, or lymph nodes upon biopsy

○ Low or absent NK cell activity

○ Soluble CD25 (soluble IL-2 receptor) >2,400 U/mL

21. What are the causes of secondary HLH?

● Secondary HLH has been described in the setting of infection (bacterial, fungal, parasitic, or viral, including EBV, CMV, HIV, and influenza), malignancy (hematologic malignancies such as lymphoma or leukemia, as well as solid tumors), during chemotherapy exposure, and in association with autoimmune disorders (including SLE, vasculitis, and adult onset Still disease). HLH in the setting of an underlying autoimmune disorder is referred to as macrophage activation syndrome (MAS-HLH).

22. What gene mutations are associated with primary HLH?

● Primary HLH is characterized by the finding of a germline mutation in any one of a number of genes. As further mutations are characterized, many cases of HLH previously described as of "secondary" or "unknown" etiology may now be classified as primary HLH.

○ Among the genes with mutations in primary HLH characterized to date are *FHL2, FHL3, FHL4, FHL5, XLP1, RAB27A* (Griscelli Syndrome type 2), *LYST* (Chediak-Higashi Syndrome), *XLP2, NLRC4, SLC7A7,* and *HMOX1*.

○ Patients with germline mutations predisposing to primary HLH may not present until adulthood, so testing for the above mutations by gene panel is recommended regardless of age at time of HLH diagnosis

23. How is HLH treated in the frontline setting?

● Frontline treatment of HLH includes treatment of underlying conditions/infections in the secondary form, as well as use of chemotherapy in both the primary and secondary forms of the disease. Standard frontline therapy for both primary and secondary HLH follows the HLH-94 protocol, with use of an 8-week induction course of IV etoposide and dexamethasone.

○ Patients with documented CNS involvement or progressive neurological symptoms receive IT methotrexate throughout the treatment course.

○ Although early cyclosporine was also used in the original HLH-94 protocol, this has begun to be removed in current practice.

24. What is the role of allogenic stem cell transplant in the treatment of HLH?

● Although use of allo-HCT in the treatment of adults with HLH has not yet been validated, it is generally recommended if any of the following features of disease are present:

○ Relapsed or refractory disease following or during frontline treatment

○ CNS involvement

○ Underlying hematologic malignancy

○ Primary HLH diagnosis per germline mutation finding as above

DENDRITIC CELL NEOPLASMS

1. What is a dendritic cell?

● Dendritic cells are antigen-presenting cells of the innate immune system and are present in both blood and in tissues.

○ Dendritic cells in tissue are small and have a "star-shaped" appearance due to the presence of dendritic processes, unlike histiocytes/macrophages, which are large, round cells.

○ Circulating dendritic cells do not show dendritic processes and may morphologically resemble monocytes (mDC) or plasma cells (pDC).

2. What is the origin of dendritic cells?

● Dendritic cells may derive from myeloid or lymphoid progenitors. They are classified as "myeloid" dendritic cells, mDC (CD1c+ or CD141+, secreting IL-12) or "plasmacytoid" dendritic cells, pDC (CD303+, secreting IFN-alpha).

3. What is blastic plasmacytoid dendritic cell neoplasm (BPDCN)?

● BPDCN is a rare and aggressive hematologic malignancy of the pDC population characterized by skin and bone marrow involvement. The disease has undergone many name changes, with "BPDCN" established by the 2008 WHO classification system.

4. What is the epidemiology of BPDCN?

- Although data are sparse, case series suggest that BPDCN makes up approximately 0.44% of all hematological malignancies, with a male female ratio of 2.5:1. Median age of onset is 60–70 years, and risk factors are unknown. 10% to 20% of cases may be associated with an additional hematological malignancy (e.g., MDS, CML, or AML).

5. What are the clinical findings of BPDCN?

- Patients typically present initially with skin lesions, which may be solitary or multiple, with variability in size (few millimeters to 10 cm), shape (papules, nodules, or plaques), and color. The lesions may show overlying erythema or ulceration. If marrow is involved at time of diagnosis, patients may also show cytopenias and/or presence of circulating blasts.

6. How is BPDCN diagnosed?

- The malignant cells in BPDCN obtained via skin or bone marrow biopsy show a characteristic immunophenotype. They are CD4 and CD56 positive, as well as positive for more specific markers of pDCs—CD123 (IL3RA), TCL1, and CD303. Myeloid, monocytic, T-, or B-lymphoid markers are typically absent. Most cases of BPDCN show clonal chromosomal abnormalities and/or gene mutations; however, none are diagnostic of the disease.

7. What is the prognosis of BPDCN?

- Prognosis of BPDCN has historically been very poor, with median overall survival (OS) in the 12–16 months range based on small series. The disease is characterized by initial response to treatment, followed by relapse and refractoriness.

8. How is BPDCN treated?

- Frontline treatment for BPDCN has been variable, partly due to uncertainty regarding the lineage of origin of the pDCs. As a result, both lymphoid- and myeloid-type chemotherapy regimens have been used. Outcomes appear to be better with use of lymphoid-type chemotherapy regimens.
  - Non-Hodgkin lymphoma (NHL)-type treatment has been used (e.g., CHOP or EPOCH) with complete remission rates in the 40% to 50% range, but with very short durations of CR.
  - In fit patients, there is an increasing tendency to use acute lymphoblastic leukemia (ALL)-type regimens; however, even with these aggressive therapies, patients achieving a CR have a 60% relapse rate.
  - As in ALL, CNS involvement is seen in BPDCN both at diagnosis and, especially, at relapse. Therefore, CNS prophylaxis is typically administered as per ALL regimens.
  - Patients who are elderly or not otherwise candidates for aggressive cytotoxic chemotherapy may receive palliative XRT or steroids for skin lesions, with considerations of low-dose chemotherapy such as oral etoposide or CHOP with non-curative intent.

9. **What is the role of stem cell transplant (SCT) in treatment of BPDCN?**
   - Patients who are fit candidates have shown a survival benefit in BPDCN with use of allogenic stem cell transplant, and this is considered the best option for long-term remission in patients achieving a CR with frontline therapy. The potential role of auto-SCT remains unclear.

10. **What targeted therapies exist for treatment of BPDCN?**
    - Aside from the cytotoxic and transplant regimens noted above, targeted therapies for BPDCN are also being developed:
      ○ Presence of *IDH1/2* or *TET2* mutation at time of diagnosis may prompt use of IDH-inhibitors or hypomethylating agents.
      ○ There have been reports of BPDCN shown to carry a *FLT3-ITD* mutation with sensitivity to *FLT3* inhibitors.
      ○ BPDCN has been shown to be sensitive to the BCL2 inhibitor venetoclax.
      ○ The current focus for targeted therapy in BPDCN is on use of SL-401, which is a fusion of diphtheria α-toxin to recombinant IL-3A. The drug-protein conjugate takes advantage of the characteristic expression of IL-3A receptor (CD123) on the surface of pDCs to target cytotoxicity.
      ○ SL-401 has been studied in the relapsed and refractory setting, with patients showing promising results in terms of major objective responses and CR rates. Studies are ongoing for use of SL-401 in the consolidative setting post-frontline chemotherapy or to clear minimal residual disease prior to allo-SCT.

11. **What are the typical side effects of SL-401?**
    - Typical side effects with SL-401 treatment include infusion reactions (amenable to premedication), capillary leak syndrome, transaminitis, thrombocytopenia/neutropenia, hypoalbuminemia, and hyponatremia.

12. **What other dendritic cell neoplasms exist?**
    - There are other, rare dendritic cell neoplasms, including indeterminate dendritic cell tumor (IND-DCT), interdigitating dendritic cell sarcoma (IDCS), and follicular dendritic cell sarcoma (FDCS).

MYELOID AND LYMPHOID NEOPLASMS WITH EOSINOPHILIA

1. **What are myeloid and lymphoid neoplasms with eosinophilia?**
   - Beginning with the WHO 2008 classification, a group of diseases with shared molecular features have been placed in a novel category based on recurrent cytogenetic abnormalities with treatment implications:

Gene Fusion	Diagnostic Criteria
FIP1L1-PDGFRA	• A myeloid or lymphoid neoplasm
	• Prominent eosinophilia (usually)
	• Presence of *FIP1L1-PDGFRA* fusion or variant fusion involving *PDGFRA* (can perform FISH for *CHIC2* deletion at fusion site)

(continued)

Gene Fusion	Diagnostic Criteria
ETV6-PDGFRB	• A myeloid or lymphoid neoplasm
	• Prominent eosinophilia (usually)
	• Neutrophilia or monocytosis (sometimes)
	• Presence of t(8;12) or demonstration of *ETV6-PDGFRB* or variant fusion involving *PDGFRB*
FGFR1 rearrangement	• MPN or MPN/MDS
	• Prominent eosinophilia
	• Neutrophilia or monocytosis (sometimes)
	OR
	• AML or T-ALL or B-ALL/lymphoma or mixed phenotype acute leukemia (usually associated with peripheral blood or marrow eosinophilia)
	AND
	• t(8;13) or variant translocation leading to *FGFR1* rearrangement
PCM1-JAK2 (provisional entity)	• A myeloid or lymphoid neoplasm
	• Prominent eosinophilia (usually)
	• Presence of t(8;9) or a variant translocation leading to *JAK2* rearrangement

2. What is the incidence of this group of diseases?

- 10% or less of patients with primary hypereosinophilia are found to have *PDGFRA* rearrangements, with data lacking on incidence of the other fusions.

3. How are the myeloid/lymphoid neoplasms with eosinophilia diagnosed?

- Patients undergoing work-up for eosinophilia in which secondary causes have been ruled out (i.e., diagnosed with primary eosinophilia) should undergo testing for the above fusions/rearrangements given therapeutic and prognostic implications
- Patients diagnosed with another hematologic disorder (myeloid or lymphoid) with a component of eosinophilia should also undergo testing for the above fusions/rearrangements

4. How are the myeloid/lymphoid neoplasms with eosinophilia treated?

- Patients with disease involving fusions of *PDGFRA* and *PDGFRB* are exquisitely sensitive to Imatinib. Diseases with the classical rearrangements can often be treated in the frontline setting with excellent response to imatinib at 100 mg PO daily (for *PDGFRA*) or 400 mg PO daily (for *PDGFRB*), although variant translocations or acquired resistance mutations may require higher dosing.

- Patients with *FGFR1* typically have an aggressive disease course with early progression to AML, and their disease is not responsive to imatinib therapy. Treatment involves cytotoxic agents with goal of CR to be followed by allogeneic HCT or use of novel FGFR1 inhibitors in the clinical trial setting.
- Patients with *JAK2* rearrangements are typically treated with JAK-inhibitors (e.g., ruxolitinib), often as a bridge to allo-HCT given relatively short duration of response.
- Supportive care (e.g., steroids) given for end-organ damage (e.g., cardiomyopathy) related to hypereosinophilia

QUESTIONS

1. An 85-year-old male with congestive heart failure, hypertension, and type II diabetes mellitus presents with a painful, ulcerated erythematous plaque measuring 5 × 5 cm to the skin of his right pectoral region. Biopsy of the lesion reveals skin infiltrated by immature-appearing cells which are CD4+, CD56+, and CD123+. Complete blood count (CBC) shows normal peripheral blood counts. Which of the following treatments would be a reasonable management option?
   A. Surgical excision
   B. Chemotherapy with cyclophosphamide, doxorubicin, vincristine, prednisone (CHOP)
   C. Systemic steroids
   D. Local radiation therapy

2. A 35-year-old male with no past medical history presents to the local ER with 3 days of fever to 39°C and significant malaise. Laboratory analysis is notable for a ferritin of 2,000 ng/mL, left upper quadrant tenderness with palpable spleen tip, neutropenia to absolute neutrophil count (ANC) of 800, and thrombocytopenia to a platelet count of 90,000. A bone marrow biopsy is performed, which shows hemophagocytosis. Which of the following additional laboratory abnormalities would be necessary to make a clinical diagnosis of hemophagocytic lymphohistiocytosis (HLH)?
   A. Elevated natural killer (NK) cell activity
   B. Low NK cell activity
   C. Low soluble IL-2R level
   D. Elevated antinuclear antibodies (ANA)

3. An otherwise healthy 50-year-old male undergoes routine complete blood count (CBC) at his primary care doctor's office and is found to have an elevated white blood cell (WBC) count to 15,000 with normal hemoglobin and platelet count. Differential shows a hypereosinophilia (75% eosinophils). There is no evidence of end-organ-damage per chest x-ray (CXR) or troponin. Work-up for secondary causes of hypereosinophilia is negative, and the patient is felt to have a primary hypereosinophilia. A bone marrow biopsy is performed with conventional karyotype analysis, fluorescence in situ hybridization

(FISH) panel, and Next Generation Sequencing. Which of the following results would predict that his disease would NOT be responsive to a commercially available tyrosine kinase inhibitor?

A. *PDGFRA* gene rearrangement per karyotype
B. *CHIC2* deletion by FISH
C. *FGFR1* rearrangement per karyotype
D. *PDGFRB* rearrangement per karyotype
E. *JAK2* rearrangement per karyotype

4. A 22-year-old female has been diagnosed with hemophagocytic lymphohistiocytosis (HLH) and is 2 weeks into her induction course with etoposide/dexamethasone with early addition of cyclosporine per HLH-94 protocol. She has never had a lumbar puncture (LP) or shown neurological symptoms. The patient suffers a generalized tonic-clinic seizure. EEG upon recovery shows non-specific slow wave. MRI shows decreased signal on T1-weighted images and hyperintense T2 abnormalities in the posterior occipital lobes bilaterally. An LP is performed, with normal cerebrospinal fluid analysis. Appropriate anti-epileptic therapy has been started. What would be the appropriate next step in management?

A. Administer IT methotrexate
B. Stop cyclosporine
C. Continue current treatment
D. Continue current treatment and begin work-up for allogeneic hematopoietic cell transplant

5. A 45-year-old female treated for blastic plasmacytoid dendritic cell neoplasm (BPDCN) with an ALL induction regimen followed by allo-HCT has relapsed 120 days posttransplant. She has enrolled on a clinical trial to receive a drug-conjugate called SL-401. What is the targeting mechanism of this drug in BPDCN?

A. Binding to CD123 on pDC cell surface
B. Binding to CD4 on pDC cell surface
C. Binding to CD56 on pDC cell surface
D. Binding to CD303 on pDC cell surface

6. A 55-year-old male presents with 3 months of progressive right thigh pain. Plain films reveal a lytic bone lesion to the right femur. A PET/CT is performed, showing fluorodeoxyglucose (FDG)-avidity to the site. No other sites of disease are noted per PET. The patient undergoes extensive work-up for plasma cell dyscrasia, which is negative. Ultimately, a biopsy of the right femur lesion is performed. Histology reveals infiltration of the osteolytic lesion by cells with tennis-racket shaped granules, which are positive per immunohistochemistry for CD14. Which of the following would be an appropriate initial treatment strategy?

A. Systemic chemotherapy with vinblastine
B. Systemic chemotherapy with cytarabine
C. IV bisphosphonate therapy
D. Local radiation therapy (XRT) to the femoral lesion

7. **Which of the following is true?**
   A. Langerhans cell histiocytosis (LCH) risk organs are: bone marrow, liver, spleen, and possibly lung
   B. The M histiocyte group includes familial and sporadic Rosai-Dorfman Diseases.
   C. The most common endocrinopathy associated with LCH is primary adrenal insufficiency.
   D. In LCH, biopsy of a lesion demonstrates cells positive for CD1a, negative for S100 and positive for CD207.

8. **Which of the following is true?**
   A. Patients with *FGFR1* rearrangement and eosinophilia have a higher likelihood of response to imatinib than patients with *PDGFRA* or *PDGFRB* rearrangements.
   B. Clonal eosinophilia can be caused by *PCM1-JAK2* rearrangement.
   C. Patients with *ETV6-PDGFRB* rearrangements have deletion of the *CHIC2* gene.
   D. Patients with *ETV6-PDGFRB* rearrangements and eosinophilia should be treated with a JAK-inhibitor.

9. **What of the following is true about hemophagocytic lymphohistiocytosis (HLH)?**
   A. Allogeneic stem cell transplant is indicated in the following situations: relapsed/refractory disease following or during frontline treatment, central nervous system (CNS) involvement, underlying hematologic malignancy, primary HLH due to a germline mutation.
   B. HLH can be due to/co-occur with a variety of infections, malignancy, autoimmune disease, and can be due to somatic mutations but cannot be due to a germline mutation.
   C. Increased natural killer (NK) cell activity is one of the criteria for diagnosing HLH.
   D. Low triglycerides is one of the criteria for diagnosing HLH.

ANSWERS

1. **D. Local radiation therapy.** This is an elderly patient with multiple comorbidities with blastic plasmacytoid dendritic cell neoplasm (BPDCN). He has an isolated skin lesion and no evidence (yet) of hematologic involvement. Prompt palliative benefit would be expected with radiation therapy to the isolated skin lesion, with the understanding that disease will likely progress in the near future. Given sensitivity to radiation therapy, surgical excision would not be recommended. Given age and comorbidities, chemotherapy with CHOP and systemic steroids would likely have increased morbidity risk.

2. **B. Low NK cell activity.** HLH is associated with low-to-absent NK cell activity, which is one of the eight diagnostic criteria for the disease. Elevated soluble IL-2R level is another diagnostic criterion. Elevated ANA may suggest a secondary etiology of the HLH but is not a diagnostic criterion.

3. **C. *FGFR1* rearrangement per karyotype.** The above gene rearrangements are associated with myeloid/lymphoid neoplasms with eosinophilia, which is in the differential for any patient with primary hypereosinophilia. *PDGFRA* and *PDGFRB* rearrangements are sensitive to imatinib, with *CHIC2* deletion by FISH a surrogate marker for *PDGFRA* rearrangement. Disease with *JAK2* rearrangement is sensitive to ruxolitinib, although duration of response is limited. Disease with *FGFR1* rearrangement is not sensitive to imatinib. Clinical trial development of *FGFR1* inhibitors is ongoing.

4. **B. Stop cyclosporine.** The MRI findings are consistent with a diagnosis of PRES (Posterior Reversible Encephalopathy Syndrome), with negative CSF arguing against HLH involvement of the central nervous system (CNS) and precluding need for IT methotrexate course. PRES has been associated with HLH treatment and remains unclear whether it is related to the disease itself or to the treatment modalities used. There is a suggestion that cyclosporine may increase risk of developing PRES and is therefore recommended to be held. Current treatment of HLH is tending to not include frontline use of cyclosporine. Transplant is not indicated at this time without further information regarding the patient's disease (e.g., primary versus secondary), but she would not appear to have CNS involvement of HLH as an indication for proceeding to transplant.

5. **A. Binding to CD123 on pDC cell surface.** All of the above choices are markers found on plasma cells (pDC) and in BPDCN. CD123 is IL-3A receptor, and is the target of the drug SL-401, which is diphtheria toxin conjugated to recombinant IL-3A.

6. **D. Local XRT to the femoral lesion.** All of the above choices are therapies used in management of Langerhans cell histiocytosis (LCH), including bone involvement. Given the unifocal nature of the patient's disease, however, systemic treatment could most likely be avoided with use of localized XRT alone.

7. **A. LCH risk organs are: bone marrow, liver, spleen, and possibly lung.**
The R histiocyte group includes familial and sporadic Rosai-Dorfman
Diseases, while the M group contains primary malignant histiocytoses and
secondary malignant histiocytoses associated with another hematologic
neoplasm. The most common endocrinopathy associated with LCH is
central diabetes insipidus. In LCH, biopsy of a lesion demonstrates cells
positive for CD1a, positive for S100, and positive for CD207.

8. **B. Clonal eosinophilia can be caused by *PCM1-JAK2* rearrangement.**
Patients with *FGFR1* rearrangement and eosinophilia have a lower likelihood of response to imatinib than patients with *PDGFRA* or *PDGFRB*
rearrangements. Patients with *FIP1L1-PDGFRA* rearrangements have
deletion of the *CHIC2* gene. Patients with *ETV6-PDGFRB* rearrangements
and eosinophilia are treated with imatinib.

9. **A. Allogeneic stem cell transplant is indicated in the following situations: relapsed/refractory disease following or during frontline treatment, CNS involvement, underlying hematologic malignancy, primary
HLH due to a germline mutation.** HLH can be due to germline mutations. Decreased NK cell activity is one of the criteria for diagnosing HLH.
Hypertriglyceridemia is one of the criteria for diagnosing HLH.

Hematologic Emergencies and Supportive Care

Angel Qin and Brian Parkin

Hematologic Emergencies

TUMOR LYSIS SYNDROME

1. **What is tumor lysis syndrome?**
   - Metabolic derangements due to tumor breakdown and release of intracellular potassium, phosphate, and nucleic acids into the systemic circulation

2. **What are the risk factors for tumor lysis syndrome?**
   - Highly proliferative malignancies (e.g., acute lymphoblastic leukemia, Burkitt's lymphoma/leukemia)
   - Elevated LDH
   - High tumor burden (e.g., hyperleukocytosis)
   - High sensitivity to cytotoxic chemotherapy
   - Preexisting hyperuricemia, renal insufficiency, and hypovolemia

3. **What are the laboratory features associated with tumor lysis syndrome?**
   - HIGH: potassium, phosphate, and uric acid
   - LOW: calcium

4. **In addition to electrolyte abnormalities, what are the signs, symptoms, and manifestations of tumor lysis syndrome?**
   - Nausea, vomiting, diarrhea, lethargy
   - Muscle cramps, paresthesias, tetany
   - Acute renal failure (defined as serum creatinine >1.5x the institutional upper limit of normal)
   - Confusion, hallucinations, seizures, syncope
   - Cardiac arrhythmias, heart failure
   - Sudden death

5. **What is the treatment for tumor lysis syndrome?**
   - Aggressive IV fluid hydration (with diuresis as needed to maintain adequate output)
   - Urinary alkalinization with sodium bicarbonate is controversial
   - Electrolyte repletion/removal; renal replacement therapy PRN
   - Hypouricemic agents

○ Allopurinol
  ■ Xanthine analog, which competitively inhibits xanthine oxidase
  ■ Decreases formation of new uric acid, does not reduce preexisting level
  ■ Needs to be renally dosed
  ■ Reduces degradation of other purines (6-mercaptopurine and azathioprine)
  ■ Adjust doses of medications also metabolized by the P450 system
○ Rasburicase
  ■ Recombinant urate oxidase, which catalyzes uric acid to allantoin
  ■ Decreases serum concentration of uric acid
  ■ Cannot be used in pregnant women or in G6PD deficiency (causes severe hemolysis and methemoglobinemia)
○ Febuxostat
  ■ Can use in the instance of allopurinol allergy

HYPERLEUKOCYTOSIS AND LEUKOSTASIS

1. **What is hyperleukocytosis?**
   - White blood cell (WBC) counts $>100 \times 10^9$/L
   - Seen in 5% to 20% of patients with acute leukemia
   - Risk factors: young age, monocytoic differentiation subtypes, certain cytogenetic abnormalities

2. **What is leukostasis?**
   - Increased viscosity due to elevated number of WBCs, which are less deformable compared to red blood cells (RBCs), and which induce endothelial expression of adhesion molecules
   - Aggregation of blasts leads to vascular occlusion

3. **What are the signs and symptoms of leukostasis?**
   - Pulmonary: dyspnea, hypoxia, ± diffuse alveolar infiltrates
   - Neurologic: headache, visual changes, confusion, somnolence, and coma
   - Less common: ECG signs of myocardial ischemia or right ventricular overload, renal insufficiency, priapism, acute limb ischemia, and bowel infarction
   - Can manifest in AML (acute myeloid leukemia) with WBC count as low as 50×10^9/L
   - Usually do not manifest in ALL (acute lymphocytic leukemia), CML (chronic myeloid leukemia), and CLL (chronic lymphocytic leukemia) until WBC $> 300 \times 10^9$/L

4. **What is the treatment for leukostasis?**
   - Aggressive hydration with IVF (intravenous fluids)
   - Leukapheresis
   - Contraindicated in acute promyelocytic leukemia (APL) due to increased risk of hemorrhage
   - Additional cytoreductive measures:

- ○ Induction chemotherapy (preferred)
- ○ Hydroxyurea (cannot be given to women who are pregnant or breastfeeding)
- Avoid blood transfusions if possible due to increased whole blood viscosity
- Monitor for/manage tumor lysis and disseminated intravascular coagulation (DIC)

URGENT/EMERGENT MANAGEMENT OF ACUTE LEUKEMIA

1. **What are the clinical signs/symptoms of newly diagnosed acute leukemia?**
   - Bone marrow failure—anemia (fatigue, shortness of breath), bleeding (petechiae, bruising), infections due to neutropenia (fever)
   - Tissue infiltration by leukemic blasts— gums, skin, meninges (most commonly associated with monocytic phenotype)
   - DIC (seen most frequently in patients with APL)
   - Leukostasis (as previously discussed)

2. **What tests do you immediately obtain in a patient whom you suspect has a new diagnosis of acute leukemia?**
   - CBC with evaluation of a peripheral smear
   - Comprehensive metabolic panel including uric acid, phosphorous, and LDH
   - Coagulation studies (in the right context)—PT/INR, PTT, fibrinogen
   - Flow cytometry

3. **What are the immediate interventions you need to start in a patient with new diagnosis of AML?**
   - IVF
   - Allopurinol
     - ○ Consider rasburicase if significantly elevated serum uric acid levels (according to institutional guidelines)
   - Hydroxyurea if leukoreduction is needed
   - Leukapheresis if there is concern for leukostasis
   - ATRA (All-trans Retinoic Acid) if concern for APL
     - ○ Presence of large bundles of Auer rods, "sliding plates" appearance of bilobed nuclei
     - ○ Hypogranular variant exists that is without significant Auer rods
   - Supportive care if there is evidence of DIC
     - ○ For example, transfusion of cryoprecipitate for hypofibrinogenemia and/or fresh frozen plasma for elevated PTT or INR

FEBRILE NEUTROPENIA

1. **What is febrile neutropenia?**
   - Fever: Per IDSA (Infectious Diseases Society of America) guidelines, single temperature higher than 38.3°C (101.3°F) or sustained temperature higher than 38°C (100.4°F) for more than 1 hour

- Neutropenia: ANC (absolute neutrophil count) <500 or ANC <1,000 with predicted decline to <500 in 48 hours

2. **What are the signs and symptoms of febrile neutropenia?**
   - Signs and symptoms may be minimal or absent

3. **What should the evaluation of febrile neutropenia include?**
   - Thorough physical exam with particular attention to skin, sinuses, mouth/oropharynx, lungs, abdomen, perirectal area (avoid digital rectal exam), and indwelling catheters
   - Laboratory studies including CBC with differential, comprehensive metabolic panel, blood cultures ×2 sets (peripheral and from indwelling catheter or port if applicable), urinalysis and culture, site-specific cultures if applicable (stool, skin lesions, etc.)
   - Ideally, cultures should be obtained prior to initiating antibiotics
   - Radiologic studies, including routine chest x-ray; additional imaging for localizing symptoms as warranted

4. **What are the associated pathogens found in febrile neutropenia?**
   - Infectious source identified in approximately 30% of patients
   - Bacterial pathogens MOST common
     - Gram-negative bacilli (particularly *Pseudomonas aeruginosa*)
     - Initial increasing trend toward gram-positive organisms (*Staphylococcus* and *Streptococcus*) since 1980s has started to swing towards gram-negative organisms given the rise of multidrug resistance
   - Fungal and viral pathogens are also common; invasive fungal infections are especially prevalent in high risk neutropenia
   - Empiric treatment must provide broad coverage against gram-negatives including *Pseudomonas*; gram-positive and anaerobic coverage dependent on risk factors and presenting signs/symptoms

5. **What is the treatment for febrile neutropenia?**
   - For select patients with anticipated brief neutropenia (<7 days), few to no comorbidities or symptoms, outpatient therapy (ciprofloxacin and augmentin) with close monitoring may be acceptable. This is not commonly done.
   - High-risk patients require inpatient hospitalization with IV antibiotics
   - For uncomplicated infections, monotherapy with broad-spectrum beta-lactams with good pseudomonal coverage is as effective as combined therapy
     - Cefepime, piperacillin-tazobactam, imipenem, meropenem, and ceftazidime based on institutional susceptibilities
   - Combination therapy should be used in setting of severe sepsis/septic shock or high prevalence of MDR (multi-drug resistant) gram-negative rods
     - Typically use a beta-lactam plus an aminoglycoside or fluoroquinolone
   - Role of vancomycin:
     - Should NOT be used initially unless one or more of the following applies:
       - Clinically suspected catheter-related infection
       - Gram-positive bacteria identified on blood culture, susceptibilities pending

- Known colonization with MRSA (methillicin-resistant staph aureus)
- Severe mucositis or soft-tissue infection
- Severe sepsis or septic shock
- Role of antifungal therapy:

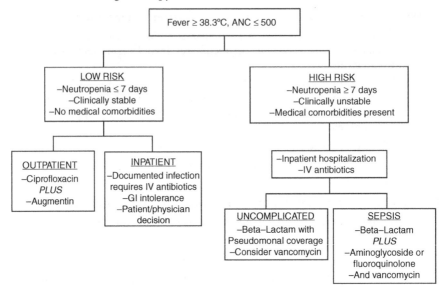

- Should be initiated for persistent fever after 4 to 7 days of broad-spectrum therapy
- Duration of antibiotics:
  - Documented infection: Treat for standard duration indicated for specific infection and/or until neutropenia resolves, whichever is longer
  - Undocumented infection: Treat until fever disappears and ANC of greater than 500 for at least 24 hours

CHEMOTHERAPY EXTRAVASATION

1. What is extravasation of chemotherapy?
- Unintended leakage of chemotherapy drug into extravascular space
- Vesicants cause tissue necrosis; irritants cause inflammation only

2. What are the common vesicant and irritant chemotherapeutic drugs?

VESICANT	COMMONLY USED TREATMENTS
Anthracyclines	• Dexrazoxane
• Daunorubicin, doxorubicin, epirubicin, idarubicin, mitomycin C	• Topical DMSO • Topical cooling
Vinca alkaloids	• Subcutaneous hyaluronidase
• Vincristine, vinblastine, vinorelbine	• Topical warming

IRRITANT	COMMONLY USED TREATMENTS
Taxanes* • Docetaxel, paclitaxel	• Topical cooling • Subcutaneous hyaluronidase
Platinums* • Carboplatin, cisplatin	
Epipodophyllotoxins • Etoposide, teniposide	• Topical warming
Topoisomerase I inhibitors • Irinotecan, topotecan	• Topical cooling

*May have vesicant properties at high volume/concentration, but generally act as irritants.

Supportive Care

ANTIMICROBIAL PROPHYLAXIS

1. **What antimicrobial precautions should be instituted in patients with neutropenia?**
   - Limit exogenous pathogen exposure
     - High-efficiency particulate air (HEPA)-filtered room
     - No sick visitors
     - If eating raw fruits or vegetables, they must be fresh and well-cleaned
     - No smoking
     - Handwashing

2. **What antimicrobial prophylaxis is recommended?**
   - Acyclovir antiviral prophylaxis is recommended for patients who are seropositive for HSV (herpes simplex virus).
   - Antibiotic prophylaxis with a fluoroquinolone is recommended if absolute neutrophil count is $<0.5 \times 10^9$/L >7 days.
   - Antifungal prophylaxis with either posaconazole or voriconazole is recommended against invasive mold infections and *Candida* spp; fluconazole would only target *Candida* and would not be adequate in these patients given their prolonged neutropenia.
   - Prophylaxis for *Pneumocystis* pneumonia (PCP) is recommended for patients receiving induction chemotherapy for ALL, patients receiving a purine analog such as fludarabine, or who will be on the dose equivalent of ≥20 mg of prednisone/day for ≥1 month.

CHEMOTHERAPY-INDUCED NAUSEA AND VOMITING

1. **What are the types of chemotherapy-induced nausea and vomiting (CINV)?**
   - **Acute:** Up to 24 hours after chemotherapy, mediated by 5-HT3 release from enterochromaffin cells

- **Delayed:** More than 24 hours after chemotherapy, mediated by NK_1 receptors
- **Anticipatory:** Occurs on the day of or some hours before the anticipated chemotherapy; typically triggered by taste, odor, sight, distressing thoughts, or anxiety

2. What is the emetogenicity of various chemotherapeutic agents?

	Risk of Emesis (w/o Antiemetics)			
	High > 90%	Moderate 31%–90%	Low 10%–30%	Minimal < 10%
IV agents	Carmustine	Alemtuzumab	Bortezomib	Cladribine
	Cisplatin	Azacytidine	Carfilzomib	Bevacizumab
	Cyclophosphamide ≥1,500 mg/m²	Bendamustine	Cytarabine ≤1,000 mg/m²	Bleomycin
		Cabazitaxel		Busulfan
	Dacarbazine	Carboplatin	Docetaxel	Cetuximab
	Dactinomycin	Clofarabine	Eribulin	Fludarabine
	Mechlorethamine	Cyclophosphamide ≤1,500 mg/m²	Etoposide	Rituximab
	Streptozotocin		5-Fluorouracil	Vinblastine
		Cytarabine >1,000 mg/m²	Gemcitabine	Vincristine
			Ixabepilone	Vinorelbine
		Daunorubicin*	Methotrexate (>1,000 mg/m²)	
		Denileukin diftitox		
		Doxorubicin*	Mitomycin	
		Epirubicin*	Mitoxantrone	
		Idarubicin*	Paclitaxel	
		Ifosfamide	Panitumumab	
		Irinotecan	PEG-liposomal doxorubicin	
		Melphalan		
		Oxaliplatin	Pemetrexed	
		Pralatrexate	Romidepsin	
		Temozolomide	Temsirolimus	
			Topotecan	
			Trastuzumab	
			Vorinostat	

(continued)

		Risk of Emesis (w/o Antiemetics)		
	High >90%	**Moderate 31%–90%**	**Low 10%–30%**	**Minimal <10%**
PO agents	Hexamethyl-melamine	Altretamine	Axitinib	6-Thioguanine
	Procarbazine	Busulfan	Bexarotene	Chlorambucil
		Crizotinib	Capecitabine	Erlotinib
		Cyclophosphamide	Cetuximab	Gefitinib
		Imatinib	Dasatinib	Hydroxyurea
		Lomustine	Estramustine	Melphalan
		Temozolomide	Etoposide	Methotrexate
		Tretinoin	Everolimus	Regorafenib
		Vandetanib	Fludarabine	Sorafenib
		Vinorelbine	Lapatinib	
			Lenalidomide	
			Nilotinib	
			Panitumumab	
			Pazopanib	
			Sunitinib	
			Tegafur uracil	
			Thalidomide	
			Topotecan	
			Vemurafenib	
			Vorinostat	

*When combined with cyclophosphamide, these anthracyclines have high emetic risk.

3. What antiemetic agents are available?

- Serotonin (5-HT$_3$) receptor antagonists
  - First generation: Dolasetron, granisetron (transdermal patch option), ondansetron (oral dissolving tablet option), tropisetron
  - Second generation: Palonosetron (higher affinity for receptor and longer half-life)
  - Oral and IV forms are similarly effective

- ○ Side effects: Headache, diarrhea, transient transaminitis, and ECG changes; prolonged QT interval seen primarily with dolasetron. Constipation with the 5-HT_3 receptor antagonists can be severe.
- NK_1 receptor antagonists
  - ○ Aprepitant and its prodrug fosaprepitant
  - ○ Potential drug interactions: moderate inhibitor of CYP3A4
- Steroids
  - ○ Oral and parenteral dexamethasone and methylprednisolone are equally effective
  - ○ Side effects: insomnia, mood changes, irritability, and hyperglycemia
- Dopamine (D_2) receptor antagonists
  - ○ Prochlorperazine, promethazine, haloperidol, and metoclopramide
  - ○ Side effects: sedation, extrapyramidal reactions, anticholinergic effects, ECG changes (haloperidol, droperidol), hypotension with rapid IV administration (phenothiazines)
- Benzodiazepines
  - ○ Lorazepam and alprazolam
  - ○ Side effects: dose-related sedation and delirium (especially in elderly patients). Benzodiazepines can potentiate the sedating effects of opioids and should be used with caution in patients receiving concomitant opioids.
- Cannabinoids
  - ○ Dronabinol and nabilone
  - ○ Side effects: sedation, confusion, dizziness, short-term memory loss, euphoria/dysphoria, ataxia, dry mouth, and orthostatic hypotension
- Antihistamines
  - ○ Diphenhydramine and hydroxyzine
  - ○ Are not useful for CINV, but helpful for motion sickness
  - ○ Side effects: sedation, dry mouth, visual changes, mydriasis, decreased GI motility, urinary changes, and increased heart rate
- Neuroleptics
  - ○ Olanzapine
  - ○ Useful for both acute and delayed CINV refractory to other treatments

4. How do you prevent nausea and vomiting?

Prophylaxis Recommended

Risk	High		Moderate		Low		Minimal	
Type	Acute	Delayed	Acute	Delayed	Acute	Delayed	Acute	Delayed
	5-HT3RA + dex + aprepitant ± lorazepam	Dex + aprepitant ± lorazepam	Anthracycline/cyclophospha mide: 5-HT3RA + dex + aprepitant ± lorazepam Others: 5-HT3RA ± dex ± lorazepam	Aprepitant ± dex ± lorazepam	Dex ± lorazepam prochlorperazine ± lorazepam Metoclopramide ± lorazepam	None	None	None

5-HT3RA, serotonin receptor antagonist; dex, dexamethasone.

5. **How do you treat breakthrough and refractory CINV?**
   - Avoid repeated dosing of agents that were given for prophylaxis and already failed.
   - Consider adding prochlorperazine, metoclopramide, a benzodiazepine, or a neuroleptic (i.e., olanzapine).

6. **What are nonpharmacologic measures for antiemetic prophylaxis?**
   - Ginger capsules or chews (prior to and during treatment cycle)
   - Cognitive distraction (i.e., playing video games during treatment)
   - Systematic desensitization (visualization and learned relaxation techniques)
   - Hypnosis
   - Acupuncture
   - Transcutaneous electrical nerve stimulation
   - Mindfulness through guided meditation

CANCER-ASSOCIATED VENOUS THROMBOEMBOLIC DISEASE

1. **What are the risk factors for VTE (venous thromboembolism)?**
   - General patient-associated risk factors
     - Active cancer
     - Advanced stage of cancer
     - Higher risk cancer types: brain, pancreas, stomach, bladder, gynecologic, lung, lymphoma, myeloproliferative neoplasms, kidney, metastatic cancers
     - Bulky regional lymphadenopathy with extrinsic vascular compression
     - Inherited and/or acquired hypercoagulable states
     - Medical comorbidities: infection, renal failure, pulmonary disease, heart failure
     - Poor performance status
     - Older age
   - Treatment-associated risk factors
     - Major surgery
     - Central venous catheter
     - Certain chemotherapies, that is, thalidomide/lenalidomide/pomalidomide and high dose dexamethasone
     - Exogenous hormonal therapy, that is, oral contraceptives and tamoxifen/raloxifene
   - Modifiable risk factors
     - Tobacco smoking
     - Obesity
     - Decreased activity/exercise

Khorana Predictive Model for Chemotherapy-Associated VTE

Patient Characteristic	Risk Score
• Site of primary cancer	2
○ Very high risk (stomach, pancreas)	1
○ High risk (lung, lymphoma, gynecologic, bladder, testicular)	1
• Prechemotherapy platelet count ≥350	1
• Hemoglobin <10 or use of ESAs	1
• Prechemotherapy leukocyte count >11	1
• BMI >35	

Total Score	Risk Category	Risk of Symptomatic VTE
0	Low	0.8%–3%
1,2	Intermediate	1.8%–8.4%
3 or higher	High	7.1%–41%

2. **When is inpatient pharmacologic VTE prophylaxis contraindicated?**
   - Absolute contraindications
     - ○ Recent CNS bleed
     - ○ Intracranial or spinal lesion at high risk for bleeding
     - ○ Major active bleeding, that is, >2U PRBC transfused in the past 24 hours
   - Relative contraindications
     - ○ Thrombocytopenia (<50K)
     - ○ Severe platelet dysfunction
     - ○ Recent major surgery at high risk for bleeding
     - ○ Coagulopathy

PAIN MANAGEMENT

1. **What are the critical features of a comprehensive pain assessment?**
   - Interview the patient to characterize the position, quality, severity, and timing of the pain. Rule out radiation or referred pain. Identify factors that provoke or palliate pain. Patients can have multiple sources of pain; each should be characterized separately.
   - Identify psychosocial factors that may interfere with treatment of pain:
     - ○ Concurrent mood disorders
     - ○ Fear of addiction or death
     - ○ Social, financial, and spiritual stressors
     - ○ Prior history of substance abuse, tobacco, or chronic opioid use
   - Inspect and palpate the site of pain, looking for associated physical signs. Rule out neurologic deficits.

- Reassess the patient when there is any change in quality or severity of pain or the consumption of pain killers.
- Severe, uncontrollable pain is a medical emergency that may require intravenous therapy and/or hospitalization.

2. **What is an appropriate approach to cancer pain management?**
   - Determine the likely mechanism of the pain. Many patients with cancer have pain that is not cancer-related and should NOT be treated with opioids.
   - Determine if the patient is a good candidate for opioids. Patients should be able to take the medication responsibly. Patients with prior history of poly-substance abuse should be provided opioids in smaller quantities (1–2 weeks at a time) and given additional supervision by staff.

		Immediate Prognosis	
		Good	**Poor**
Severity of Cancer Pain	**Mild**	NSAID and/or Acetaminophen prn	Dose find with strong, short-acting opioid prn; rotate to Strong, short acting prn + long-acting opioid over time
	Moderate–Severe	Strong, short-acting opioid prn only	

3. **What are opioid equivalences as compared with single dose morphine?**

Drug	Parenteral Dose (mg)	Oral Dose (mg)	Factor (IV ≥ PO)	Peak	Duration of Action (hours)	Starting IV Dose	Starting PO Dose
Morphine	10	30	3	PO: 1.5–2 hr IV: 20 min	3–4	2–4 mg q2–4 hr	15 mg immediate release q4 hr
Hydromorphone	1.5	7.5	5	PO and IV: 1 hr	2–3	0.2–2 mg q2 hr	2–4 mg q4–6 hr
Fentanyl	100 mcg	–	–	IV: 1–5 min Transdermal: 24 hr	1–3	0.25–1 mcg/kg prn	Transdermal: 12–25 mcg/hr q72 hr
Levorphanol	2	4	2	PO: 1 hr IV: 20 min	3–6	1 mg q3–6 hr	2 mg q6–8 hr
Oxycodone	–	15–20	–	1–2 hr	3–5	–	5–10 mg q4–6 hr
Hydrocodone	–	30–45	–	2 hr	3–5	–	5–10 mg q4–6 hr
Oxymorphone	1	10	10	PO: 1 hr	3–6	0.5 mg q4 hr	5–10 mg immediate release q4 hr
Codeine	–	200	–	1.5 hr	3–4	–	30–60 mg q4 hr
Tramadol	–	50–100	–		3–7	–	50–100 mg q4–6 hr

Methadone's conversion ratio to oral morphine equivalents is dose-dependent.

4. What opioid do you choose?

- Short-acting opioids are indicated for intermittent or breakthrough pain.
- Long-acting opioids are indicated when patients are taking short-acting opioids round-the-clock.
- Compounded opioids should be avoided in patients whose pain condition is likely to worsen over time as there is a ceiling level, preventing upward titration.
- Choice of opioid depends upon the severity of the pain as well as the patient's past trials of opioids.
- First line:
  - Mild pain: hydrocodone
  - Moderate to severe pain: oxycodone or morphine
- Some situations merit specific opioids:
  - Poor compliance or mild cognitive impairment: transdermal fentanyl
  - Intractable constipation: transdermal fentanyl
  - Neurotoxicity: hydromorphone, oxycodone, or methadone
  - Renal impairment: buprenorphine, fentanyl, and methadone (if patient is not on dialysis)
  - Liver impairment: oxycodone
  - Opioid tolerance: hydromorphone
  - Complex pain (with heavy neuropathic component): methadone

5. How do you initiate short-acting opioids?

- For patients who are opioid-naïve, begin opioids at the lowest recommended dose (see table in question 3); consider even lower doses for older patients or patients with renal or liver disease.
  - Effectiveness of a given dose can be gauged within 1 hour of taking an oral opioid and 15 minutes of taking an IV opioid
- For ambulatory patients with pain but not in crisis, start opioids as above have them keep a diary, and follow-up within a week. When pain control is not achieved, increase dose in increments by 30% to 50%.
- For ambulatory patients in a pain crisis, start opioids as recommended above, have them keep a diary, and reassess within 24 hours. When pain is not controlled, increase dose by 100% and reassess again within 24 hours.
- Patients in crisis whose pain cannot be controlled at home with oral opioids should be admitted to the hospital for IV treatment. IV is preferred for patients who have malabsorption or intractable vomiting.

6. How do you initiate long-acting opioids?

- Patients should not be started on a long-acting opioid without "dose finding" with a short-acting opioid first to determine the TDD (total daily dose).
- Once the TDD is known, divide the TDD by the number of times the patient will be taking the long-acting opioid per day. For example, for BID long-acting morphine, 50% of the TDD should be given in the morning and 50% of the TDD should be given in the evening.

- Try to use the short- and long-acting forms of the same opioid. Rarely is a combination of different opioids helpful.
- When converting a patient from one opioid to another (e.g., morphine to oxycodone), calculate the TDD of the initial opioid and convert to the equivalent TDD of the replacement opioid using the equianalgesic doses (see table in question 3). Account for incomplete cross-tolerance by decreasing the TDD of the new opioid by 25% to 50%. Then convert into long- and short-acting forms.

7. **What is appropriate dosing for breakthrough pain medication?**
   - Once patients are on a long acting opioid, the short acting breakthrough opioid should be dosed at 10% to 20% of the TDD.
     ○ For example, if a patient is taking 40 mg long-acting oxycodone twice daily, then an appropriate dose of breakthrough medication would be 5–10 mg oxycodone every 4 hours as needed.
   - Oral opioids may be safely dosed as often as every 1 to 2 hours during a pain crisis.
     ○ Short-acting opioids given orally reach peak effect at 1 hour and last no more than 4 hours.

8. **What are common side effects of opioids?**
   - All patients on opioids get constipation.
   - Other common side effects include delirium, myoclonus, urinary retention, sedation, nausea and vomiting, pruritus, and respiratory depression. Tolerance develops over time for all these effects **except delirium, myoclonus, and urinary retention**; these side effects and hypersensitivity reactions require switching to a different opioid.
   - Prevent constipation in patients on opioids by administering a motility agent (bisacodyl or senna) daily.
     ○ Titrate the dose every 2 to 3 days for a bowel movement at least once every 48 hours.
     ○ Avoid constipating agents (e.g., fiber, anticholinergics, haldol, calcium channel blockers, iron, anticonvulsants, ondansetron).

9. **What are risks of long-term opioid use?**
   - Addiction: malingering for opioids is rare in patients with active cancer but can be seen among patients whose cancers are in remission, especially those with a preceding history of polysubstance abuse. Every effort should be made to titrate patients entirely off opioids once their cancer is in remission.
   - Dependence: manifests as withdrawal symptoms (nausea, chills, sweats) at cessation or dose reduction
   - Tolerance: all patients taking opioids regularly develop tolerance; providers should expect that TDD will go up over time, even when disease is stable.
   - Hyperalgesia: increased pain sensitivity that develops with regular, long-term opioid use; precise mechanism is poorly understood; escalating the opioid dose may paradoxically increase the level of pain.

10. **How does one terminate opioid therapy?**
    - Decrease TDD by 10% to 20% daily or more slowly if withdrawal develops.
    - Treat withdrawal: loperamide (for diarrhea), prochlorperazine (for nausea/vomiting), clonidine (for sweats)

11. **What are examples of adjuvant analgesics?**
    - Anticonvulsant medications
      - Gabapentin, pregabalin, lamotrigine, topiramate, carbamazepine, valproic acid, and phenytoin
    - Antidepressants
      - SNRIs, SSRIs, and TCAs
      - Useful as singular agents in patients without cancer
      - For patients with cancer, they should be added once opioids have been initiated. Patients should be monitored for anticholinergic side effects. Avoid TCA use in elderly.
    - Bisphosphonates
      - Pamidronate, ibandronate, and zoledronate
      - Effective for treating bone pain related to metastases (i.e., in multiple myeloma)
      - Also used to decrease the incidence of myeloma-related skeletal events in patients with existing skeletal lesions and those who are at increased risk for skeletal events (i.e., baseline osteopenia/osteoporosis)
      - Local anesthetics (i.e., lidocaine patch)
      - Effective for treating localized, superficial neuropathic and somatic pain syndromes
    - Corticosteroids
      - Effective for pain and weakness associated with nerve impingement or boney metastases
    - Antispasmodics (i.e., dicyclomine)
      - Effective for visceral pain
    - Interventional pain clinic
      - Referral for nerve/plexus blocks, infusion pumps, stimulation units, kyphoplasty/vertebroplasty

12. **What are examples of nonpharmacologic pain therapy?**
    - Acupuncture
    - Relaxation/biofeedback
    - Recreation/art/music therapy
    - Transcutaneous electrical nerve stimulation
    - Myofascial trigger release
    - Massage, healing touch
    - Behavioral counseling

CANCER CACHEXIA

1. What is cancer cachexia?

- Characterized by loss of appetite, chronic nausea, fatigue, and weight loss (≥6% decrease over 6 months). Thought to be secondary to:
  - Proinflammatory cytokines (TNF, IL-1, IL-6, IFN), which lead to hypermetabolism and anorexia (from changes in ghrelin, leptin, and serotonin production)
  - Tumor production of proteolysis-inducing factor and lipid-mobilizing factor causes fat and muscle loss
  - Inefficient energy metabolism and insulin resistance leads to further lean body mass depletion
- Cancer cachexia is an independent predictor of early mortality.
- Overfeeding may lead to further metabolic derangement without resultant weight gain.

2. What are appropriate interventions for anorexia/cachexia?

- Treat reversible causes: e.g., nausea and vomiting, xerostomia, mucositis, dental issues, dysgeusia, dysphagia, early satiety, bowel obstruction, constipation, pain, and depression.
  - Rule out endocrine abnormalities.
- Review and eliminate medications that interfere with appetite.
- Rule out social and economic factors.
- Nutrition consultation to help identify barriers to increased intake or recommend dietary modifications.
- Caloric supplementation:
  - Increased intake does not result in improved survival or tumor response
  - Enteral feeding is preferred (less infection risk, decreased catabolic hormones, improved wound healing, shorter hospital stays, and maintenance of gut integrity).
  - Parenteral nutrition (rarely indicated unless patient is NPO)
- Pharmacological interventions:
  - Metoclopramide helps treat nausea as well as delayed gastric emptying in patients who complain of early satiety. Watch for EPS.
  - Glucocorticoids help to increase appetite, but should be used for short periods of time due to the long-term effects.
  - Megestrol works like steroids and is rarely effective if the patient has not responded to steroids in the past. Do not give megestrol concurrently with steroids. Note: Megestrol can increase risk for thromboembolic events.
  - Mirtazapine
  - Dronabinol is not effective for increasing appetite in cancer patients.

DYSPNEA

1. What is an appropriate approach to the management of dyspnea?

- Assess and identify the causes of the dyspnea

- Treat reversible causes:
  - Infection: antibiotics as indicated
  - Anemia: transfuse as needed
  - Bronchospasm
  - Pneumothorax
  - Pulmonary embolus: anticoagulation if possible
  - Airway mechanical obstruction (e.g., mass)
  - Effusions (pleural and pericardial): thoracentesis and pleurodesis
  - Airway obstruction: bronchoscopic interventions and/or radiation
    - Comorbid COPD: inhaled corticosteroids and bronchodilators
- Relieve symptoms
  - Nonpharmacologic
    - Fans (for patients without COPD [chronic obstructive pulmonary disease] or CAD [coronary artery disease]), cooler temperatures, stress management, and relaxation therapy
    - Supplemental oxygen for hypoxia (SaO_2 < 90%) or subjective relief
    - Emotional, psychosocial, and educational support
  - Pharmacologic
    - Low-dose opioids (i.e., 2.5–5 mg morphine q2–4 hr) to reduce air hunger
    - Anxiolytics to reduce the anxiety that coexists with dyspnea (use with caution in patients who are taking concomitant opioids)
    - Expectorants (i.e., guaifenesin) to thin secretions
    - Antitussives (i.e., dextromethorphan, codeine, and hydrocodone) to reduce frequency of cough
    - Anticholinergics (i.e., atropine and hyoscine) to control secretions
  - Noninvasive positive pressure ventilation (CPAP and BiPAP)

PSYCHIATRIC SYNDROMES

1. **What are common psychiatric syndromes seen in cancer patients?**
   - Adjustment disorder
   - Major depression
   - Anxiety
   - Delirium

2. **What is adjustment disorder?**
   - Time-limited, maladaptive reaction to a specific stressor (e.g., cancer diagnosis and treatment)
   - Onset within 3 months of stressor, duration <6 months
   - Lack neurovegetative signs and suicidal ideation
   - Treatment directed at crisis intervention, brief psychotherapy, and symptom management

3. **What are the diagnostic criteria for major depressive disorder (MDD)?**
   - Persistently low mood or anhedonia plus five of the following for at least 2 weeks:
     ○ Sleep disturbance
     ○ Loss of interest
     ○ Feelings of hopelessness, helplessness, or guilt
     ○ Low energy
     ○ Poor concentration
     ○ Appetite disturbance
     ○ Psychomotor retardation/agitation
     ○ Suicidal or homicidal ideation
   - Screen using the PHQ-2, and assess using the PHQ-9
   - Rule out pseudo-depression

4. **What are some causes of pseudo-depression?**
   - Uncontrolled pain
   - Hypothyroidism
   - Medications (steroids, certain chemotherapies such as interferon)
   - Metabolic abnormalities (electrolytes, B12, or folate deficiency)
   - Organic brain disease (metastatic brain involvement, endocrinopathies, etc.)
   - Dementia
   - Substance abuse
   - Adjustment disorder
   - Fatigue
   - Personality disorders

5. **What is the treatment of MDD?**
   - Psychotherapy
   - Pharmacotherapy
     ○ SSRIs and SNRIs are especially useful in patients who also have neuropathic pain. Can take 4 to 8 weeks to see full benefit
     ○ Methylphenidate has a shorter duration of action, but should be avoided in anyone who has insomnia, agitation, active CAD, or anxiety
     ○ TCAs should be avoided in patients over age 65
     ○ Mirtazapine is a good option for patients with cancer anorexia and/or insomnia
     ○ Antidepressants should be continued for 12 months from the point of remission if first episode of MDD

6. What are commonly used antidepressants?

Class	Name	Dose Range (mg)	Side Effects
SSRI	Fluoxetine	5–60	GI symptoms, weight changes, sleep disruption, sexual dysfunction, dry mouth, hyponatremia
	Paroxetine	10–60	
	Sertraline	12.5–200	
	Citalopram	10–60	
	Escitalopram	5–40	
Mixed agents	Venlafaxine	18.75–300	GI symptoms, sexual dysfunction, anticholinergic effects, hypertension w/doses > 225 mg, reduces hot flashes
	Bupropion	37.5–450	GI symptoms, tremor, lowers seizure threshold
	Duloxetine	20–60	GI symptoms, headache, dizziness; also indicated for neuropathic pain
	Mirtazapine	7.5–45	Sedation, dry mouth, increased appetite and weight gain
	Trazodone	25–200	Sedation, orthostatic hypotension, priapism
Tricyclic antidepressants	Amitriptyline	25–150	Dry mouth, sedation, weight gain, GI symptoms, ECG changes, orthostatic hypotension, anticholinergic effects
	Nortriptyline	25–150	
	Desipramine	25–150	
	Doxepin	10–150	
Psychostimulants	Methylphenidate	2.5–60*	Hypertension, tachycardia, anxiety
	Dextroamphetamine	10–60	

*For off-label use in depression, maximum dose is 20 mg and sustained release product is not recommended. For stimulant use, maximum daily dose is 60 mg.

7. What is the management of anxiety?

- Rule out reversible causes
  - Poorly controlled symptoms
  - Metabolic disturbances (e.g., hypercalcemia, hypoglycemia, and carcinoid syndrome)
  - Medications (e.g., thyroxine and phenothiazines)

- Nonpharmacologic treatment
  - ○ Behavioral therapy and psychotherapy
- Pharmacologic treatment
  - ○ Benzodiazepines (e.g., lorazepam, alprazolam, and clonazepam)
  - ○ Antidepressants (e.g., SSRIs and mixed agents)
  - ○ Neuroleptics (e.g., haldol and atypical antipsychotics) for severe and persistent anxiety
  - ○ Other drugs: buspirone, propranolol (for autonomic symptoms), sedative hypnotics (for insomnia)

8. What is delirium?

- Acute confusional state characterized by fluctuating course of cognitive impairment, perceptual disturbances, delusions, mood changes, and disruption of sleep–wake cycle
- May be hyperactive (agitated) or hypoactive (quiet)

9. What is the management of delirium?

- Identify and treat precipitating factors
  - ○ Direct CNS causes
    - ■ Brain tumor
    - ■ Brain metastases
    - ■ Seizures
  - ○ Indirect causes
    - ■ Metabolic encephalopathy
    - ■ Electrolyte imbalance
    - ■ Medications (steroids, narcotics, anticholinergics, antiemetics)
    - ■ Infection
    - ■ Hematologic abnormalities
    - ■ Nutritional deficiencies
    - ■ Paraneoplastic syndromes
- Pharmacologic treatment
  - ○ Neuroleptics (e.g., haloperidol)
    - ■ Side effects: sedation, EPS, hypotension, QT prolongation
  - ○ Atypical neuroleptics (e.g., olanzapine, quetiapine, and risperidone)
    - ■ Side effects: sedation, weight gain, metabolic syndrome, and QT prolongation
  - ○ Benzodiazepines (e.g., lorazepam, midazolam)
    - ■ Should not be prescribed in patients with delirium
  - ○ Palliative sedation (only for terminal delirium, with patient and/or surrogate consent)
    - ■ Propofol 10–70 mcg/hour
- Environmental modification

○ Keep the environment calm and quiet with adequate, but soft, indirect light and limit noise levels.

○ Provide glasses and hearing aides to maximize sensory perception.

○ Consider the use of night lights to combat nighttime confusion.

○ Use music which has an individual significance to the confused and agitated client to prevent the increase in or decrease agitated behaviors.

QUESTIONS

1. A 28-year-old otherwise healthy male presents with malaise and fevers and a routine complete blood count (CBC) reveals elevated white blood cells (WBCs) of 20 × 10⁹/L, a hemoglobin of 8.3g/dL, and a platelet count of 58 × 10⁹/L. A peripheral smear reveals shows large, immature appearing WBCs that are concerning for acute leukemia. Flow cytometry yields the diagnosis of acute lymphoblastic leukemia (ALL). After a thorough evaluation has been obtained, it is recommended that he begin induction chemotherapy with a pediatric-inspired protocol. What atypical infection does he require prophylaxis for?
   A. Human immunodeficiency virus (HIV)
   B. Hepatitis C
   C. Pneumocystis pneumonia
   D. Neisseria meningitis

2. You are on the inpatient hematology/oncology service and are taking care of a 66-year-old female with diffuse large B-cell lymphoma (DLBCL) status post her first cycle of R-CHOP chemotherapy. She presented 4 days ago with fevers (Tmax 101.2F) and was found to be neutropenic with absolute neutrophil count (ANC) of 0.4 × 10⁹/L. She complained of general malaise and myalgias but did not have any localizing symptoms. Chest x-ray and urinalysis at the time of admission were unremarkable. After blood cultures were obtained, she was started on empiric therapy with piperacillin-tazobactam. Vancomycin was then added given that she does have a port in place. It is now day 5 and she is still persistently febrile with Tmax of 100.9°F. Her vitals are otherwise stable and she continues to not have any localizing symptoms. Her cultures have thus far been negative. Her ANC is now 0.25 × 10⁹/L. What medication changes would you consider making next?
   A. Discontinue piperacillin-tazobactam and start meropenem
   B. Add amikacin
   C. Discontinue vancomycin and start daptomycin
   D. Add fluconazole

3. A 60-year-old male with history of stage III chronic kidney disease secondary to a history of poorly controlled type II diabetes as well as essential hypertension is started on "7+3" induction chemotherapy with daunorubicin and cytarabine for a newly diagnosed acute myeloid leukemia with t(8;21). His baseline labs include a white blood cell (WBC) count of 65 × 10⁹/L, hemoglobin of 8.9 g/dL, a platelet count of 45 × 10⁹/L, serum sodium 138 mmol/L, serum potassium 4.3 mmol/L, serum creatinine of 1.7 mg/dL, serum calcium 9.7 mg/dL, serum

phosphorous 5.0 mg/dL, and serum albumin 3.8 g/dL. He has already been started on IV fluids and allopurinol. 24 hours later, you note an improvement in his WBC to 25 × 10⁹/L, but his serum creatinine is now 3.5 mg/dL, serum potassium is 6.0 mmol/L, serum calcium is 7.4 mg/dL, and serum phosphorous is 6.2 mg/dL. He continues to have adequate urine output and his physical exam does not reveal signs of fluid overload. You check a serum uric acid, which was not checked at baseline, and it is 13 g/dL. What intervention should you consider?

A. Administer a 1-liter bolus of normal saline
B. Administer rasburicase
C. Consult nephrology for the initiation of dialysis
D. Add febuxostat

4. As the hematology consult fellow, you are asked to evaluate a 35-year-old female in the emergency department. She is otherwise healthy and has no medical problems. Her only medication is a daily multivitamin. She presented for evaluation in the emergency room as she noted the development of a petechial rash in her bilateral lower extremities. She has also noted that her current menstrual cycle is characterized by significantly heavier bleeding without any personal history of menorrhagia. Routine blood work in the emergency department revealed a white blood cell (WBC) count of 8.5 × 10⁹/L, a hemoglobin of 6.3 g/dL, and a platelet count of 38 × 10⁹/L. Coagulation tests reveal that she has an elevated PTT, PT, as well as a low fibrinogen at 82 mg/dL. A serum pregnancy test is negative. You reveal the peripheral blood smear and see the presence of large, immature appearing WBC with many dense blue cytoplasmic granules. The nuclei also appear to be bilobed. In addition to initiating supportive care, what other treatment would you recommend STAT?

A. Hydroxyurea
B. All-trans retinoic acid (ATRA)
C. Daunorubicin and cytarabine
D. Dexamethasone

5. A 63-year-old otherwise healthy female is referred to you for new diagnosis of standard-risk IgG Kappa multiple myeloma. This was recently diagnosed after she experienced pain in her right arm after a mechanical fall. X-ray obtained at the time had revealed the presence of a lytic lesion in her right humerus which prompted further evaluation. A skeletal survey done as part of her evaluation revealed additional lytic lesions in her calvarium, left humerus, and right iliac bone. She is currently without any pain and does not use any analgesics. You recommend initiation of treatment with lenalidomide, bortezomib, and dexamethasone. In addition to discussing venous thromboembolism (VTE) prophylaxis and shingles prophylaxis, what other supportive measures would you recommend at this time?

A. Radiation to bone lesions
B. Prophylactic intravenous immunoglobulin (IVIG) infusions given her increased risk for infection

C. Initiation of bisphosphonates

D. Instruct her to avoid exercise given that she has lytic lesions

6. You are seeing a 25-year-old female with Hgb SS disease. She is currently on oxycodone 5 mg as needed for pain control and is compliant with her hydroxyurea and folic acid supplementation. Her pain has been managed well as an outpatient and she is rarely admitted for pain crises. She reports that she is needing the oxycodone 6 times a day which controls her pain at a 3/10, which she states is tolerable. She is on an appropriate bowel regimen and is not having any constipation. She is concerned about the frequency at which she is needing to take the oxycodone, especially as she wakes up at night to take her medication and is inquiring regarding long acting pain medication. You recommend:

   A. MS Contin 30 mg every 12 hours with 5 mg oxycodone PRN for breakthrough

   B. Oxycontin 15 mg every 12 hours

   C. Oxycontin 15 mg every 12 hours with 5 mg oxycodone PRN for breakthrough

   D. Oxycontin 30 mg every 12 hours with 5 mg oxycodone PRN for breakthrough

7. You are called by the emergency department to evaluate a 57-year-old otherwise-healthy male who was brought in for evaluation of progressive confusion. According to his wife, her husband had complained of a worsening generalized headache since yesterday and found him acutely confused this morning. He has no history of alcohol or substance abuse and had otherwise not had any complaints prior to this. In the emergency department, a routine complete blood count (CBC) showed a white blood cell (WBC) count of 112×10^9, hemoglobin of 11 g/dL, and platelet count of 89×10^9. The preliminary differential on the CBC reports 63% blasts. A CT of the head without contrast does not reveal any acute intracranial process. When you evaluate the patient at the bedside, he is difficult to arouse, unable to follow commands, and unable to cooperate with a neuro exam. His vital signs are otherwise stable. You review his peripheral smear under the microscope and the blasts appear to be consistent with acute myeloid leukemia (AML) without features to suggest acute promyelocytic leukemia (APL). In addition to recommending aggressive IV hydration, what other intervention should you consider for this patient at this time?

   A. MRI of the brain with gadolinium

   B. Administering hydroxyurea

   C. Performing a lumbar puncture

   D. Initiation of leukapheresis

8. You are seeing your patient who was recently diagnosed with stage III diffuse large B-cell lymphoma (DLBCL) receiving chemotherapy with RCHOP. She is a 62-year-old female whose only other medical prob-

lem was a history of anxiety. She was very apprehensive to initiate chemotherapy given her concerns for side effects. You had received several calls given her concerns about nausea that were controlled with prochlorperazine and ondansetron. She is now in your office for evaluation prior to cycle 2 of chemotherapy. She states that she tolerated cycle 1 better than anticipated; no fevers, chills, and some mild fatigue that improved on its own. She did not have any emesis and nausea was well controlled with around the clock prochlorperazine and ondansetron. She states that she is continuing to take those medications given her fear of nausea. Her chief concern today is constipation, reporting not having had a bowel movement for 3 days. She states that this is very atypical for her. She does not take any opiate medications. In addition to her anti-emetics, her only other medications are prednisone (as part of RCHOP) and alprazolam. She has not noticed any significant change in her diet. Her vital signs are stable and her physical exam is otherwise benign. What is the most likely cause of her constipation?

A. Ondansetron
B. Large bowel obstruction
C. Side effect of chemotherapy
D. Alprazolam

ANSWERS

1. **C. Pneumocystis pneumonia.** The patient is receiving induction chemotherapy for ALL, which incorporates long term use of high-dose steroids, especially in the pediatric-inspired protocols. Therefore, prophylaxis for pneumocystis pneumonia is indicated.

2. **D. Add fluconazole.** The patient is persistently febrile despite being on appropriate broad spectrum antibiotics. It is appropriate to consider adding antifungal coverage in this patient given her increased risk for fungemia.

3. **B. Administer rasburicase.** The patient has evidence of tumor lysis syndrome with a rise in serum potassium and phosphorous as well as a decrease in serum calcium. He is also noted to have a very elevated serum uric acid. His rising creatinine suggests that he is developing renal impairment, likely secondary to tumor lysis syndrome, compounded by poor baseline renal function. At this time, administering additional intravenous fluid (IVF) or adding febuxostat is not likely to significantly improve his renal function. He does not have any obvious indication for dialysis, though a nephrology consultation should be considered if his renal function continues to deteriorate. Administering rasburicase should be considered in this patient to reduce serum uric acid, thereby limiting further damage to the renal tubules.

4. **B. All-trans retinoic acid (ATRA).** The patient presents with classic findings suspicious for acute promyelocytic leukemia (APL), including the finding of disseminated intravascular coagulation (DIC) on blood work as well as blasts with bilobed nuclei and cytoplasm filled with dense granules which are likely Auer rods. The initiation of timely therapy is crucial for the outcomes of these patients. In addition to treating the DIC, the patient should also be started on ATRA. She should have a thorough evaluation including diagnostic testing that will confirm the diagnosis of APL, but one should not wait for the results of these studies prior to initiation of ATRA.

5. **C. Initiation of bisphosphonates** following dental evaluation. Bisphosphonates are indicated to decrease the incidence of myeloma-related skeletal events, especially as this patient already has known lytic lesions. Radiation is currently not indicated as the patient is asymptomatic; should the patient develop significant pain associated with her bone lesions, radiation can certainly be considered. While patients with multiple myeloma are considered immune-compromised, there is no role for treatment with IVIG (which is sometimes considered in CLL). Finally, there is no evidence to suggest that exercise increases the risk for adverse skeletal events, especially as this patient will be starting on a bisphosphonate.

6. **C. Oxycontin 15 mg every 12 hours with 5 mg oxycodone PRN for breakthrough.** To convert from short acting opioids to long act-

ing opioids, you calculate the total daily dose (TDD) and divide it by the frequency at which it will be taken. In the example of this patient, her TDD of oxycodone is 6 × 5 mg = 30 mg. Oxycontin is prescribed every 12 hours, so her AM and PM doses should be 15 mg. While BID Oxycontin may be sufficient for her pain control, breakthrough short acting pain medciations at 10% to 20% of her TDD is still recommended. Finally, if possible, the long acting and short acting formulation should be of the same opioid.

7. **D. Initiation of leukapheresis.** This patient's altered mental status is likely due to leukostasis which he is at risk for given his elevated WBC in the setting of likely a new diagnosis of AML. Signs and symptoms of leukostasis are attributable to increased viscosity and resultant vascular occlusion. It is important to avoid leukapheresis in patients with APL as this increases the patient's risk for hemorrhage. Patients receiving leukapheresis should be monitored closely given the risk for development of DIC.

8. **A. Ondansetron.** Ondansetron is a first generation 5-HT3 receptor antagonist. This class of drugs is very effective for the treatment of chemotherapy-induced nausea and vomiting (CINV). However, a known side effect is constipation, which can be severe. It is very important when starting patients on these medications to educate them on preventing constipation (i.e., increased fiber intake, appropriate bowel regimen). In the case of this patient, she is continuing to take her ondansetron well after the expected time frame of CINV and it is important to discuss with her how to appropriately take this drug.

Transfusion Medicine

Radhika Gangaraju and Daniel Couriel

Blood Products and Transfusion

DIAGNOSTIC CRITERIA

1. **How is the ABO blood type determined and what are the clinical implications of blood type?**
   - ABO type of a person is determined by the group of carbohydrate antigens on the red cells defined by their terminal saccharide moiety.
   - Group A or group B antigens are formed by the addition of N–acetylgalactosamine or galactose to the subterminal galactose of red blood cells (RBCs) respectively.
   - AB individuals express both sugars, whereas individuals who express neither of these sugars are group O.
   - Isohemagglutinins directed against the respective ABO antigens that are not present on their own cells occur naturally. These are of the IgM type, can fix complement, and cause intravascular hemolysis leading to shock, renal failure, disseminated intravascular coagulation, and death.
   - Group A individuals have anti-B antibodies, group B individuals have anti-A antibodies, group O individuals have anti-A and anti-B antibodies, and group AB individuals have neither. Type O individuals also have anti-A,B, which cross-reacts with both type A and type B RBCs, and is predominantly of the IgG isotype. Hence these antibodies may cross the placenta and cause ABO hemolytic disease of the fetus and newborn in blood group O mothers with non–blood group O fetuses and newborns.

SIGNS AND SYMPTOMS

1. **How do you treat an Rh negative woman during pregnancy to prevent hemolytic disease of the new born?**
   - Rh (D) – immune globulin is 99% effective in preventing maternal alloimmunization when given at a dose of 300 mcg at 28 weeks of pregnancy.
   - It is repeated again at delivery if the newborn is Rh positive (dose calculated depending on the amount of feto-maternal hemorrhage).

2. **What is Rh null phenotype?**
   - Rh system is comprised of several different antigens encoded by two genes, *RHD* and *RHCE*. Absence of Rh antigens on red cell surface results in Rh null phenotype and causes low grade hemolytic anemia with stomatocytic erythrocytes.

3. **What is McLeod phenotype?**
   - Weakened expression of Kell antigens due to deficiency of a protein called Kx.
   - This results in spur cells (acanthocytes).
   - X-linked recessive *disorder* that may affect the *blood, brain, peripheral nerves, muscle,* and *heart.*
   - Common features include *peripheral neuropathy, cardiomyopathy,* and *hemolytic anemia.* Other features include limb *chorea,* facial *tics, seizures, dementia,* and behavioral changes.

4. **What are Donath-Landsteiner antibodies?**
   - Cold reacting IgG autoantibodies against the P antigen found in paroxysmal cold hemoglobinuria (normally cold reacting antibodies are IgM).
   - Paroxysmal cold hemoglobinuria is an acquired hemolytic anemia associated with childhood viral infections and syphilis.
   - The autoantibody binds to red blood cell (RBC) at cold temperatures and fixes complement, but the RBCs are lysed upon warming to 37°C.
   - Lab tests are consistent with intravascular hemolysis, direct antiglobulin test (DAT) is usually positive for C3, negative for IgG.
   - The Donath-Landsteiner test is a hemolytic assay in which the patient's serum is incubated with normal RBCs and complement at 0–4°C to allow the early components of complement to be fixed. The specimen is then incubated at 37°C in order to allow the later components of complement to be activated and lyse the RBCs.
   - Blood warmer can be used during transfusion, although not supported by data.
   - Management of underlying infection helps in resolution of the hemolysis.

5. **What are the indications for RBC transfusion?**
   - To provide increased oxygen carrying capacity
   - To increase blood volume in a bleeding patient and hypovolemia

6. **What are the RBC transfusion thresholds?**
   - There is no fixed hemoglobin (Hb) target or threshold for transfusion of RBC and restrictive transfusion strategies are recommended in most clinical situations.
   - The need for transfusion depends on patients underlying clinical condition, age, comorbidities (especially cardiac), and rapidity of anemia. Clinical judgment rather than following a Hb target is important.
   - Hemodynamically stable patients in the ICU could be safely transfused for a Hb <7 gm/dl.
   - In patients with symptomatic autoimmune hemolytic anemia, transfusion should not be withheld due to lack of compatible units, as all units will be cross-match incompatible.

7. **What are the common tests that are performed prior to blood transfusion?**
   - ABO grouping (forward and reverse) and RhD typing

- Antibody screen: Test patient serum versus RBCs from fully phenotyped group O individuals (reagent RBCs)
- Crossmatch is used to determine compatibility between recipient serum and donor RBCs
- Crossmatch is required before transfusion of any product that contains at least 2 mL of RBCs and is needed for transfusion of whole blood, RBCs, and granulocyte concentrate but not for plasma, platelets, or cryoprecipitate.
- New sample for compatibility testing is required every 3 days.
- Infectious disease screening is done on the donated products for the following agents: HIV-1, HIV-2, human T- lymphotropic virus (HTLV)-I, HTLV-II, hepatitis C virus, hepatitis B virus, West Nile virus, *Treponema pallidum*, *Trypanosoma cruzi* (Chagas disease, only required to be performed on the first donation by a particular donor), and Zika virus.
- All apheresis platelet units are tested for bacterial contamination by an automated culturing technique, 24 hours after collection.

8. **What are the thresholds for transfusion of platelets?**
   - Risk of spontaneous bleeding increases with platelet count <5,000/microL.
   - In patients with hematologic malignancies no prophylactic transfusion is inferior to prophylaxis, with a platelet target of 10,000/microL.
   - In patients with fever or sepsis, aim for a platelet count of 20,000/microL, as platelet recovery is decreased in these conditions.
   - In patients with active bleeding, DIC, and prior to procedures such as lumbar puncture, aim for platelet count of 50,000/microL.
   - Intracranial or intraocular bleeding, and prior to CNS surgeries, aim for higher count of 70,000–100,000/microL.

9. **What are the types of platelet products?**
   - Single donor apheresis platelets contain at least 3×10^{11} platelets.
   - Platelet concentrates prepared from multiple single units of whole blood must contain 5.5×10^{10} platelets per unit of blood utilized and are called random donor platelets.

10. **What is platelet transfusion refractoriness?**
    - One unit of apheresis platelets typically increases the counts by 30,000–50,000/microL. This response may not be seen in patients with splenomegaly, DIC, active bleeding, anti-HLA, and anti-platelet antibodies.
    - Post-transfusion platelet count increment <10,000/microL in two consecutive transfusions indicates platelet transfusion refractoriness.
    - Corrected count increment adjusts for body size and the amount of platelets actually infused, and <5,000/microL indicates refractoriness, and anti-HLA antibodies should be tested.
    - Human leukocyte antigen (HLA) matched platelets (matched for H or platelet crossmatching) should be requested for these patients.
    - For special products and indications, see the following.

11. **What is the common shelf life and temperature of storage for different blood products?**
    - Shelf life of RBC depends on the additive solution used. AS-1 is the commonly used solution and RBCs can be stored for 42 days at 4°C.
    - Platelet are stored at room temperature with mild agitation, and have a shelf life of 5 days.
    - Plasma is frozen at less than –18°C and can be stored for up to 1 year. Shelf life after thawing is 24 hours at 1–6°C.
    - FFP contains physiologic concentrations of all coagulation and anticoagulation factors.
    - Cryoprecipitate is prepared by thawing FFP at 1–6°C and must be frozen within 1 hour.
    - Cryoprecipitate contains only fibrinogen, factor VIII, factor XIII, fibronectin, and von Willebrand factor.
    - Granulocytes are stored at 20–24°C without agitation. Shelf life is 24 hours.

12. **How do you calculate the dose of cryoprecipitate to replace fibrinogen?**
    - Blood volume is calculated as: Weight in kg × 70 ml/kg
    - Plasma volume is: blood volume (ml) × (1 – hematocrit)
    - Fibrinogen dose (in mg) = (desired fibrinogen level in mg/dl – initial level) × plasma volume/ 100 ml/dl
    - Number of bags needed = mg fibrinogen needed/ 250 mg fibrinogen per bag.

13. **What are the common changes that occur in stored RBC products (storage lesions)?**
    - The storage lesion refers to changes in red cells during storage.
    - Over time, glucose in stored blood is consumed, levels of 2,3-diphosphoglycerate (DPG) and ATP decrease. This causes an increase in the oxygen affinity of Hb leading to shift of the oxygen dissociation curve to the left, and reduction in oxygen delivery to the peripheral tissues.
    - Lipid peroxidation, oxidative stress to band 3 structures, and other structural molecular changes also occur leading to spheroechinocytes and osmotic fragility.
    - Free Hb (from in-bag hemolysis) can scavenge nitric oxide, which may increase vascular tone.
    - The sodium–potassium pump becomes inactive and allows potassium ions to exit the cell and sodium ions to enter.
    - No major differences in morbidity or mortality have been demonstrated in randomized controlled trials that have been undertaken to know the outcomes in different patient populations after transfusion of older versus fresh RBC.

Special blood products and their indications:

Product	Indications
Leukocyte reduced (contains < 5 × 10^6 leukocytes per unit)	• Reduces febrile non-hemolytic transfusion reactions, cytomegalovirus (CMV) infection, HLA alloimmunization
Irradiation (decreases risk of transfusion associated graft versus host disease [GVHD])	• All BMT patients • All HLA matched and crossmatched platelets for intended recipients • Patients with congenital immune deficiency like DiGeorge syndrome • Intrauterine transfusions and infants under 4 months of age • Patients receiving purine analogs, fludarabine, clofarabine, nelarabine • All directed donations from relatives
Washed products (must be transfused within 24 hours)	• Severe allergic or anaphylactic reactions • IgA deficiency when IgA deficient donor is not available • Neonatal or intrauterine transfusions, especially after irradiation to prevent hyperkalemia
CMV negative products (leukocyte reduction decreases the risk of transmission and are considered CMV safe)	• Lung and heart transplant patients who are CMV negative • BMT patients when the recipient is CMV negative • Intrauterine and neonatal exchange transfusions • Infants up to 4 months age

RISKS ASSOCIATED WITH TRANSFUSION OF BLOOD PRODUCTS

1. **What are the common transfusion reactions and how do you diagnose them?**
   - **Acute transfusion reactions**
     - ○ Acute hemolytic transfusion reactions
       - ■ Caused by ABO mismatch
       - ■ Patients develop fever, chills, dyspnea, hypotension, DIC, red or brown urine, chest/flank/abdominal pain, nausea, pain at IV infusion site, oliguria, anxiety.
       - ■ In anesthetized patients, hypotension and dark urine may be the only manifestations

- Labs show falling hematocrit, increased LDH, decreased haptoglobin, positive DAT, hemolyzed plasma, hemoglobinuria.
- Repeating ABO testing in pre- and post-transfusion sample and checking patient information to see if the correct unit was transfused helps in diagnosis.
- Treatment is symptomatic: pressors to treat hypotension, pain medications, keep urine output >1ml/kg/hr. Blood components may be needed to treat the bleeding.
- Febrile nonhemolytic transfusion reactions
  - Defined as ≥1°C rise in temperature above 37°C that is associated with transfusion for which no other cause is identifiable.
  - Occurs due to the accumulated cytokines and from the leukocytes in blood product.
  - Treat with antipyretics, incidence decreases with prestorage leukocyte reduced blood products.
- Allergic reactions
  - Common transfusion reaction occurring due to antibody to donor plasma proteins.
  - Symptoms include urticaria, itching, rash, flushing.
  - Treat with antihistamines.
  - May restart transfusion slowly if symptoms are mild and resolve with treatment.
- Anaphylactic reactions
  - Occur due to antibody to donor plasma proteins (IgA, haptoglobin, C4), and cytokines.
  - Patients develop symptoms of anaphylaxis including hypotension, bronchospasm, respiratory distress, edema, anxiety, and urticaria.
  - Rule out hemolysis and testing for IgA and anti-IgA should be performed.
  - Symptomatic treatment for anaphylaxis with fluids, antihistamines, epinephrine, corticosteroids, beta 2 agonists.
  - IgA deficient blood components or washed products should be provided for patients with IgA deficiency.
- Transfusion-related acute lung injury (TRALI)
  - Caused by antibodies to human leukocyte antigens (HLAs) or human neutrophil antigens (HNAs) in the transfused blood product given to a patient whose leukocytes express the cognate antigen.
  - Occurs within 6 hours of transfusion
  - Patients have dyspnea, oxygen saturation <90%, fever, chills, hypotension (PaO_2/FiO_2 ≤300 mmHg), pulmonary artery pressure ≤18 mmHg. May also have transient leukopenia.
  - Chest x-ray shows bilateral pulmonary infiltrates.
  - Treatment is symptomatic.
  - Implicated donors should be deferred from future donations.

○ Transfusion associated circulatory overload (TACO)
  ■ Volume overload due to transfusion.
  ■ Occurs commonly in older patients, patients with cardiac, renal problems and if transfusion was given rapidly.
  ■ Dyspnea, orthopnea, cough, tachycardia, hypertension, headache are the common symptoms.
  ■ Chest x-ray (CXR), increased pro-BNP help in diagnosis.
  ■ Oxygen and diuretics to treat.
○ Transfusion associated sepsis
  ■ Bacterial contamination more common with platelets as they are stored at room temperature.
  ■ Most commonly with gram positive cocci, like coagulase negative staphylococci.
  ■ Sepsis due to RBC transfusion is commonly due to gram negative organisms, especially Yersinia enterocolitica.
  ■ Fever, chills, hypotension are common findings.
  ■ Rule out hemolytic reaction.
  ■ Positive culture identifying same organism from patient and the transfused unit is diagnostic.
  ■ Treat with broad spectrum antibiotics.
○ Non-immune hemolysis
  ■ Rare and occurs due to physical or chemical destruction of blood components, due to heating, freezing, addition of hemolytic drug or solution.
  ■ Test the unit for hemolysis.
○ Other reactions which are commonly seen with massive transfusion include citrate toxicity, hypokalemia, hypothermia, coagulopathy, and volume overload.
● **Delayed transfusion reactions**
○ Alloimmunization
  ■ Can occur to red cell antigens, and HLA antigens on WBC and platelets.
  ■ Red cell alloimmunization can be detected by antibody screen and positive DAT.
    • Commonly seen in patients with hemoglobinopathies, MDS, aplastic anemia who are transfusion dependent.
    • Avoid unnecessary transfusions.
  ■ Platelet refractoriness due to alloimmunization can be reduced by leukoreduced products and avoiding unnecessary transfusions.
○ Delayed hemolytic transfusion reaction
  ■ Hemolysis occurring 5–14 days after transfusion due to anamnestic immune response to red cell antigens that the patient was previously exposed to.
  ■ Fever, decreasing Hb, newly positive antibody screen, positive DAT, increased LDH and bilirubin.
  ■ Can transfuse compatible RBC units if clinically indicated.

- Iron overload
  - Each RBC unit has about 200–250 mg of iron.
  - Iron overload commonly occurs in patients with hemoglobinopathies, MDS, aplastic anemia, hemolytic anemia, and sideroblastic anemia, and can be seen after transfusion of 10–15 units of RBC in some patients.
  - Causes diabetes, cirrhosis, cardiomyopathy.
  - Routinely monitor with iron studies (serum ferritin).
  - Liver iron is the best marker of total body iron, and biopsy or MRI are used to assess this.
  - MRI can also be used to quantitate cardiac iron. Patients with T2* >20 msec (no detectable cardiac iron) do not typically develop heart dysfunction, while patients with T2* <10 msec are at a higher risk for cardiac dysfunction.
  - Iron chelators and phlebotomy are used for treatment.
- Transfusion associated graft-versus-host disease
  - Lymphocytes from the donor engraft in the host and mount an immune response.
  - Develop maculopapular rash, diarrhea, hepatitis, pancytopenia, fever, anorexia, nausea, vomiting.
  - Irradiation of blood products prevents development.
- Post-transfusion purpura
  - Rare complication occurring 5–14 days after transfusion, due to recipient antibodies against platelet antigens, most commonly to HPA-1a.
  - Present with thrombocytopenia, mostly severe and with bleeding.
  - Platelet antibody screen is done to identify the condition.
  - Treated with intravenous immunoglobulin (IVIG) and plasmapheresis.
  - HPA-1a negative platelets should be transfused.
- Infections
  - The risk of acquiring HIV, hepatitis B and C has decreased considerably with screening.
  - Other organisms which can be transmitted through transfusion include HTLV, West Nile virus, parvo virus B19, CMV, Trypanosoma cruzi, malaria, babesiosis (common in New England region), and Borrelia.

APHERESIS

What are the commonly performed apheresis procedures?

- Apheresis is a procedure in which blood of the patient or donor is passed through a medical device which separates out one or more components of blood and returns remainder with or without extracorporeal treatment or replacement of the separated component.
- Therapeutic Plasma exchange (TPE) is a therapeutic procedure in which the plasma is removed and replaced with a crystalloid/colloid solution.
- RBC exchange is a therapeutic procedure in which blood of the patient is passed through a medical device which separates RBCs from other components of

blood; the RBCs are removed and replaced with donor RBCs alone and colloid solution.

- Leukocytapheresis is a procedure in which blood of the patient or the donor is passed through a medical device which separates out WBCs (e.g., leukemic blasts or granulocytes), and returns remainder of the blood with or without addition of replacement colloid and/or crystalloid solution. This procedure can be used therapeutically or in preparation of blood components.
- Platelet apheresis is a procedure in which blood of the donor is passed through a medical device which separates out platelets, collects the platelets, and returns remainder of the donor's blood.
- Extracorporeal photopheresis (ECP) is a therapeutic procedure in which buffy coat, separated from patient's blood, is treated extracorporeally with a photoactive compound (e.g., psoralens), exposed to ultraviolet A light, and subsequently reinfused to the patient during the same procedure.

Common indications for apheresis procedures:

TPE	• Hyperviscosity in monoclonal gammopathies
	• TTP
	• Inflammatory and demyelinating neuropathies
	• Myasthenia gravis
	• Antiglomerular basement membrane disease with diffuse alveolar hemorrhage
	• Focal segmental glomerulosclerosis
	• Wilsons disease, fulminant
	• Desensitization prior to ABO incompatible liver and kidney transplants
RBC exchange	• Acute stroke in sickle cell anemia
	• Stroke prophylaxis and iron overload prevention in sickle cell anemia
Leukocytapheresis	• Symptomatic hyperleukocytosis in acute leukemias
	• Stem cell collection
Platelet apheresis	• Symptomatic thrombocytosis with acute thromboembolism or hemorrhage in myeloproliferative disorders
ECP	• Chronic GVHD
	• Cutaneous T cell lymphoma

RISKS ASSOCIATED WITH THERAPEUTIC APHERESIS PROCEDURES

1. **Electrolyte abnormalities**
   - Hypokalemia, hypomagnesemia, hypokalemia due to citrate used for anticoagulation

2. ACE inhibitor related complications
   - Flushing and hypotension occurs due to inhibited bradykinin metabolism with infusion of bradykinin (negatively charged filters) or activators of prekallikrein
   - Discontinue ACE inhibitors, and avoid albumin replacement for plasma exchange and avoid bedside leukocyte filters.

3. Hypotension due to fluid shifts from intravascular space.

4. Coagulation factor and immunoglobulin depletion.

5. Complications due to vascular access like infection, bleeding.

6. Other complications similar to blood product transfusion when plasma or RBCs are used during the procedure.

QUESTIONS

1. A false statement concerning red cell exchange in sickle cell disease is:
   A. Red cell units used for exchange should be screened for hemoglobin S (HbS)
   B. The red cells should be matched with the sickle cell patient for all known red cell antigens
   C. Post procedure HbS should be 30% or less
   D. It is not desirable to have the final hematocrit above 30%

2. A 45-year-old male patient is admitted due to confusion, anemia, and thrombocytopenia. He was diagnosed with thrombotic thrombocytopenic purpura (TTP) and undergoes therapeutic plasma exchange. During the procedure, he develops perioral numbness and a funny sensation in his legs. What is the next step in management?
   A. Reassure the patient that his symptoms are due to TTP and will subside with time
   B. Discontinue the procedure
   C. Order MRI brain to diagnose a stroke
   D. Administer calcium
   E. Administer IV fluids as his symptoms are due to hypovolemia

3. A 72-year-old male patient is admitted with fatigue and shortness of breath and was found to have hemoglobin (Hb) of 6.2 gm/dl. He was admitted a week ago with gastrointestinal (GI) bleed when he was transfused 2 units of red blood cells (RBCs) and the Hb at the time of discharge was 7.4 gm/dl. His current labs show elevated lactic acid dehydrogenase (LDH) and bilirubin in addition to anemia. What is the next step in diagnosis?
   A. Order a direct antiglobulin test (DAT)
   B. Proceed with colonoscopy
   C. Peripheral smear
   D. Chest x-ray

4. A 63-year-old male with multiple myeloma was noted to have progression of disease and started treatment with daratumumab 2 months ago. He is now admitted with gastrointestinal (GI) bleeding with Hb of 6.9 gm/dl, and the treating physician orders transfusion of 1 unit of red blood cells (RBC). His antibody screen returns positive and compatible blood was not found.
   What is the reason for positive antibody screen?
   A. Warm autoimmune hemolytic anemia
   B. Interference from daratumumab
   C. Cold autoimmune hemolytic anemia
   D. Alloimmunization from previous transfusions

5. A 65-year-old woman was admitted with bleeding gums and extensive bruising of her extremities and was noted to have a platelet count of 10,000/microL. She had a normal white blood cell (WBC) count and Hb of 10 gm/dl. She was discharged from the hospital 7 days ago when she was admitted for a gastrointestinal (GI) bleed from diverticulosis and received 2 units red blood cells (RBC). She has four children and was never transfused prior to this episode. What is the cause of her thrombocytopenia?
   A. TTP
   B. Post transfusion purpura
   C. Drug induced thrombocytopenia
   D. DIC

6. A 75-year-old man was admitted with melena and was found to have an Hb of 6.2 gm/dl. He has a history of hypertension (HTN), diabetes mellitus (DM), and follicular lymphoma which was treated with fludarabine, cyclophosphamide, and rituximab. Two units of red blood cells (RBC) were ordered. Which modification of blood products is needed for this patient?
   A. Irradiation
   B. Washed blood products
   C. Leukoreduced products
   D. Cytomegalovirus (CMV) negative products

ANSWERS

1. **B. The red cells should be matched with the sickle cell patient for all known red cell antigens.** The goal of red cell exchange in sickle cell patients is to reduce the amount of HbS to less than 30%, and hence it is important to use HbS negative units for this purpose. It is impossible to match the units for all the red cell antigens and only ABO, D, C, E, Kell are commonly matched. Aiming for a normal hematocrit can increase the viscosity and trigger sickling due to poor perfusion.

2. **D. Administer calcium.** Citrate is used as an anticoagulant during apheresis procedures as it is short acting and is rapidly reversible. Citrate chelates calcium ions causing hypocalcemia. Commonly seen symptoms include perioral paresthesias, shivering, lightheadedness, twitching, tremors, hypotension, seizures, tetany, and carpopedal spasm. Treatment includes slowing the reinfusion rate, to allow for dilution of citrate and metabolism of calcium citrate complex and replacement of calcium.

3. **A. Order a DAT.** The patient developed delayed hemolytic transfusion reaction due to anamnestic response to red cell antigens that he was exposed to during the last transfusion. DAT and repeating the antibody screen will help in diagnosis.

4. **B. Interference from daratumumab.** Daratumumab binds to CD38, a protein that is expressed on RBCs, causing the false positive antibody screens. It is recommended to do blood typing before starting medication.

5. **B. Post transfusion purpura.** This patient has post transfusion purpura due to development of anti-platelet antibodies from anamnestic response to platelet antigens, most likely to HPA-1a. Treatment of choice is intravenous Immunoglobulin (IVIG) 1 gm/kg/day for 2 days. Plasmapheresis can also be used. Washed RBC can be ordered for future RBC transfusions.

6. **A. Irradiation.** Irradiated blood products should be given to patients who received fludarabine to prevent graft versus host disease.

Stem Cell Biology and Hematopoiesis

22

Morgan Jones, Richard King, J. Matthew Hancock,
and Monalisa Ghosh

1. How many blood cells are produced every day?

- Humans produce approximately 300–500 billion blood cells per day.

2. What is hematopoiesis?

- Hematopoiesis is the process by which blood cells are produced.
- Hematopoietic stem cells (HSCs) differentiate into the various cellular components of blood.
- Hematopoiesis begins in gestational weeks 4–5 in the human embryo in the ventral wall of the dorsal aorta in an area called the aorto-gonad-mesonephros.
- In adults, hematopoiesis occurs primarily in the bone marrow of the pelvis, ribs, vertebrae, sternum, and skull.

3. What are HSCs?

- HSCs represent 1 in 10–20,000 cells in the bone marrow.
- HSCs can self-renew and differentiate into multiple types of precursor cells.
- They are pluripotent and can give rise to all mature blood cell types.
- HSCs can differentiate into lineage-committed precursors, which can then differentiate into erythrocytes, lymphocytes, platelets, neutrophils, eosinophils, basophils, natural killer cells, dendritic cells, and monocytes.

4. How do HSCs differentiate into mature blood cells?

- HSCs, hematopoietic growth factors (erythropoietin, thrombopoietin, and G-CSF) nutrients, and the bone marrow microenvironment are all essential for normal blood production.
- Signaling through transcription factors and growth factors regulates HSC differentiation and self-renewal.
- Furthermore, specific driver mutations in these transcription factors, such as GATA2, RUNX1, Ikaros, CEBPA, and PAX5, are pathogenic in malignant hematologic diseases such as leukemia and lymphoma.

5. How are HSCs identified?

- Most HSCs express the cell surface marker CD34, which is a marker of immaturity.
- HSCs can be identified and selected by analyzing characteristic surface markers using flow cytometry.
- The most common cell surface marker phenotype of HSCs is: CD34+, CD38+, CD45RA–, CD90+.

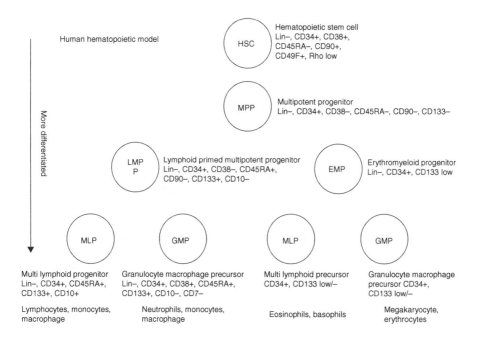

6. **Where are HSCs located?**
   - In the developing fetus, HSCs are found in the liver, spleen, and thymus.
   - In the adult, HSCs are found in the bone marrow.

7. **What is the stem cell niche?**
   - The bone marrow is composed of fat, hematopoietic cells, and vascular sinuses. Mature cells can exit the bone marrow through thin-walled sinusoids lined by endothelial cells. The bone marrow stem cell niche is located near the perivascular space which is close to the endosteal surface.
   - HSCs have complex interactions with osteoblasts, neurons, macrophages, reticular cells, endothelial cells, mesenchymal cells, and adipocytes, among other cells. These interactions all contribute to hematopoiesis.

8. **How do HSCs home to the sinusoid venous system?**
   - HSCs can leave the bone marrow, circulate through the systemic vasculature, and then either enter other organs or return through the circulation to the bone marrow.
   - HSCs interact with adhesions molecules and chemokines to determine where to travel.
   - Areas of high chemokine expression attract HSCs. Such areas include sites of constitutive chemokine production (bone marrow, secondary lymph organs, and sites of inflammation).
   - Chemokines interact with cell surface receptors to promote cellular homing
   - Two important subfamilies of chemokines are the CXC and CC
     - CXC: important for neutrophil migration and activation
     - CC: important for monocyte and lymphocyte homing

- The interaction between CXCL12 (also known as SDF-1α) and CXCR4 is particularly important in HSC homing and homeostasis in the marrow
  - CXCL12 is produced by reticular cells of the bone, sinus endothelial cells, and cells in the perivascular space
  - CXCR4 is expressed on HSCs, mature blood cells, and on endothelial cells
  - Stem cells can be mobilized using the drug Plerixafor, which is an inhibitor of CXCR4, or granulocyte colony-stimulating factor (G-CSF)
- CXCL12-mediated HSC homing through the marrow sinusoid endothelial cells occurs via two main mechanisms:
  - Integrin binding: α4β1 integrin (also known as very-late antigen [VLA] 4) on HSCs binds to VCAM-1 on the marrow venous sinus endothelial cells. Other integrins also play supporting roles.
  - Selectin ligands: P-selectin glycoprotein ligand-1 (PSGL-1) binds to P-selectin. L-selectin and E-selection ligands bind to E-selectin on marrow venous sinus endothelial cells

9. **How do HSCs migrate within the marrow space?**
   - Once HSCs traverse the sinus endothelial layer into the marrow space, they migrate to two main HSC niches in the marrow in response to CXCL12:
     - The perivascular niche contains HSCs that are more likely to proliferate, differentiate, and move into the blood stream
       - HSCs home to marrow reticular areas with the most CXCL12 abundant reticular cells
       - The perivascular space contains high concentrations of CXCL12 abundant reticular cells
       - Endothelial cells express CXCR4 and bind circulating CXCL12. Expression of CXCR4 by endothelial cells increases during stress leading to increased binding of CXCL12 and which then attracts more HSCs
     - The endosteal niche is an area where HSCs are mainly quiescent
       - HSCs home here due to proximity to the perivascular areas and because osteoblasts and osteoclasts produce high levels of CXCL12
       - CXCL12 expression may be potentiated by the relative hypoxia in this area
       - HSCs from the endosteal and central areas of the marrow provide the best reconstitution for transplant
       - The HSCs here can be mobilized to the peripheral blood stream by G-CSF
       - When transplanted, the HSCs must home back to the marrow and return to quiescence

10. **What are some mechanisms by which HSCs are stabilized in the bone marrow?**
    - Annexin II is important in initial adhesion of HSCs in the niche.
    - Mesenchymal stromal cells (MSCs) promote engraftment when transplanted with HSCs.
    - Osteoblasts with parathyroid hormone receptor produce factors that promote engraftment including annexin, VCAM-1, intracellular adhesion molecule-1, CD44, CD164, and osteopontin.

- Stem cell factor (SCF) is secreted in the marrow matrix and expressed on stromal cells
- CD44 on HSCs binds to elements in the marrow matrix.
- The calcium-sensing receptor on HSCs is important for collagen binding.
- The Tie-2 receptor on HSCs is involved in fibronectin binding.

11. **How are HSCs and other cells from the bone marrow released into the circulation?**
    - HSCs pass through a series of steps to leave the bone marrow:
      ○ Detach from the niche, at least in part due to proteolytic cleavage
      ○ Travel between adventitial cells
      ○ Attach to endothelial cells of the marrow sinusoidal network at adhesion proteins, such as VCAM-1, ICAM-1, E-selectin, and P-selectin
    - Several factors promote release of HSC into the blood stream. Most mechanisms involve reversal or inhibition of the process of how HSC home and stay in the marrow:
      ○ G-CSF
        - Likely has a direct impact on the CXCR4-CXCL12 interaction and may trigger neutrophil-mediated proteolysis of adhesion molecules.
        - Takes several days for maximal effect
      ○ Plerixafor
        - Small molecule antagonist of CXCR4
        - Rapidly mobilizes HSCs for peripheral blood collection for transplant and is thus used when rapid mobilization is needed
      ○ Alpha-4 integrin binding blockade
        - Disrupts VLA-4 activity
        - Causes HSC mobilization

12. **What is the bone marrow examination?**
    - Bone marrow examination is used to diagnose and stage disorders affecting the bone marrow and to assess hematopoiesis.
    - The bone marrow is assessed for cellularity, cell morphology, and cell maturation. More specialized testing such as flow cytometry, cytogenetic analysis, and molecular testing can be performed on bone marrow specimens.
    - Bone marrow examination consists of bone marrow biopsy (trephine biopsy) and aspiration.
    - Bone marrow is usually taken from the posterior iliac spine using a Jamshidi¨ needle.
    - A bone marrow examination should include analysis of the following:
      ○ Percent cellularity—an estimate of expected cellularity can be calculated by subtracting the patient's age from 100
      ○ Myeloid:erythroid ratio—which is normally 2–4:1
      ○ Myeloid and erythroid maturation

- Stages of Myeloid maturation include myeloblast → promyelocyte → myelocyte → metamyelocyte → band cell → mature myeloid cell (basophil, neutrophil, eosinophil)
- Stages of erythroid maturation include proerythroblast → basophilic erythroblast → polychromatophilic erythroblast → orthochromatic erythroblast → polychromatic erythrocyte (reticulocyte) → erythrocyte
  - Dysplasia in the erythroid and myeloid elements and megakaryocytes
    - Evidence of erythroid dysplasia: nuclear cytoplasmic dyssynchrony and the presence of multinucleated erythroid precursors
    - Evidence of myeloid dysplasia: hyper- or hyposegmented neutrophils or hypogranular neutrophils
  - Characterization of lymphocytes, lymphoid aggregates, megakaryocytes, and plasma cells to identify abnormal populations
  - Determination of iron stores by iron staining and assessment for "ringed sideroblasts"
  - Other findings might include infiltration by carcinoma, bacterial infections, fungal infections, intracellularyeast, or hemophagocytosis

13. What can HSCs be used for?

- HSCs can be transplanted between individuals for a variety of therapeutic uses.
- HSCs are able to traffic into and out of the bone marrow niche. They are able to engraft in the recipient's bone marrow.
- GCSF is used to stimulate HSC mobilization from the bone marrow niche into the peripheral blood where they can be collected to be used for HSC transplantation.
- In clinical practice, isolation of 100% pure stem cells is not necessary for bone marrow transplantation. It is possible to safely use only CD34+ purified grafts for stem cell transplant.
- HSC transplantation can be utilized for the following therapeutic indications:
  - Bone marrow failure or genetic disorders that cause bone marrow failure
  - Malignant disease (mostly hematologic malignancies)—for reconstitution of hematopoiesis following high doses of chemotherapy and/or radiation
  - Gene therapy for various genetic disorders including X-SCID, chronic granulomatous disease, or Wiskott–Aldrich Syndrome—normal gene copies can be inserted into genetically defective stem cells

14. What are the sources of stem cells and progenitor cells for HSC transplantation?

- Donor sources
  - Bone marrow or peripheral blood stem cells can be obtained from matched sibling, matched unrelated, or haplo-identical donors
  - Umbilical cord blood can be obtained from donors
- Bone marrow

- Collection of stem cells from the bone marrow is a more invasive procedure compared to collection of stem cells from other sources
- Engraftment usually occurs between 18–21 days after transplantation
- Collection process:
  - Collection occurs in the operating room under general anesthesia
  - Both posterior iliac crests are used to collect 50–100 aspirations on each side
  - The goal is to collect at least 2×10^8 nucleated marrow cells per kilogram body weight of the recipient
- Peripheral blood
  - Collection of stem cells from peripheral blood is as less invasive procedure than collection of stem cells from bone marrow
  - Engraftment usually occurs between 12–15 days after transplantation
  - Contains more T-cells than bone marrow collections
  - Collection process:
    - G-CSF at a dose of 10 mcg/kg once daily is usually used to mobilize HSCs from the bone marrow
    - Peripheral blood stem cells (PBSCs) are collected by apheresis starting on day 5 of G-CSF injections
    - The adequacy of the collection is determined by measuring the absolute number of CD34+ cells per kilogram of recipient body weight
    - The minimal acceptable dose is usually $> 2 \times 10^6$ CD34+ cells per kilogram of recipient body weight for adults (maximum of 8–9×10^6 CD34+ cells per kilogram of recipient body weight)
    - The optimal dose is $\geq 4 \times 10^6$ CD34+ cells per kilogram of recipient body weight
    - Some studies have shown that doses of $> 8 \times 10^6$ CD34+ cells per kilogram are associated with high rates of chronic graft versus host disease (GvHD) in matched sibling donor allogeneic transplants
    - There is no evidence of additional benefit from doses $> 9 \times 10^6$ CD34+ cells per kilogram in matched unrelated donor allogeneic transplants
    - Higher doses of CD34+ cells are associated with earlier engraftment
    - Lower doses of CD34+ cells are correlated with delayed platelet recovery
    - If insufficient numbers of CD34+ cells are collected, then Plerixafor (CXCR4 antagonist) can be used for further mobilization
- Umbilical cord blood
  - Collection and procurement of umbilical cord blood is easiest amongst the different options
  - Engraftment time is variable, but is generally longer than engraftment after using bone marrow or PBSC sources. Platelet recovery often takes longer.
  - Contains fewer T-cells than PBSC collections. Often, only a 4/6 HLA-match is needed.
  - The risk of infection is higher because immune cells from UCB are immunologically naïve and CD8+ T-cell recovery is delayed in patients receiving

umbilical cord blood transplant compared to patients receiving bone marrow or PBSC transplant

- ○ Collection process:
  - Umbilical cord blood is rich in HSCs
  - Cells are collected from umbilical blood vessels in the placenta during delivery, then cryopreserved for future use
  - Each collection tends to have a relatively smaller number of HSCs compared to other sources. Therefore, to obtain enough HSCs for an adult, two sources of cord blood are usually needed.
  - The optimal collection is approximately 2.5×10^7 total nucleated cells/kilogram of recipient body weight or $\geq 2 \times 10^5$ CD34+ cells/kilogram of recipient body weight
  - If there is HLA-mismatch, then higher cell doses are needed
    - 5/6 HLA match: $> 4 \times 10^7$ nucleated cells/kilogram of recipient body weight
    - 4/6 HLA match: $> 5 \times 10^7$ nucleated cells/kilogram of recipient body weight
- Comparison of stem cell sources
  - ○ Engraftment
    - PBSCs engraft more rapidly than bone marrow
    - Engraftment time is variable for umbilical cord stem cells
  - ○ GvHD
    - PBSC collections can have 10-fold higher amounts of T-cells than marrow collections
    - GvHD, especially chronic GvHD, occurs at higher rates in allogeneic transplants using PBSCs than in allogeneic transplants using bone marrow
    - Umbilical cord collections have fewer T-cells. Rates of GvHD are lower than in transplants using PBSCs.
  - ○ Graft versus tumor effect
    - There is increased graft versus tumor effect in allogeneic transplants using PBSCs than in allogeneic transplants using bone marrow due to the increased number of T-cells in PBSC collections
  - ○ Survival
    - Overall, there is not much evidence of difference in survival rates in patients receiving transplants with bone marrow versus PBSCs or umbilical cord blood cells

15. How do the recipient and donor cells interact?

- Recipient immune system
  - ○ If the recipient's immune system is intact, the recipient T-cells and NK cells will reject the allograft (donor cells)
  - ○ Pre-transplant conditioning of the recipient with chemotherapy and/or radiation, plus post-transplant immunosuppression is used to keep the recipient's immune system from rejecting the allograft

- Allograft
  - ○ Donor T-cells help facilitate HSC engraftment
  - ○ Depletion of T-cells from the allograft results in increased rates of graft rejection and decreased graft versus tumor effect
- HLA matching
  - ○ Human leukocyte antigens (HLA) are encoded on chromosome 6
    - ■ Major histocompatibility complex (MHC)
      - • Class I
        - – HLA-A, HLA-B, HLA-C
        - – Present on all cells
      - • Class II
        - – DR, DQ, DP, DM, DO
        - – Present on immune antigen presenting cells
    - ■ Minor histocompatibility antigens
      - • Also play a role in allo-immune response
  - ○ Chance that a full sibling matches to a recipient is slightly less than 25%
  - ○ Matched unrelated donors
    - ■ Match at HLA-A, HLA-B, HLA-C, DRB1 and DQB1
    - ■ More likely to be a mismatch at minor histocompatibility antigens
      - • Increased risk of GVHD
      - • Increased chance of GVT
- Graft versus tumor effect
  - ○ Graft T-cells and NK cells recognize residual host tumor cells and eradicate them
    - ■ CD8+ cytotoxic T-cells recognize tumor antigens in context of MHC class 1 antigens
    - ■ CD4+ T-cells recognize tumor-associated antigens in context of MHC class II antigens
      - • Th1 cytokines, such as IFN-γ and IL-2, upregulate expression of class I MHC antigens and promote expansion and activation of CD8+ cytotoxic T-cells
    - ■ NK cells recognize stress ligands and cells lacking MHC expression
  - ○ T-cell depletion of allograft increases the rate of relapse
  - ○ Donor lymphocyte infusions consisting primarily of T-cells are often used to treat relapsed malignant disease after allogeneic transplantation
- Graft versus host disease
  - ○ Develops due to a complex interaction of donor T-cells in the allograft and host antigens
  - ○ T-cells in the allograft target MHC molecules of the recipient
  - ○ T-cells in the allograft become activated by antigen presenting cells, T-cell receptor and MHC interactions, and interaction with vascular endothelial cells

○ Damage to host tissues from chemotherapy and radiation helps to potentiate the activation of donor T-cells

○ Activated T-cells and other immune cells release inflammatory cytokines such as tumor necrosis factor-alpha, IL-6, and IL-1, which mediate the graft versus host reaction leading to tissue damage and inflammation

○ GvHD can be treated with suppression of the host immune system and activated T-cells by using immunosuppressive and T-cell targeted drugs

QUESTIONS

1. **What is the immunophenotype for human hematopoietic stem cells (HSCs)?**
   A. Lin− CD34+, CD38+, CD45RA−
   B. Lin+, CD34−, CD38+, CD45RA−
   C. Lin−, CD34+, CD38−, CD45RA+
   D. Lin+, CD34+, CD38+, CD45RA+
   E. None of the above

2. **Genetic alterations in which of these transcription factors that are important in hematopoiesis has NOT been implicated in human leukemia?**
   A. CEBPA
   B. RUNX1
   C. GATA1
   D. Pax5
   E. None of the above

3. **Embryonic hematopoietic activity is first found in which of these areas in the developing human embryo?**
   A. The neural crest
   B. The notocord
   C. The aorta gonad mesonephros
   D. The embryonic ectoderm
   E. The embryonic endoderm

4. **A person undergoes stem cell mobilization with granulocyte colony-stimulating factor (G-CSF). The absolute CD34+ cell count is checked during peripheral blood cell collection and is found to be 1.5 × 10⁶ CD34+ cells per kilogram. The decision is made to add Plerixafor (AMD3100) to increase the yield. This agent works primarily through:**
   A. Disruption of VLA-4 activity
   B. Antagonism of CXCR4
   C. Impact on CXCR4-CXCL12 interaction and possible triggering of neutrophil-mediated proteolysis of adhesion molecules

5. **Which of the following methods of donor stem cell collection results in a product with the most T-cells?**
   A. Bone marrow aspiration
   B. Peripheral blood apheresis
   C. Umbilical cord blood collection

6. The human leukocyte antigens (HLAs) are encoded on chromosome 6 and include class I (HLA-A, -B, -C) and class II (HLA-DR, -DQ, -DP, -DM, -DO) molecules. The chance that a full sibling is an exact HLA match is approximately:
   A. 12.5%
   B. 25%
   C. 50%
   D. 75%
   E. 100%

ANSWERS

1. **A. Lin– CD34+, CD38+, CD45RA–.** Current evidence suggests that HSC are Lin–, CD34+, CD38+, CD45RA–. HSC used for transplant are taken from a pool of CD34+ cells. CD34 is a marker of immaturity.

2. **E. None of the above.** CEBPA, RUNX1, GATA1 and Pax5 are all implicated in human leukemia. In addition, SCL/TAL1, MLL, LMO2, PU.1, E2A have all been implicated in human leukemia.

3. **C. The aorta gonad mesonephros.** Although the earliest primitive hematopoiesis occurs in the embryonic yolk sac, the first embryonic hematopoiesis is detected in the mesoderm, specifically in the area around the ventral wall of the dorsal aorta. This is detected at 4–5 weeks of gestation.

4. **B. Antagonism of CXCR4.** Plerixafor (AMD3100) is a small molecule that acts as an antagonist on CXCR4 and can be used to increase the yield when G-CSF alone results in a suboptimal number of CD34+ cells in the collection. Alpha-4 integrin binding blockade disrupts VLA-4 binding. G-CSF has numerous effects on the bone marrow environment and is thought to cause stem cell mobilization through effects on CXCR4-CXCL12 interaction and stimulation of neutrophil-mediated proteolysis of adhesion molecules.

5. **B. Peripheral blood apheresis.** Peripheral blood collections have 10-fold higher amounts of T-cells than marrow collections. Umbilical cord blood has fewer T-cells compared to peripheral blood collections. The higher amounts of T-cells are thought to contribute to higher rates of graft-versus-host disease (GvHD) seen in donations from peripheral blood collections compared to bone marrow collections.

6. **B. 25%.** Each individual has two HLA haplotypes. Thus, offspring from two individuals have a 25% chance of sharing the same 2 haplotypes, 50% chance of sharing 1 haplotype, and 25% of sharing no haplotypes.

Hematopoietic Cell Transplant In the Management of Hematologic Disease

23

Lyndsey Runaas and Mary Mansour Riwes

1. How are hematopoietic cell transplants (HCTs) classified?

	Autologous
Modality	Patient's own stem cells transplanted
	Allogeneic
	Stem cells from a human leukocyte antigen (HLA) matched donor transplanted
	Syngeneic
	Stem cells from an HLA identical donor transplanted (i.e., identical twin)
For allogeneic HCT only…	
Donor Source	**Matched related**
	Related donor who is at least an 8/8 HLA match with recipient (HLA-A, HLA-B, HLA-C, and HLA-DRB1 identical)
	Matched unrelated
	Unrelated donor who is at least an 8/8 HLA match with the recipient
	Mismatched
	Donor who is less than an 8/8 HLA match with the recipient
	Haploidentical
	A related donor who is mismatched at as many as 3/6 HLA loci (HLA-A, HLA-B, and HLA-DR)
	Umbilical cord blood
	Stem cells collected from umbilical cord and placenta after baby is born. Immaturity of immune system allows for level of HLA mismatch that would otherwise be prohibitive from other sources. Requires at least 4/6 HLA match at HLA-A, HLA-B, and HLA-DRB1.

(continued)

	Autologous
Stem Cell Source	**Peripheral blood stem cells**
	Stem cells are collected from donor using peripheral blood pheresis procedure. Stem cells are mobilized using either a chemokine-based or chemotherapy-based regimen.
	Bone marrow
	Stem cells are collected directly from the bone marrow. Typically does not require any pre-procedure mobilization but does typically occur in the operating room with general anesthesia.
Preparative Regimen	**Myeloablative**
	Conditioning regimen is expected to destroy stem cells with usually irreversible and often fatal pancytopenia unless rescued with HCT. Typically total body irradiation ≥5 Gy in a single dose of busulfan >8 mg/kg.
	Nonmyeloablative
	Conditioning regimen with less cytopenia but with significant lymphopenia. Would not require stem cell rescue. Example includes fludarabine and cyclophosphamide, TBI ≤2 Gy.
	Reduced intensity
	Intermediate between myeloablative and nonmyeloablative. For example, busulfan ≤8 mg/kg or melphalan ≤140 mg/m2.

2. How many HCTs occur in the United States yearly?

- In 2015, nearly 14,000 autologous and over 8,000 allogeneic transplants were performed in the United States.
- Among allogeneic transplants, the most common donor source was unrelated, followed by related, haploidentical, and umbilical cord blood.

3. What are the indications for an autologous stem cell transplant?

- Malignant:
  - *Myeloma*:
    - In 2014, approximately 7,000 autologous stem cell transplants were performed for myeloma in the United States.
    - There is high-quality evidence to support autologous HCT following induction chemotherapy for all eligible patients with symptomatic myeloma.
    - Commonly used conditioning regimen is melphalan.
  - *Other plasma cell dyscrasias*:
    - Autologous HCT can also be considered for primary amyloidosis and plasma cell leukemia.

○ *Non-Hodgkin lymphoma*:
- Autologous HCT recommended for relapsed *diffuse large B cell lymphoma*.
- There is no convincing evidence for its use in high-risk disease in first complete remission (CR).
- Commonly used conditioning regimens include BEAM (BCNU, etoposide, cytarabine, and melphalan) and cyclophosphamide/TBI.
- Autologous HCT is recommended as consolidative therapy for fit patients with aggressive stage II bulky-stage IV *mantle cell lymphoma*. There is no consensus regarding its use in the relapsed setting.
- Autologous HCT is recommended as consolidative therapy for fit patients with *peripheral T cell lymphoma* (PTCL) in first CR.
- Autologous HCT can be considered for relapsed *follicular lymphoma* on an individualized basis.

○ *Hodgkin lymphoma:*
- Autologous HCT is recommended for *relapsed* and *primary refractory* disease, though benefit is limited to progression-free and not overall survival.
- Common conditioning regimens include BEAM or cyclophosphamide/TBI.

○ *Relapsed germ cell tumors:*
- High dose chemotherapy with autologous HCT can be considered for certain individuals with relapsed germ cell tumors.

○ *Acute promyelocytic leukemia (APL):*
- Consolidative therapy with an autologous HCT is standard of care for fit patients with relapsed APL in a molecular remission after repeat induction therapy.

- **Benign:**
  ○ *Autoimmune conditions:*
  - Autologous HCT is being investigated for a variety of nonmalignant conditions including multiple sclerosis, scleroderma, and systemic lupus erythematosus, among others.

4. What are the indications for an allogeneic stem cell transplant?

- **Malignant:**
  ○ *Acute myeloid leukemia (AML):*
  - Allogeneic HCT is recommended as the standard of care for eligible patients with AML and the following features: CR1 and intermediate or high-risk features (see Chapter 11), including secondary or therapy-related AML-CR2
  - Allogeneic HCT can also be considered for certain patients in CR3+ or not in remission at the time of transplant.
  ○ *Acute promyelocytic leukemia (APL):*
  - Allogeneic HCT is recommended for patients with APL not in molecular remission after induction therapy in CR2. It can also be considered for patients who relapse after prior autologous HCT.

○ *Acute lymphoid leukemia (ALL):*

- Allogeneic HCT continues to play a role in management of patients with ALL but selecting the appropriate patients remains challenging and controversial. It can be considered standard of care in CR1 for eligible high-risk patients as well as all eligible patients in CR2. Defining risk remains challenging as testing and treatment strategies evolve. In general, consider allogeneic HCT in CR1 for patients with Philadelphia chromosome or Philadelphia chromosome like positivity, patients with t(4;11), and patients with minimal residual disease.

○ *Myelodysplastic disease/myeloproliferative neoplasms:*

- Allogeneic HCT recommended for eligible patients based on various risk calculations that assess risk for mortality from disease and risk for transformation to AML. In general, higher risk features include blast percentage, poor-risk cytogenetics, and transfusion dependency.

○ *Chronic myeloid leukemia (CML):*

- Prior to the advent of tyrosine kinase inhibitors (TKIs), CML was a common indication for allogeneic HCT. Now, it is considered standard of care only for those patients presenting in accelerated or blast phase or for those patients refractory to or intolerant of TKIs.

○ *Chronic lymphocytic leukemia (CLL):*

- Allogeneic HCT can be considered for transplant-eligible patients with CLL and high-risk features, such as TP53 mutations. However, how this is incorporated into today's treatment paradigm with the advent of drugs such as ibrutinib and other targeted agents remains unclear.

○ *Myeloma:*

- Allogeneic HCT should still be considered experimental as an upfront treatment strategy in patients with myeloma. However, it can be carefully considered for eligible patients who relapse after autologous transplant or in the refractory setting.

○ *Non-Hodgkin lymphoma:*

- Allogeneic HCT can be considered for relapsed follicular, large cell, or mantle cell lymphoma after a prior autologous HCT. It can also be considered for these patients with primary refractory disease.

○ *Hodgkin lymphoma:*

- Allogeneic HCT can be considered for relapsed Hodgkin lymphoma after a prior autologous HCT.

- **Benign:**

○ *Aplastic anemia:*

- Allogeneic HCT, utilizing bone marrow as a stem cell source, should be considered as the upfront standard of care for eligible young patients (~<40 years old) with a new diagnosis of severe aplastic anemia and with an available related donor. Allogeneic HCT can be considered after failure of immunosuppressive therapy for older patients or for patients without a matched related donor.

○ *Congenital marrow failure syndromes:*

■ While rare, allogeneic HCT can be considered for patients with a variety of congenital marrow failure syndromes including but not limited to Fanconi's anemia and dyskeratosis congenita. Conditioning must be carefully considered in these patients due to their underlying congenital abnormalities.

○ *Hemoglobinopathies:*

■ Allogeneic HCT can be considered for selected patients with sickle cell disease. Patients with a matched related donor should be considered for indications including but not limited to stroke, acute chest syndrome, pulmonary hypertension, and sickle nephropathy. Indications for patients without a related donor generally become more stringent, such as recurrent stroke despite adequate chronic transfusion strategy. Allogeneic HCT remains in development for patients with thalassemia.

5. **What is the Hematopoietic Comorbidity Index (HCT-CI)?**

● The HCT-CI was developed to assess relevant comorbidities in allogeneic HCT patients and allow for appropriate risk assessment prior to transplant. It considers such factors as hepatic disease, pulmonary disease, cardiac disease, psychiatric disturbance, prior malignancy, and inflammatory bowel disease (IBD) among others. A score of 5 is considered high risk for nonrelapse mortality, with an estimated 2-year nonrelapse mortality of 41% versus a 2-year overall survival of only 34%.

Comorbidity	Definition	HCT-CI Score
Arrhythmia	Atrial fibrillation or flutter, sick sinus syndrome, any ventricular arrhythmia	1
Cardiac	CAD, CHF, MI, or EF <50%	1
Inflammatory Bowel Disease	Crohn's or ulcerative colitis	1
Diabetes	Requiring treatment with insulin or oral agent	1
Cerebrovascular Disease	TIA or CVA	1
Psychiatric disturbance	Depression/anxiety requiring psychiatric consult or treatment	1
Hepatic, mild	Chronic hepatitis, bilirubin >ULN to 1.5 x ULN or AST/ALT >ULN to 2.5 x ULN	1
Obesity	BMI >35	1
Infection	Documented infection or FUO requiring antimicrobial treatment before, during, and after the start of conditioning	1
Rheumatologic	SLE, RA, polymyositis, mixed CTD, polymyalgia rheumatica	2
Peptic ulcer	Requiring treatment	2

(continued)

Comorbidity	Definition	HCT-CI Score
Moderate/ severe renal	Cr >2 mg/dL, on dialysis or prior renal transplant	2
Moderate pulmonary	DL_{co} and/or FEV_1 >65–80% or dyspnea or slight activity	2
Prior solid tumor	Treatment at any time in past history, excludes nonmelanoma skin cancer	3
Heart valve disease	Except mitral valve prolapse	3
Severe pulmonary	DL_{co} and/or FEV_1 ≤65 or dyspnea at rest or requiring oxygen	3
Moderate/severe hepatic	Cirrhosis, bilirubin >1.5 x ULN or AST/ALT >2.5 x ULN	3

BMI, body mass index; CAD, coronary artery disease; CHF, congestive heart failure; Cr, creatinine; CTD, connective tissue disorder; CVA, cerebral vascular accident; DLco, Diffusing lung capacity corrected; EF, ejection fraction; FEV1, forced expiratory volume in 1 second; FUO, fever of unknown origin; MI, myocardial infarction; RA, rheumatoid arthritis; SLE, systemic lupus erythematosus; TIA, transient ischemic attack; ULN, upper limit of normal

QUESTIONS

1. **A 58-year-old man is diagnosed with stage III mantle cell lymphoma. He is treated with 6 cycles of R-CHOP (rituximab, cyclophosphamide, doxorubicin, vincristine, prednisone) chemotherapy, which he tolerated well. Imaging suggests he is in a complete remission. He has two human leukocyte antigen (HLA) matched sisters. Which of the following would you offer at this time?**
   A. Rituximab maintenance
   B. Allogeneic hematopoietic cell transplant (HCT) utilizing one of his HLA matched siblings
   C. Observation
   D. High dose chemotherapy and autologous HCT

2. **A 28-year-old man with no prior medical history is diagnosed with Philadelphia chromosome like acute lymphoid leukemia (ALL). He begins induction chemotherapy and achieves a complete hematologic remission. What is the most appropriate consolidative therapeutic approach?**
   A. Allogeneic hematopoietic cell transplant (HCT) using his identical twin brother
   B. POMP (6-mercaptopurine, vincristine, methotrexate, prednisone) maintenance chemotherapy
   C. Matched unrelated allogeneic HCT
   D. High dose chemotherapy and autologous HCT

3. A 77-year-old woman with a history of type 2 diabetes mellitus, previously treated breast cancer, and depression is diagnosed with high-risk myelodysplastic syndrome (MDS). She has RAEB-2 based on her marrow blast percentage as well as complex cytogenetics consistent with a therapy-related MDS. She is transfusion dependent for red blood cells (RBC). Her ECOG PS (Eastern Cooperative Group Performance Status) is 1 and she has a human leukocyte antigen (HLA) matched related sibling. What would you recommend?
   A. Treatment with 5-azacitidine
   B. Treatment with 3 + 7 standard induction chemotherapy
   C. Reduced intensity allogeneic hematopoietic cell transplant (HCT)
   D. Lenalidomide

4. A 60-year-old man is diagnosed with stage IV, double-hit diffuse large B cell lymphoma. After treatment with multi-agent chemotherapy, he achieves a complete remission based on imaging. What further therapy do you recommend at this time?
   A. Allogeneic hematopoietc cell transplant (HCT) using a matched unrelated donor
   B. Rituximab maintenance
   C. Observation
   D. High dose chemotherapy and autologous HCT

5. Which of these patients would not be recommended to undergo an allogeneic hematopoietic cell transplant (HCT) in first complete remission?
   A. Fit 45-year-old man with acute myeloid leukemia (AML) demonstrating t(8;21)
   B. Fit 45-year-old man with AML demonstrating normal karyotype and *FLT-3 ITD* mutation
   C. Fit 45-year-old man with relapsed acute promyelocytic leukemia (APL) who has not achieved a complete molecular remission after repeat induction
   D. Fit 45-year-old man with a history of testicular cancer for which he received chemotherapy, now with AML

6. A 43-year-old man with high-risk acute myeloid leukemia (AML) achieves a complete remission following induction chemotherapy. He has a human leukocyte antigen (HLA) matched sibling. His HCT-CI is 0. What would you recommend for consolidation therapy?
   A. Autologous stem cell transplant
   B. High dose cytarabine chemotherapy for 4 cycles
   C. Matched related allogeneic stem cell transplant with fludarabine and cyclophosphamide (nonmyeloablative regimen)
   D. Matched related allogeneic stem cell transplant with busulfan and cyclophosphamide conditioning (myeloablative regimen)

7. A 49-year-old woman with inv(16) acute myeloid leukemia (AML) is treated with standard induction chemotherapy, 3 + 7, and achieves a complete remission. She receives 4 cycles of high dose cytarabine consolidation. Unfortunately, 14 months after completing therapy she suffers a relapse. She undergoes repeat induction chemotherapy using fludarabine, cytarabine, granulocytic colony-stimulating factor (G-CSF), and idarubicin and achieves a second complete remission. What should now be offered to consolidate her remission?
   A. Allogeneic stem cell transplant
   B. Autologous stem cell transplant
   C. High dose cytarabine chemotherapy
   D. Hypomethylating agent for 4 cycles

ANSWERS

1. **D. High dose chemotherapy and autologous HCT.** Autologous stem cell transplant (SCT) is recommended in first complete remission (CR) for eligible patients with mantle cell lymphoma. Rituximab maintenance can be considered post HCT but should not be chosen in place of HCT for eligible patients. Allogeneic HCT is reserved for patients with mantle cell lymphoma who have primary refractory or relapsed disease. Observation alone would be insufficient for this patient.

2. **C. Matched unrelated allogeneic HCT.** Philadelphia chromosome-like ALL is considered a poor prognostic feature. As such, allogeneic HCT is recommended in CR1. Syngeneic HCT, that is, using his identical twin brother, is not recommended when transplant is utilized for malignant conditions as there is a higher risk of relapse. POMP maintenance and autologous HCT are both inappropriate choices for this high-risk disease in a transplant eligible, fit young man.

3. **A. Treatment with 5-azacitidine.** Despite having high-risk MDS, the patient is elderly with significant comorbidities giving her a Hematopoietic Comorbidity Index (HCT-CI) score of 5. The HCT-CI was developed to assess relevant comorbidities in allogeneic HCT patients and allow for appropriate risk assessment prior to transplant. It considers such factors as hepatic disease, pulmonary disease, cardiac disease, psychiatric disturbance, prior malignancy, and IBD among others. A score of 5 is considered high risk for nonrelapse mortality, with an estimated 2 year nonrelapse mortality of 41% versus a 2 year overall survival of only 34%. Therefore, allogeneic HCT would not be recommended. Lenalidomide could be considered for the 5q minus syndrome, which this patient does not have. 5-azacytidine has been demonstrated to improve survival in patients with high-risk MDS.

4. **C. Observation.** At this time, there is insufficient evidence to suggest upfront autologous HCT for patients with diffuse large B-cell lymphoma (DLBCL), even those with adverse prognostic features such as double hit. Autologous HCT would be recommended in the setting of relapsed disease. Allogeneic HCT is rarely considered for patients with primary refractory DLBCL, which this patient fortunately does not have. There is no role for rituximab maintenance in DLBCL.

5. **A. Fit 45-year-old with AML demonstrating t(8;21).** This patient has a core-binding factor leukemia, which is considered favorable risk disease. These patients should undergo consolidation with chemotherapy alone and allogeneic HCT should be reserved only for CR2. All of the other patients listed have an indication to proceed with allogeneic HCT at this time.

6. **D. Matched related allogeneic stem cell transplant with busulfan and cyclophosphamide conditioning (myeloablative regimen).** Patients with high-risk AML who are fit are recommended to undergo allogeneic

stem cell transplant in first complete remission to minimize risk of disease relapse and improve overall survival. Given his low HCT-CI, recommendation would be for a myeloablative over a nonmyeloablative conditioning regimen for improved leukemia-free survival.

7. **A. Allogeneic stem cell transplant.** For young, fit patients who have a late relapse from initial AML therapy treatment options include clinical trials or chemotherapy followed by an allogeneic stem cell transplant. This patient is young and should be considered for an allogeneic stem cell transplant in second complete remission.

Complications After Hematopoietic Cell Transplantation

24

Nguyen H. Tran and Mary Mansour Riwes

MARROW ENGRAFTMENT FAILURE

1. What is graft failure? How common is it?

- Graft failure is the term used when donor stem cells are not engrafted within the host marrow and are failing to produce the necessary hematopoietic elements. This may be demonstrated by either failure of the donor stem cells to ever engraft (primary graft rejection), or loss of donor cells after initial engraftment (secondary graft rejection).
- The causes of graft failure may be rejection, an immunologic phenomenon, or other causes including infection and drugs.
- The risk of graft rejection is related to degree of human leukocyte antigens (HLA) incompatibility, stem cell source, and intensity of conditioning—with higher risk of rejection with increased HLA incompatibility, cord blood, and reduced intensity conditioning. Graft failure remains relatively rare, occurring in approximately 5% of transplants.

GRAFT VERSUS HOST DISEASE (GVHD)

1. What is GVHD? How common is it?

- GVHD is an immunological phenomenon where donor lymphocytes respond to polymorphic HLAs present in host tissues, and mount an attack against these tissues. The resulting clinical syndrome is best described as an inflammatory response predominantly involving the skin, intestine, and liver. The interactions between donor lymphocytes and polymorphic HLAs on host tissue are amplified by the significant tissue injury that occurs during the conditioning regimen.
- The risk of GVHD depends on many factors, including degree of HLA compatibility, stem cell source, conditioning regimen, etc. Acute GVHD can be estimated to occur in 40% to 50% of patients undergoing an HLA-matched related stem cell transplant and 50% to 70% of patients undergoing an unrelated donor stem cell transplant. Chronic GVHD occurs in more than 50% of all patients who undergo an allogeneic stem cell transplant and the majority of patients who develop acute GVHD.

2. What are the organs affected in acute GVHD?

- Acute GVHD classically affects the skin, gastrointestinal tract, and the liver.
  - Skin involvement is typically a maculopapular rash that may be painful or pruritic upon first development. In severe cases, rash may cover the whole body and be associated with bullae, vesicles, and desquamation.

○ Gut involvement can be either upper or lower gastrointestinal (GI) tract with symptoms most typically being diarrhea but can also include abdominal pain, nausea, vomiting, or ileus.

○ Liver involvement is typically recognized by hyperbilirubinemia.

3. How is acute GVHD quantified?

Stage	Skin	Liver (bilirubin)	Gut (stool output/day)
0	No GVHD rash	<2 mg/dl	<500 mL/day
1	Maculopapular rash <25% BSA	2–3 mg/dl	500–999 mL/day OR Persistent nausea, vomiting, anorexia with a positive upper GI biopsy
2	Maculopapular rash 25%–50%	3.1–6 mg/dl	1,000–1,500 mL/day
3	Maculopapular rash >50%	6.1–15 mg/dl	>1,500 mL/day
4	Generalized erythroderma (>50% BSA) *plus* bullous formation and desquamation >5% BSA	>15 mg/dl	Severe abdominal pain with or without ileus, or grossly bloody stool (regardless of stool volume)

- Overall clinical grade:
  - ○ Grade 0: No stage 1–4 of any organ
  - ○ Grade I: Stage 1–2 rash and no liver or gut involvement
  - ○ Grade II: Stage 3 rash, or Stage 1 liver or Stage 1 gut
  - ○ Grade III: Stage 0–3 skin, with Stage 2–3 liver or Stage 2–3 gut
  - ○ Grade IV: Stage 4 skin, liver, or GI involvement

4. What organs are typically affected in chronic GVHD?

- A multitude of organs can be affected by chronic GVHD. Typically, the following organs are considered:
  - ○ Skin: Variety of skin changes can be seen including atrophic changes, lichen sclerosis like changes, sclerotic changes, hypo- or hyper-pigmentation. Changes can include hair and nails.
  - ○ Eyes/Mouth: Lichenoid changes of oropharynx, leukoplakia, xerostomia, dry eye, photophobia.
  - ○ Liver: Elevated bilirubin, alkaline phosphatase, or aminotransferases.
  - ○ Lungs: Patients with lung chronic GVHD may present with dyspnea or wheezing. Pulmonary function tests (PFTs) demonstrate obstructive or restrictive changes. Lung biopsy can confirm bronchiolitis obliterans.
  - ○ Musculoskeletal: Fasciitis, joint stiffness, or contractures.

5. **How is chronic GVHD graded?**
   - Chronic GVHD is graded by the NIH grading system: Each organ is given a score of 0–3. A score of 0 is no GVHD manifestations and a score of 3 is the most severe GVHD manifestations.
   - Mild disease involves only 1 or 2 organs or sites, with no lung involvement and a max score of 1 at each involved site.
   - Moderate disease involves at least one site with a max score of 2 or 3 or more organs with a score of 1. A lung score of 1 will also be considered moderate disease.
   - Severe disease is when any organ or site is scored as 3 or a lung score of 2 or greater.

6. **What measures are used to prevent GVHD?**
   - Nonpharmacologic preventative measures include use of properly matched donors, T cell depletion, and minimizing pretransplant organ damage.
   - Medications used to prevent GVHD vary by transplant center, preparative regimen, and donor source but common agents include methotrexate, tacrolimus, mycophenolate, cyclosporine, and sirolimus.

7. **What medications are used to treat acute GVHD?**
   - First-line therapy for acute GVHD depends on the initial GVHD grade:
     - For grade 1 (skin stage 1), topical steroids are recommended.
     - For grades II–IV, topical therapy in addition with high dose IV steroids (Methylprednisolone 2 mg/kg/day) is recommended.
   - If GVHD is progressing after 3 days of therapy, or if there is no response to treatment after 5 days of therapy, second-line therapies should be considered. There is no standard second-line therapy and decisions should be tailored to the patient and clinical scenario. Options include infliximab, etanercept, mycophenolate, anti-thymocyte globulin, sirolimus, alemtuzumab, and octreotide.

8. **What medications are used to treat chronic GVHD?**
   - First-line therapy for chronic GVHD typically consists of prednisone at a dose of 1 mg/kg/day for moderate or severe disease.
   - Second-line treatment should be considered if there is progression of chronic GVHD despite optimal first-line treatment for 2 weeks or if there is no improvement after 4–8 weeks of sustained therapy or if there is an inability to taper prednisone. Second-line therapies include phototherapy, tacrolimus, cyclosporine, mycophenolate, sirolimus, and rituximab.

OPPORTUNISTIC INFECTIONS

1. **What are the infectious risks associated with stem cell transplant?**
   - Infectious risks are distinct depending on the phase of transplant.
   - *In the pre-engraftment period (approximately day 0 through 30 days posttransplant):* The major risk is related to neutropenia, altered barriers (mucositis and diarrhea), and vascular devices. Thus, bacterial organisms from skin, oral and GI flora are the most common sources of infection. Invasive fungal infections and HSV, typically reactivation, can be seen in this time period as well.

- *In the post-engraftment period (approximately day 30 through day 100 post-transplant)*: Severe neutropenia is resolved and barrier defenses are healing. However, patients remain immunosuppressed due to impaired cell mediated immunity, humoral immunity, and decreased phagocyte function. If acute GVHD has occurred, this can impair immune function and damage immune barriers, in addition to the immunosuppressive effects of the GVHD directed therapies, thereby multiplying the immunocompromised state of patients. Overall, bacterial infections become less common during this period. Instead, viral infections are the most common infections encountered in this period of time. Specific pathogens of note include cytomegalovirus (CMV), adenovirus, community-acquired respiratory viruses, enterovirus, HHV-6, and BK virus. Invasive fungal infections can continue to occur, especially in those patients with GVHD. In addition, parasitic infections with *Pneumocystis jiroveci* can occur in this time period, necessitating prophylaxis to prevent this infection.

- *In the late posttransplantation period (>100 days posttransplant)*: Cellular mediated immunity and humoral immunity recovers. Immunosuppressive therapy is slowly withdrawn. Without GVHD, infection is unusual in this period. However, with chronic GVHD, there remain defects in both cellular and humoral immunity as well as deficits in the barrier function of the skin, oropharynx, and GI track. Infections during this period tend to localize to the skin, and upper, and lower respiratory tract. Pathogens tend to be viral, especially Varicella zoster virus (VZV) and CMV, followed by bacterial. Patients with chronic GVHD tend to have functional asplenia and therefore have increased susceptibility to encapsulated bacteria.

HEPATIC SINUSOIDAL OBSTRUCTION SYNDROME

1. What is hepatic sinusoidal obstruction syndrome?

- Sinusoidal obstruction syndrome (SOS) is characterized by painful hepatomegaly, ascites, jaundice, and weight gain, and can lead to fulminant liver failure. This is seen in patients undergoing hematopoietic cell transplantation but can also be seen in patients ingesting large quantities of herbal tea containing pyrrolizidine alkaloids, receiving high-dose radiation therapy to the liver without cytoreductive chemotherapy, and after liver transplantation. The mechanism of injury begins in the hepatic venous endothelium, with progressive occlusion of the venules and sinusoids leading to widespread liver disruption and hemorrhagic necrosis.

- Patients with preexisting liver disease are at increased risk of SOS due to abnormalities in hepatic endothelial cells, which can be more susceptible to cytoreductive regimen. Other risk factors leading to development of SOS include viral hepatitis, choice of conditioning therapy, source of graft, patient age, and poor baseline performance status.

- SOS typically occurs 3 to 21 days posttransplant with abnormal weight gain, and may be followed by liver abnormalities, painful hepatomegaly, and ascites. Diagnosis is often made clinically. Severe cases are often fatal.

2. How is SOS prevented and treated?

- The risk of developing severe SOS is decreased by minimizing risk factors including exposure to hepatotoxic agents (i.e., abused substances, over-the-counter medications, prescribed drugs with hepatotoxic side effects, certain herbal remedies), considering preparative regimen with reduced intensity conditioning protocols, and choosing the appropriate GVHD prophylaxis. In patients undergoing myeloablative allogeneic hematopoietic cell transplantation (HCT), ursodeoxycholic acid (UDCA) (12 mg/kg daily, divided in two doses) can be used as prophylaxis prior to the preparative regimen and continued for 3 months posttransplant.

- Treatment of SOS depends on severity of the disease. Mild to moderate cases may be treated with supportive care alone with special attention to fluid balance, maintaining intravascular volume, and renal perfusion. In severe cases, defibrotide (6.25 mg/kg every 6 hours for 21 days) is approved for use. Transjugular intrahepatic portosystemic stent-shunt has been performed in a small number of patients with SOS.

MANAGEMENT OF RELAPSE

1. What options are available after relapse?

- Relapse occurs in 40% to 75% of patients undergoing autologous HCT and 10% to 40% of those undergoing an allogeneic HCT. Donor lymphocyte infusions (DLI) can be used to treat relapse following an allogeneic HCT. The infusions allow expansion of the antileukemic cell population with increased antileukemic effect. The efficacy of DLI depends on the underlying malignancy, the dose of infused lymphocytes, and degree of host lymphodepletion. Best outcomes have been seen in patients with chronic phase chronic myeloid leukemia (CML), followed by lymphoma, multiple myeloma, and acute myeloid leukemia. Risks associated with DLI include emergence of GVHD and myelosuppression. Current investigative therapies include immunotherapy, antigen-pulsed dendritic cells, and chimeric antigen receptor T cells.

LATE EFFECTS

1. What are some common complications seen in long-term survivors following HCT?

- Late relapse of primary disease and chronic GVHD are the most common causes of death after allogeneic HCT.
- Late infection in the absence of chronic GVHD also contributes to nonrelapse-related death.
- Higher incidence of cardiovascular diseases including ischemic heart disease, cardiomyopathy, heart failure, rhythm disturbance.
- Pulmonary toxicities including chronic respiratory failure and inflammatory pneumonitis.
- Renal dysfunction related to radiation injury, immunosuppression use, and their toxicities.
- Endocrinopathies including type 2 diabetes mellitus, hypothyroidism, osteopenia, hypogonadism, infertility, and hypoadrenalism.
- Treatment related myelodysplasia/secondary leukemia
- Increased risk for secondary solid tumors such as melanoma, cancer of the buccal cavity, liver, brain.

QUESTIONS

1. A 45-year-old woman underwent a matched related full intensity conditioning stem cell transplant 50 days ago for Philadelphia chromosome positive acute lymphoblastic leukemia (ALL) in first complete remission. Her transplant course had been smooth and she was discharged home on day 20. She remains on full dose tacrolimus for graft versus host disease (GVHD) prophylaxis and continues to take acyclovir, fluconazole, oral and IV magnesium, trimethoprim/sulfamethoxazole, and ursodiol. Her tacrolimus level is therapeutic. However, over the past 2 days she has had loss of appetite, mild epigastric pains and 6–8 episodes of non-bloody diarrhea daily. What is the next step in management?
   A. Increase tacrolimus dose
   B. Start mycophenolate motifil
   C. Start photopheresis
   D. Obtain both upper and lower endoscopies with biopsies

Questions 2 and 3 refer to the following scenario.
A 60-year-old man is 120 days from a matched unrelated stem cell transplant for acute myeloid leukemia. His early transplant course was complicated by gastrointestinal (GI) acute graft versus host disease (GVHD), which was treated with steroids with good improvement. He presents to clinic today complaining of blurry vision, skin changes on both of his arms, as well as muscle and joint tightness. His exam is notable for a mild weight loss of 2 kg, irritation of bilateral sclera, and shiny/indurated skin on both of his arms. He has moderate limited range of motion of both his elbows but no muscle tenderness on exam. He remains on tacrolimus for GVHD prophylaxis but this has been tapered. In addition, he continues to take acyclovir, fluconazole, and trimethoprim/sulfamethoxazole for infectious disease prophylaxis.

2. What is the most likely diagnosis?
   A. Chronic GVHD
   B. Side effects from tacrolimus
   C. Infection with cytomegalovirus (CMV)
   D. Sjogren's syndrome

3. What is the next step in management for this patient?
   A. Stop tacrolimus
   B. Start prednisone 1mg/kg/day
   C. Skin biopsy
   D. Start Ibrutinib

4. A 57-year-old man with chronic myeloid leukemia (CML) intolerant to tyrosine kinase inhibitors (TKIs) underwent a matched unrelated transplant in second chronic phase. Posttransplant course has been complicated by acute mild skin graft versus host disease (GVHD) that responded to steroid treatment, and an admission for pneumonia. He is currently taking tacrolimus for GVHD prophylaxis. He presents at 1 year follow-up with evidence of relapse. What is the best option?
   A. Initiate tyrosine kinase inhibitor
   B. Donor lymphocyte infusion

C. Reduce immunosuppression
D. Both B and C

5. **A 55-year-old woman with Hepatitis B and acute myeloid leukemia (AML) in first remission underwent a myeloablative transplantation conditioning regimen with busulfan and cyclophosphamide, followed by infusion of matched unrelated peripheral blood stem cells 15 days ago. Graft versus host disease (GVHD) prophylaxis has consisted of tacrolimus and methotrexate. She now presents with 7 kg weight gain over 2 days. She is noted to have tender hepatomegaly with ascites. Laboratory testing is notable for a total bilirubin of 5.0 mg/ dL and transaminases that are 5-fold above baseline. Which is the most likely explanation for her current condition?**
A. Engraftment syndrome
B. Hepatic sinusoidal obstruction syndrome (SOS)/hepatic veno-occlusive disease (VOD)
C. Methotrexate toxicity
D. Right heart failure

6. **Donor lymphocyte infusion is a good option in patients with relapsed disease following allogeneic hematopoietic cell transplantation (HCT). Which disease has donor lymphocyte infusions (DLI) been shown to have the greatest response?**
A. Acute lymphoblastic leukemia (ALL)
B. Acute myeloid leukemia (AML) without minimal residual disease (MRD) status
C. Chronic myeloid leukemia (CML)
D. Multiple Myeloma

7. **A 45-year-old man with multiple relapsed classical Hodgkin disease underwent full human leukocyte antigen (HLA)-matched unrelated donor transplant. He is currently receiving methotrexate and cyclosporin immunosuppression. Posttransplant course has been complicated by mild skin graft versus host disease (GVHD). At 3 months after transplant, he developed gross hematuria with dysuria. His laboratory work demonstrates only mild anemia to 11.1 g/dL and no abnormalities in kidney or liver function. BK virus quantification is 100,000 in the urine. What is your next step?**
A. Start Cidofovir
B. Check cytomegalovirus (CMV) polymerase chain reaction (PCR), Adenovirus serum PCR, and BK serum PCR
C. Stop immunosuppression
D. Start intravenous immunoglobulin (IVIG)

8. **A 65-year-old woman presents for 1-year follow up after receiving matched unrelated donor allogeneic stem cell transplantation for high risk primary myelofibrosis. What vaccination is appropriate at this time?**

A. Hepatitis B, DTaP, Haemophilus influenzae type b (Hib)
B. Pneumococcal conjugate, pneumococcal polysaccharide, polio-live vaccine
C. Measles, mumps, and rubella
D. Varicella zoster virus (VZV)

ANSWERS

1. **D. Obtain both upper and lower endoscopies with biopsies.** This
patient is developing symptoms concerning for acute GVHD and should
obtain endoscopies with biopsies to confirm the diagnosis. Optimal first-
line therapy for treating acute GVHD involving the gastrointestinal tract
is steroids, typically prednisone with methylprednisolone reserved for
patients who cannot tolerate oral therapy. It is critical to recognize and
initiate therapy promptly. There is no role for increasing tacrolimus when
levels are already therapeutic as there is significant risk for toxicity with
limited increasing therapeutic effect. Photopheresis and mycophenolate
can both be effective therapies for GVHD but are typically reserved for
patients who are not responding to steroids.

2. **A. Chronic GVHD.** His symptoms of blurry vision and skin changes with
joint tightness are symptoms of chronic GVHD. This is illustrated by his
exam as well. This is an appropriate time frame for chronic GVHD to
begin and his history of prior acute GVHD and his unrelated donor transplant are both risk factors for development of chronic GVHD. Sjogren's
syndrome typically presents with dry eyes and dry mouth, but his skin
finding is not consistent with this diagnosis. Viral etiologies can certainly
have a protean presentation of symptoms, but would not explain skin
changes. Tacrolimus does not cause dry eyes, mouth, or arthralgias. More
commonly, it results in renal wasting of magnesium and rarely microangiopathic hemolytic anemia, neurologic changes, or renal dysfunction. More
importantly, the patient's tacrolimus is being tapered, suggesting her
symptoms are related to the withdrawal of this immunosuppressant—i.e.,
GVHD—and are not a symptom of the medication itself.

3. **B. Start prednisone 1mg/kg/day.** This patient has evidence of moderate chronic GVHD with 3 organs involvement (eyes, skin, and joints) with
one organ being moderately affected (limited range of motion [ROM]
of the elbow joints). His physical exam findings are distinctive of chronic
GVHD and a skin biopsy is not needed. For moderate disease, he requires
systemic therapy with glucocorticoids. It is inappropriate to stop tacrolimus as this would further exacerbate his symptoms. Ibrutinib is currently
approved for chronic GVHD after failure of 1 or more lines of systemic
therapy.

4. **D. Both B and C.** This patient has completed allogeneic HCT with
evidence of relapse at 1 year. All patients with CML with relapse after
transplant should be considered for treatment with a TKI. The stem of the
question indicated he was intolerant to TKIs and thus this is not a good
option. Both reduction of immunosuppression and DLI should be incorporated into the initial management unless there is concern regarding
GVHD or intolerable myelosuppression.

5. **B. Hepatic sinusoidal obstruction syndrome (SOS)/hepatic veno-occlusive disease (VOD).** The patient's signs and symptoms are most suggestive of hepatic SOS/VOD as demonstrated by the rapid weight gain

with ascites and/or peripheral edema, tender hepatomegaly, and rapid rise in liver function tests (LFT). Her history of hepatitis B and myeloablative preparative regimen placed her at increased risk of developing SOS. Most commonly this condition is seen 3—21 days after transplant. Severe cases are almost universally fatal but most patients with mild to moderate disease will recover with only supportive care. Engraftment syndrome more typically presents with fevers and a cytokine release syndrome. It would be unlikely to result in such significant LFT abnormalities. While methotrexate can cause LFT abnormalities, typically this is not associated with tender hepatomegaly. Right heart failure may present similarly with edema and weight gain; however, patients typically have cardiac history which she does not.

6. **C. CML.** Donor lymphocyte infusion has shown the greatest efficacy in patients with CML in chronic phase following relapse after transplant. Multiple myeloma cases have shown moderate response. The response is less robust in AML and even less in ALL. This is due to the rapid proliferative nature of malignant cells in AML and ALL. Full response to DLI can take months.

7. **B. Obtain CMV PCR, Adenovirus serum PCR, and BK virus serum PCR.** This patient is presenting with symptoms concerning for hemorrhagic cystitis, which can be caused by BK virus or adenovirus in posttransplant patients. It is important, prior to starting treatment, to check for concomitant infections. Treatment for BK virus infection typically involves the use of IVIG, which has antibodies against BK virus, in addition to decreased immunosuppression. Stopping immunosuppression abruptly at this time is not appropriate and will increase his risk for GVHD.

8. **A. Hepatitis B, DTaP, Haemophilus influenzae type b (Hib).** Following autologous and allogeneic stem cell transplants, patients are susceptible to infection with encapsulated organisms and certain viral infections. Vaccinations for hepatitis B, acellular tetanus and diphtheria, and hemophilus influenzae type B should be administered at 12, 14, and 24 months. Pneumococcal pneumonia should also be administered at 12 and 24 months after transplantation, and influenza should be given at least 6 months after transplantation. Live vaccines such as measles, mumps, and rubella are given after at least 24 months after transplantation. VZV and live polio vaccines at present are not recommended in these patients.

Biostatistics

Alexander T. Pearson and Emily Bellile

BASIC CONCEPTS AND DEFINITIONS

1. **What is a *p-value* and what does it mean?**
   - The *p*-value assumes a null hypothesis (often, the null hypothesis is that two measurements or datasets are equal) and describes the probability that an observed difference between them is due to chance or random variation alone. Generally, a *p*-value <.05 (5%) is considered sufficient to indicate that the null hypothesis can be rejected because the difference between two datasets is not due to chance alone.

2. **What do the terms *incidence* and *incidence proportion* mean?**
   - Incidence is the number of new cases that occur over a specific period of time.
   - Incidence proportion refers to the total number of new cases in a population over a given time divided by the total number of people at risk initially.

3. **What does the term *prevalence* mean?**
   - The total number of cases in a population at a given point in time

4. **What is a *relative risk*?**
   - The probability (incidence proportion) of an event in patients exposed to a variable (treatment, exposure) divided by the probability (incidence proportion) of an event in patients not exposed to that variable. Also called *risk ratio*. Often used in randomized controlled studies and cohort studies.

5. **What is an *odds ratio*?**
   - The odds ($p/[1 - p]$, where p is probability) of an event (condition/diagnosis) occurring in one group divided by the odds of the event (condition/diagnosis) occurring in another group. The odds ratio measures the strength of an association between a condition/diagnosis and other variables. Because of its connection with logistic regression analysis, it is used with multivariable analysis and case-control studies.

6. **What is *absolute risk reduction*?**
   - Absolute risk reduction is the change in incidence attributable to an exposure or treatment. This rate is calculated by subtraction of the incidence proportion of a condition in an exposed group from the incidence proportion in a control population over a specific period of time.

7. **How is *number needed to treat* calculated?**
   - Number needed to treat is the number of patients needed to treat with a given intervention to prevent one event. It is calculated by: 1/(event rate in control group – event rate in intervention group).
   - Example: 50% to 30% = 20% or 0.2. 1/0.2 = 5. The number needed to treat is 5.

DIAGNOSTIC TESTS

1. **What is *sensitivity*?**
   - Sensitivity is the number of patients who have a positive test with the disease divided by the total number of patients with the disease, that is, what proportion of the total population with a disease is detected by the test.
   - See Figure 25.1.

Test results	Condition or disease: Positive	Condition or disease: Negative	
Positive	A	B	Positive predictive value = A/(A + B)
Negative	C	D	Negative predictive value = D/(C + D)
	Sensitivity = A/(A + C)	Specificity = D/(B + D)	

FIGURE 25.1 ■ Sensitivity and specificity calculations.

2. **What is *specificity*?**
   - Specificity is the number of patients who have a negative test and do not have the disease divided by the number of patients who do not have the disease.
   - See Figure 25.1.

3. **What is *positive predictive value* (PPV)?**
   - PPV represents the likelihood that a patient with a positive test will actually have the disease. It incorporates the overall incidence of the disease.
   - See Figure 25.1.

4. **What is the *negative predictive value* (NPV)?**
   - NPV represents the likelihood that a patient with a negative test does not actually have the disease. It incorporates the overall incidence of the disease in the population.
   - See Figure 25.1.

5. **What is a *likelihood ratio* in diagnostic testing?**
   - Likelihood ratio is an aggregate of sensitivity and specificity for a given test and reflects whether a test result changes the probability that a condition exists. Positive likelihood ratio = sensitivity/(1 – specificity) is used for a positive test result. Negative likelihood ratio = (1 – sensitivity)/specificity is used for a negative test result.

CLINICAL TRIALS

1. What is a confidence interval?

- A confidence interval refers to the range of values most likely to incorporate the true value in a population and is based on the concept of repeat sampling. This range incorporates the number of observations sampled and the variance within the sample dataset. The range will narrow as variability decreases and the number of observations increases.

2. What is a type 1 error (alpha)?

- A type 1 error is commonly referred to as the significance of a test and refers to the probability of rejecting the null hypothesis when the null hypothesis is true, that is, finding a significant difference when there is no difference but that from chance alone. The p-value for any hypothesis test is the alpha level at which we are on the borderline of accepting or rejecting a null hypothesis. If a test between two groups in a data set has a p-value of .05, then there is a 5% chance that the difference found could occur by chance.

3. What is a type 2 error (beta)?

- Type 2 error refers to the probability that a study will not detect a true difference between two datasets when a difference truly exists. The power of a study is a function of the type 2 error.

4. What is the "power" of a study?

- Power refers to the probability that a given study will detect a difference between two populations if one actually exists. It is calculated by 1-beta. Power is influenced by the magnitude of the difference, the number of subjects included in the study, the population variance, and the significance level of the test desired.

5. What is multivariate analysis?

- Multivariate analysis (technically called multivariable analysis) is a statistical method of analysis to control for multiple variables that could contribute to an outcome.

6. What is a Kaplan–Meier Survival Analysis?

- This analysis generates predicted probabilities of survival by calculating the number of surviving patients divided by the number of patients at risk at each time point, allowing for varying follow-up times. When plotted over time, a characteristic survival curve is generated. A log-rank test is often used to test survival differences between two groups using the Kaplan–Meier estimates.

7. What is a Cox Proportional Hazards Analysis?

- A Cox proportional hazards model is a way of analyzing survival or time-to-event data. Similar to multivariate analysis, this analysis can take multiple variables into account in predicting outcome. The models generate hazard ratios, which indicate the magnitude of increased risk of the event attributable to a given variable.

8. **What is a cohort study?**
   - A form of longitudinal study where a group of patients is followed and associations between differential exposures and outcome can be compared. Study can be completed retrospectively or prospectively.

9. **What is a case-control study?**
   - A type of observational study where a group of patients with a disease is compared to a similar control group without the disease.

10. **What is a randomized controlled study?**
   - A type of experiment where subjects are randomly allocated to receive one or another treatment under study, then followed in exactly the same way. The advantage of randomized studies is that it minimizes allocation bias and provides balance in the comparison groups on prognostic factors known and unknown that could influence outcome.

STUDY BIASES

1. **What is a reporting bias?**
   - Reporting bias is a shift in outcomes resulting from a selective inclusion or exclusion of results. A subtype of reporting bias is publication bias, wherein positive study results preferentially appear in the literature and negative studies are suppressed.

2. **What is lead time bias?**
   - Lead time bias is a false extension of the time length between disease diagnosis and time of death resulting from improvements in disease screening, which do not impart an improvement in the length of life but change the date of diagnosis.

3. **What is length time bias?**
   - Length time bias is an underestimation of cancer mortality rate incurred when deaths are estimated from disease prevalence at a single point in time. Rapidly progressive cancers are less likely to be captured on a single day, and thus slowly progressive tumors are overemphasized, thereby biasing the time survival time for disease longer.

4. **What is centripetal bias?**
   - Centripetal bias is when a specific individual or institution draws a cohort of patients that are unlike the population at large, thereby changing the generalizability of outcome results produced from clinical studies. For example, patients who are fit enough to travel long distances to see an expert are more likely to live longer while participating in a clinical study, independent of the true effectiveness of the intervention.

QUESTIONS

1. **Which of the following quantities is not used when a power calculation is performed?**
   A. The magnitude of the expected difference between groups
   B. The number of subjects or events to be included in the study

C. Statistical alpha
D. The cost of the study
E. The amount of statistical variance expected in the data

2. **The Kaplan–Meier statistic requires which of the following quantities to calculate median leukemia specific survival?**
   A. Length of participating individuals' time in the study
   B. Number of participating individuals' deaths occurring during study
   C. Participating individuals' date of leukemia diagnosis
   D. A + B
   E. B + C

3. **Which of the following combinations represents the best evidence for strong association?**
   A. $r = -.8$, $p = .001$
   B. $r = -.08$, $p = .001$
   C. $r = .08$, $p = .008$
   D. $r = .8$, $p = .008$
   E. $r = .8$, $p = .8$

4. **Which of the following statements regarding 95% confidence intervals is correct?**
   A. The width of the confidence interval is dependent only on data variability
   B. The confidence interval does not necessarily contain the true value
   C. It is narrower than the 90% confidence interval holding other parameters equal
   D. If this experiment was repeated on 20 samples, 19 of these intervals would contain the true value

5. **A new public health surveillance testing initiative is most likely to induce which of the following:**
   A. Lead time bias
   B. Sampling bias
   C. Centripetal bias
   D. Bogus control bias

6. **100 men are tested for a disease. 20 people have the disease, but only 15 of them test positive for it. Of those who don't have the disease, 40 tested positive. Calculate the sensitivity.**
   A. 50%
   B. 75%
   C. 25%
   D. 37.5%
   E. 67%
   F. 20%
   G. 43%
   H. 92%

7. 100 men are tested for a disease. 20 people have the disease, but only 15 of them test positive for it. Of those who don't have the disease, 20 tested positive. Calculate the specificity.
   A. 50%
   B. 75%
   C. 25%
   D. 37.5%
   E. 67%
   F. 20%
   G. 43%
   H. 92%

8. 100 men are tested for a disease. 20 people have the disease, but only 15 of them test positive for it. Of those who don't have the disease, 20 tested positive. Calculate the positive predictive value.
   A. 50%
   B. 75%
   C. 25%
   D. 37.5%
   E. 67%
   F. 20%
   G. 43%
   H. 92%

9. 100 men are tested for a disease. 20 people have the disease, but only 15 of them test positive for it. Of those who don't have the disease, 20 tested positive. Calculate the negative predictive value.
   A. 50%
   B. 75%
   C. 25%
   D. 37.5%
   E. 67%
   F. 20%
   G. 43%
   H. 92%

ANSWERS

1. **D. The cost of the study.** While the number of events and number of individuals in a study are important, the cost of the study is not required for a power calculation. In a power calculation, four of the following are held constant and the fifth is calculated for: statistical alpha, statistical beta, amount of variance, magnitude of expected variance, and number of subjects/events.

2. **D. A + B.** The Kaplan–Meier method can calculate the median survival for a clinical study that enrolls participants beginning at different time points but will only require each participant's time on the study and his or her event class (e.g., withdrawal from study, death, etc.).

3. **A. $r = -.8$, $p = .001$.** For the correlation coefficient r, associations are measured between -1 and 1. Stronger associations are farther from 0, whether positive or negative. For p-values, lower p-values imply stronger evidence that associations are not due to random variation.

4. **B. The confidence interval does not necessarily contain the true value.** Confidence intervals are a mechanism for calculating the amount of variability around a point estimate of a parameter. The calculation is based on the quantity and variability of data used in calculation. Confidence intervals with higher degrees of confidence (such as 95% vs. 90%) must be wider to accommodate more variability. A confidence interval does not necessarily contain the true value being estimated, and when repeating the study there is no guarantee for the number of successful estimations.

5. **A. Lead time bias.** Lead time bias defines the time between when a disease is detected by preventative screening and when it would be detected by clinical symptoms. Sampling bias defines the deviations from reality induced when a sample is collected nonrepresentatively. Centripetal bias is the deviation from a representative population caused by a patient population seeking a particular type of medical institution (e.g., a tertiary care center).

6. **B. 75%.** The sensitivity is true positive/number of patients with the disease × 100 = 15/20 × 100 = 75%.

7. **B. 75%.** The specificity is number of patient who have a negative test and do not have the disease/number of patients who do not have the disease × 100 = 60/80 × 100 = 75%.

8. **G. 43%.** The positive predictive value is the likelihood that a patient with a positive test will actually have the disease × 100 = 15/35 × 100 = 43%.

9. **H. 92%.** The negative predictive value is the likelihood that a patient with a negative test does not actually have the disease × 100 = 60/65 × 100 = 92%.

Index